AMERICAN PSYCHIATRIC ASSOCIATION

MOC

FOCUS

Major Depressive Disorder
Maintenance of Certification Workbook

Editors *FOCUS* Journal

Deborah J. Hales, M.D.
Mark Hyman Rapaport, M.D.

Editors MOC Workbooks

Deborah J. Hales, M.D.
Mark Hyman Rapaport, M.D.
Kristen Moeller

AMERICAN PSYCHIATRIC ASSOCIATION

AMERICAN PSYCHIATRIC ASSOCIATION

MOC

FOCUS

Major Depressive Disorder
Maintenance of Certification Workbook

MOC Activities approved by ABPN for
MOC Part 2 – Self-Assessment
MOC Part 4 – Performance in Practice

Editors

Deborah J. Hales, M.D.
Mark Hyman Rapaport, M.D.
Kristen Moeller

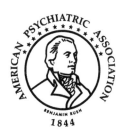

American Psychiatric Association
1000 Wilson Boulevard
Arlington, VA 22209-3901
www.psych.org

Table of Contents

*Laura J. Fochtmann, M.D., Farifteh F. Duffy, Ph.D., Joyce C. West, Ph.D.,
M.P.P., Robert Kunkle, M.A., and Robert M. Plovnick, M.D., M.S.*

Work Group on Major Depressive Disorder

*Gerald Gartlehner, M.D., M.P.H., Richard A. Hansen, Ph.D., R.Ph.,
Laura C. Morgan, M.A., Kylie Thaler, M.D., M.P.H., Linda Lux, M.P.A.,
Megan Van Noord, M.S.I.S., Ursula Mager, Ph.D., M.P.H.,
Patricia Thieda, M.A., Bradley N. Gaynes, M.D., M.P.H.,
Tania Wilkins, M.Sc., Michaela Strobelberger, M.A., Stacey Lloyd, M.P.H.,
Ursula Reichenpfader, M.D., M.P.H., and Kathleen N. Lohr, Ph.D.*

J. Craig Nelson, M.D., and George I. Papakostas, M.D.

Introduction

Deborah J. Hales, M.D.
Mark Hyman Rapaport, M.D.
Kristen Moeller

The FOCUS Major Depressive Disorder Maintenance of Certification (MOC) Workbook represents the first book developed by the American Psychiatric Association (APA) to provide a single comprehensive tool for the busy physician to meet the American Board of Psychiatry and Neurology (ABPN) MOC requirements. This workbook will give practicing psychiatrists the tools needed to meet Part 2, self-assessment and continuing medical education (CME) credits, and Part 4, Performance in Practice (PIP), requirements. Activities in the workbook provide up to 37 AMA PRA Category 1 credits.

Included in this workbook are a Self-Assessment ABPN approved for Part 2 of MOC), consisting of 50 multiple-choice questions on major depressive disorder, and a Performance in Practice Clinical Module (ABPN approved for Part 4 of MOC). Forms for Feedback Modules (Peer and Patient—Part 4 of MOC) are also provided. Resources for use in an improvement plan—a "Real-Time Assessment Tool for Patients with Major Depressive Disorder,"

as well as the executive summary from the APA "Practice Guideline for the Treatment of Patients With Major Depressive Disorder, 3rd Edition" and reprints of recent influential publications on depression, selected by experts—are included. Work is done both in the workbook and online in order to complete documentation of MOC activities and record CME credits in the physician's own CME transcript on the APA website/Learning Management System (www.apaeducation.org).

The goal of MOC is to improve patient care by assuring that psychiatrists keep up with advances in clinical practice. We have gathered in this workbook practical and evidence-based materials to help psychiatrists develop a sound foundation of medical knowledge and clinical recommendations to keep up-to-date. We hope that psychiatrists find the tools in this workbook to be helpful, both for improving practice and as a simple, "one-stop" way to meet MOC requirements.

How to Use This Workbook: Earning CME Credit and Fulfilling MOC Requirements

Maintenance of Certification (MOC)

MOC is an initiative mandated by the American Board of Medical Specialties (ABMS) to ensure that physician specialists offer quality patient care through an ongoing process of self-improvement and performance improvement. The American Board of Psychiatry and Neurology (ABPN), the certifying board for psychiatrists, is one of 24 member boards of the ABMS. The ABMS oversees the 24 member specialty boards and dictates the basic requirements of MOC.

Certificates issued by the ABPN after October 1, 1994, are time-limited and expire on December 31, 10 years from the year of successful board certification. For those receiving certification after 1994, MOC entails four basic components:

- Part 1—Professional standing (an unrestricted license to practice medicine)

- Part 2—Self-assessment (ABPN approved) and continuing medical education (CME)
- Part 3—Cognitive expertise (the recertification examination)
- Part 4—Performance in Practice (ABPN approved chart review and feedback modules)

The ABPN's MOC program is being phased in incrementally; current requirements and phase-in schedule for the four-part program are provided on the ABPN website (www.abpn.com) and in the appendix to this workbook. Individual ABPN diplomates can access the requirements based on their year of certification by accessing the ABPN website and clicking on **ABPN Physician Folios** at the top of the webpage. After activating the folio, diplomates can access information regarding their MOC requirements by clicking the **MOC Qualifying Status** button.

Earning CME Credit and Fulfilling MOC Requirements With This Workbook

Credit for activities in this workbook is recorded through the American Psychiatric Association's (APA's) Lifelong Learning and CME Center website (apaeducation.org), which was developed in compliance with ABPN reporting requirements and reports MOC progress to ABPN automatically for MOC activities completed through the website.

Three programs that provide MOC or CME credit are included in this workbook.

- **Self-Assessment in Major Depressive Disorder** (MOC Part 2, up to 12 American Medical Association [AMA] PRA Category 1 credits™)
- **Performance in Practice: Clinical Module for the Care of Patients with Major Depressive Disorder** (MOC Part 4, up to 20 AMA PRA Category 1 credits™)
- **Real-Time Assessment Tool for Patients with Depression** (CME Activity, 5 AMA PRA Category 1 credits™)

Target Audience

Psychiatrists participating in MOC and other psychiatrists in clinical practice; psychiatric residents and fellows; physicians who wish to improve their knowledge of clinical psychiatry and patient care in depressive disorders.

Educational Objectives

By completing the Major Depressive Disorder (MDD) programs in this workbook, physicians will

- Assess their strengths and weaknesses in the diagnosis and treatment of patients with depressive disorders.
- Evaluate their knowledge and clinical skills.
- Participate in a program of quality improvement and develop and implement their own plan of improvement.
- Advance their assessment, communication, diagnostic, and treatment skills and improve patient care for patients with MDD.

CME Credit and MOC Approval

MOC activity: **Self-Assessment in Major Depressive Disorder**

Provides up to 12 AMA PRA Category 1 credits™ and is approved by the ABPN for MOC Part 2.

> Begin date: July 2012
> End date: July 2015

Accreditation: The APA is accredited by the Accreditation Council for Continuing Medical Education (ACCME) to provide continuing medical education for physicians.

The APA designates this enduring material (the self-assessment) for a maximum of 12 AMA PRA Category 1 Credits™. Physicians should claim only the credit commensurate with the extent of their participation in the activity.

MOC activity: **Performance in Practice: Clinical Module for the Care of Patients with Major Depressive Disorder**

Provides 20 AMA PRA Category 1 credits™ for completion of three STAGES in sequence. This module is approved by the ABPN for MOC Part 4.

> Begin date: July 2012
> End date: July 2015

Accreditation: The APA is accredited by the ACCME to provide continuing medical education for physicians.

The APA designates this Performance in Practice enduring material (the Clinical Module) for up to 20 AMA PRA Category 1 Credits™. Physicians should claim only the credit commensurate with the extent of their participation in the activity.

Improvement activity: **Real-Time Assessment Tool for Patients with Depression**

Provides up to 5 AMA PRA Category 1 credits™.

> Program release date: February 2007
> Most Recent Program Review Date:
>   December 2011
> Program End Date: December 2014

Accreditation: The APA is accredited by the ACCME to provide continuing medical education for physicians.

The APA designates this enduring material for a maximum of 5 AMA PRA Category 1 Credits™. Physicians should claim only the credit commensurate with the extent of their participation in the activity.

Affiliation and Disclosure of Editors, Contributors, and Advisors to this Workbook

Editors

Deborah J. Hales, M.D., Director, Division of Education, American Psychiatric Association, Arlington, Virginia
Dr. Hales reports no competing interests.
Mark Hyman Rapaport, M.D., Chairman, Department of Psychiatry and Behavioral Sciences, Emory University

School of Medicine, and Chief of Psychiatric Services, Emory Healthcare System, Atlanta, Georgia
Scientific Advisory Board: PAX Neuroscience.
Kristen Moeller, Director of Continuing Medical Education, Division of Education, American Psychiatric Association, Arlington, Virginia
Ms. Moeller reports no competing interests.

Contributors

PIP Clinical Module and Real-Time Self-Assessment Tool Authors

Laura J. Fochtmann, M.D., Professor, Department of Psychiatry and Behavioral Science and Department of Pharmacological Sciences, State University of New York at Stony Brook, and Practice Guidelines Medical Editor, American Psychiatric Association

Robert Kunkle, M.A., Practice Guidelines Program Director, Department of Quality Improvement and Psychiatric Services, American Psychiatric Association, Arlington, Virginia

Robert M. Plovnick, M.D., M.S., Director, Department of Quality Improvement and Psychiatric Services, American Psychiatric Association, Arlington, Virginia

Farifteh F. Duffy, Ph.D., Quality Care Research Director, American Psychiatric Institute for Research and Education, Arlington, Virginia

Joyce C. West, Ph.D., M.P.P., Health Policy Research Director, American Psychiatric Institute for Research and Education, Arlington, Virginia

All authors of the PIP Clinical Module and Real-Time Self-Assessment Tool report no competing interests.

FOCUS Self-Assessment Editorial Board Contributors to the Self-Assessment

The following contributors to the Self-Assessment report no competing interests:

Robert J. Boland, M.D., Associate Professor of Psychiatry and Human Behavior, Division of Biology and Medicine, Brown University, Providence, Rhode Island

John H. Coverdale, M.D., Associate Professor of Psychiatry and Medical Ethics, Baylor College of Medicine, Houston, Texas

Arden D. Dingle, M.D., Associate Professor, Department of Psychiatry and Behavioral Sciences, and Training Director, Child and Adolescent Psychiatry, Emory University School of Medicine, Atlanta, Georgia

Suzanne Garfinkle, M.D., M.Sc., Fellow in Child and Adolescent Psychiatry, Mount Sinai School of Medicine, New York, New York

Annette M. Matthews, M.D., Portland Veterans Affairs Medical Center, Assistant Professor of Psychiatry, Oregon Health and Science University, Portland, Oregon

Deepak Prabhakar M.D., M.P.H., Child & Adolescent Psychiatry Fellow, Department of Psychiatry & Behavioral Neurosciences, Detroit Medical Center/Wayne State University, Detroit, Michigan

Brenda Roman, M.D., Assistant Dean for Curriculum Development and Professor and Director of Medical Student Education in Psychiatry, Boonshoft School of Medicine, Wright State University, Dayton, Ohio

Rima Styra, M.D., Toronto General Hospital, University Health Network, Department of Psychiatry, Toronto, Ontario, Canada

Eric R. Williams, M.D., Assistant Professor of Child and Adolescent Psychiatry, University of South Carolina School of Medicine, Columbia, South Carolina

Isaac Wood, M.D., Associate Professor of Psychiatry and Pediatrics, Associate Dean of Student Activities, and Director of Medical Student Education in Psychiatry, Virginia Commonwealth University School of Medicine, Richmond, Virginia

The following contributors to the Self-Assessment report disclosures as follows:

James W. Jefferson, M.D., Clinical Professor of Psychiatry, University of Wisconsin Medical School; Distinguished Senior Scientist, Madison Institute of Medicine, Inc.; and Director, Healthcare Technology Systems, Inc., Madison, Wisconsin
Grant/research/support: Bristol-Myers Squibb, GlaxoSmithKline, Lilly, Novartis, Pfizer, Wyeth; *Consultant:* GlaxoSmithKline; *Lecture honoraria:* Bristol-Myers Squibb, GlaxoSmithKline, Lilly, Wyeth; *Stock shareholder:* Bristol-Myers Squibb, GlaxoSmithKline, SciClone; *Principal:* Healthcare Technology Systems, Inc.

Vishal Madaan, M.D., Director, Pediatric Consultation-Liaison Psychiatry and Associate Training Director, General Psychiatry Program, University of Virginia Health System, Charlottesville, Virginia
Pediatric Advisory Board: Avanir.

David W. Preven, M.D., Clinical Professor, Department of Behavioral Sciences and Psychiatry, Albert Einstein College of Medicine, Montefiore Medical Center, Bronx, New York
Speaker: Pfizer, Forest.

Marcia L. Verduin, M.D., Assistant Professor of Psychiatry, University of Central Florida College of Medicine, Orlando, Florida
Research support: Bristol-Myers Squibb, Lilly.

How to Earn Credit for Self-Assessment in Major Depressive Disorder

This self-assessment activity enables physicians to learn about their strengths and weaknesses in a topic area and identify areas for further study. To earn AMA PRA category 1 credit™ as well as document your completion of an ABPN-approved MOC program for Self-Assessment, input your answers to the 50 multiple-choice questions online. The minimum passing score for this activity is fulfilled by your receipt of a score report and completion of all questions. In the online program, you will input your self-assessment answers, read the rationale and reference for the question, claim credit, evaluate the program, and obtain your confidential self-assessment score report and peer comparison. Your score report and peer comparison appear as the final section of the online course called "Peer Comparison Report." This report is dynamic, changing as the peer group increases, so it is recommended that you periodically access this link to see where your results stack up as compared with your peers.

How to Use the Unique Purchaser Number to Enroll Online

Go to the APA online learning center, www.apaeducation.org, and enroll in your selection of the following courses (by following the steps below):

- SA: FOCUS Major Depressive Disorder Maintenance of Certification (MOC) Workbook Self-Assessment (Unique Purchase # Prefix FMDDS-A)
- PIP: FOCUS Major Depressive Disorder Maintenance of Certification (MOC) Workbook (Unique Purchase # Prefix FMDDP-IP)
- AT: FOCUS Major Depressive Disorder Maintenance of Certification (MOC) Workbook Real Time Assessment (Unique Purchase # Prefix FMDDA-T)

On the home page, click the link "Enter CME Code for Credit" in the left navigation menu under "Books and Journals." Log in using your username and password. *If you don't have a username and password, please click the link to create a new account.* After you log in, enter the CME Code printed on the inside back cover of your book and click "Proceed to Course Enrollment." Use the unique purchaser number printed on the inside back cover of your book to enroll. Your will need to enter the Unique Purchase Number for each credit opportunity in this workbook in which you wish to participate. Confirm that the title displayed is correct—select OK. The course will appear on your Student Home page. Repeat this for each course you wish to complete.

Performance in Practice (PIP) Clinical Modules (Chart Review) Stage A, Stage B, and Stage C

The APA's PIP modules are guided practice improvement programs created for psychiatrists and designed to meet Part 4 MOC requirements for clinical modules. Modules follow a three-stage Performance Improvement CME structure that takes place within a 24-month period.

By 2017, when ABPN MOC requirements are fully in place, MOC participants will be required to complete three PIP units, each consisting of both a clinical module (chart review) and a feedback module (patient/peer survey). The PIP requirement will impact ABPN time-limited certifications starting with those preparing to re-certify in 2014. Because it may take up to 2 years to complete one clinical PIP module—and by 2017 physicians will be required by the ABPN to complete three units (which includes one clinical and one feedback module) over the 10-year MOC cycle—it is important for those preparing for recertification to start the process as early as pos-

sible within their cycle. Please note that neither clinical modules nor feedback modules are to be submitted to the ABPN. The APA CME Transcript is able to document APA-sponsored online activities by date and topic in the individual's CME online transcript at www.apaeducation.org.

In **STAGE A—Chart Review,** the physician compares his or her current practice (through a review of chart documentation) to guidelines and measures provided for the topic area. No patient/chart data needs to be submitted, but the physician must go online and evaluate the program at www.apaedcation.org so that completion of this Stage is recorded in the individual's CME transcript.

In **STAGE B—Improvement,** based on the results of chart review, the physician then selects an area where improvement is needed and documents his or her strategy for improvement. This improvement plan is for the personal use of the physician and does not need to be submitted to the

APA. Educational resources are provided in this workbook that can assist with the improvement plan; however, any educational accredited CME activities relevant to the improvement plan can be used. During STAGE B, the physician implements the educational plan for as long as the doctor deems necessary. This workbook contains basic resources, such as a real-time activity that guides the interviewer through a detailed assessment of one patient and that can be copied and used again, and the executive summary from the "Practice Guideline for the Treatment of Patients With Major Depressive Disorder, 3rd Edition." Key influential publications on aspects of depression and research into its treatment are also reprinted in the workbook. Reading and studying these papers can be part of a STAGE B Improvement plan. The physician must go online and evaluate the program at www.apaedcation.org so that completion of this stage is recorded in the individual's CME transcript.

In **STAGE C—Second Chart Review,** the physician reassesses his or her performance with review of five patient charts and determines the results of his or her performance improvement effort. These can be the same five patients or a new group of patients seen since the physician began the PIP activities. Again, the physician retains all patient/chart data. After the physician completes the CME evaluation at www.apaeducation.org, credit and completion date for the entire PIP will appear on his or her CME transcript. The complete module, three stages in sequence within 24 months, earns the participant 20 CME credits.

The APA PIP modules meet ABPN MOC and potential Maintenance of Licensure requirements. We hope this workbook not only meets certification requirements but also helps the physician maintain a solid foundation for excellent patient care.

Real-Time Assessment Tool for Patients with Major Depressive Disorder

The Real-Time Assessment Tool for Patients with Major Depressive Disorder is a CME activity that can be used as an improvement resource to gain a better understanding of detailed guideline measures. Complete the real-time activity checklist in this workbook and go online to www.apaeducation.org to evaluate the program and claim CME credit. Your use of the unique purchaser number in the back of this book creates an enrollment in this course. Access to the evaluation and claiming of credit is available through your Student Home page enrollments (see p. xii).

Performance-in-Practice Feedback Modules (Patient/Peer Survey)

Feedback modules require ABPN time-limited certificate holders participating in MOC to request personal performance feedback from at least five peers and five patients concerning the physician's clinical activity over the previous 3 years. Sample forms, developed by ABPN for obtaining feedback, are available in this workbook and also on the ABPN website (ABPN.com). These forms are not to be returned to the APA or to the ABPN, but to be kept by the psychiatrist. The physician must attest to the ABPN that the peer and patient feedback activities have been done.

Hardware/Software

This activity takes place both in the workbook and online; no special software other than a standard web browser is needed.

For questions about FOCUS MOC Major Depressive Disorder Workbook please contact:

American Psychiatric Association
Dept. of CME
1000 Wilson Blvd., Suite 1825
Arlington, VA 22209
(703) 907-8631
educme@psych.org

MOC Part 2: Self-Assessment in Major Depressive Disorder

Approved by the American Board of Psychiatry and Neurology for Maintenance of Certification (MOC) Part 2.

Up to 12 American Medical Association (AMA) PRA Category 1 credits™.

The Self-Assessment in Major Depressive Disorder is designed to test current knowledge and its clinical application. The self-assessment is a component of an individualized program of lifelong learning and is designed to identify areas in which practitioners may benefit from further study.

To earn AMA PRA category 1 credit™ as well as document your completion of an American Board of Psychiatry and Neurology (ABPN)–approved MOC program for Self-Assessment, input your answers to these 50 multiple-choice questions online at **www.apaeducation.org**. The minimum passing score for this activity is fulfilled by your receipt of a score report and completion of all questions. In the online program, you will input your self-assessment answers, read the rationale and reference for the question, claim credit, evaluate the program, and obtain your confidential self-assessment score report and peer comparison. Your score report and peer comparison appear as the final section of the course called "Peer Comparison Report." This report is dynamic, changing as the peer group increases, so it is recommended that you periodically access this link to see how you scored compared to your peer group.

Go to the American Psychiatric Association's (APA's) Lifelong Learning and CME Center (www.apaeducation.org) and enroll in the course "FOCUS: Self-Assessment in Major Depressive Disorder." Use the unique purchaser number printed on the inside back cover of your book to enroll.

On the home page, click the link **"Enter CME Code for Credit"** in the left navigation menu under "Books and Journals." Log in using your username and password. If you don't have a username and password, please click the link to create a new account. After you log in, enter the continuing medical education (CME) code printed on the inside back cover of your book and click "Proceed to Course Enrollment." Confirm that the title displayed is correct—select OK. Once you have enrolled, the course will be available from your Student Home page.

1. What proportion of patients has persistent residual symptoms and social or occupational impairment between major depressive episodes?

    A. 1%–15%.
    B. 20%–35%.
    C. 40%–55%.
    D. 60%–75%.

2. In the Sequenced Treatment Alternatives to Relieve Depression (STAR*D) study, patients with an inadequate benefit from initial treatment with citalopram had the option to switch to a different treatment. Which of the following switches produced the highest remission rate?

    A. Sertraline.
    B. Bupropion SR.
    C. Venlafaxine XR.
    D. Cognitive therapy.
    E. There was no difference.

3. An important finding of STAR*D level 2, regarding cognitive therapy versus medication in augmentation and switch strategies as second-step treatments, was that patients who received cognitive therapy either alone or in combination with citalopram had which of the following?

    A. Similar response and remission rates to patients assigned to medication strategies alone.
    B. Faster-emerging benefits with cognitive therapy, with a 20-day difference in time to remission than patients with medication strategies.
    C. Significantly greater tolerability with cognitive therapy than patients with medication strategies alone.
    D. Significantly greater reported side effects than patients with medication strategies alone.

4. Which of the following has been cleared by the U.S. Food and Drug Administration (FDA) to treat major depressive disorder in adults who have failed to respond satisfactorily to one prior adequate trial of an antidepressant?

    A. Electroconvulsive therapy (ECT).
    B. Vagus nerve stimulation (VNS).
    C. Transcranial magnetic stimulation (TMS).
    D. Deep brain stimulation (DBS).
    E. Magnetic seizure therapy (MST).

5. Which of the following is FDA approved as adjunctive treatment for major depressive disorder?

    A. Aripiprazole.
    B. Buspirone.
    C. Lithium carbonate.
    D. Methylphenidate.
    E. Thyroid hormone.

6. A 75-year-old woman with acute major depressive disorder is already taking eight medications for various medical conditions. Adding which of the following antidepressants would be LEAST likely to cause a pharmacokinetic interaction?

    A. Bupropion.
    B. Paroxetine.
    C. Duloxetine.
    D. Venlafaxine.
    E. Nefazodone.

7. A 34-year-old woman finds that her usual dose of codeine is no longer effective for treating her headaches. Having started which of the following antidepressants is most likely to account for the loss of efficacy?

    A. Mirtazapine.
    B. Escitalopram.
    C. Desvenlafaxine.
    D. Paroxetine.
    E. Nefazodone.

8. A physician plans to use triiodothyronine (T$_3$) to augment an antidepressant. Which of the following would be the most appropriate starting dose?

    A. 0.25 mg.
    B. 2.5 mg.
    C. 25 µg.
    D. 100 µg.
    E. 25 mg.

9. A 38-year-old patient with treatment-resistant major depressive disorder is to be treated with a combination of medications. Which of the following would be contraindicated because of the risk of a fatal interaction?

    A. Paroxetine and bupropion.
    B. Fluoxetine and buspirone.
    C. Tranylcypromine and T$_3$.
    D. Venlafaxine and selegiline patch.
    E. Desipramine and lithium carbonate.

10. In the STAR*D study comparing antidepressant treatments, what was a level 3 conclusion reached by the investigators? (Level 3 included patients who did not get better after two medication treatment steps and who did not withdraw from the study.)

    A. Switching to a different antidepressant medication is not a reasonable option.
    B. Adding a new medication to the existing one is a reasonable option.
    C. Treatment response differed significantly between T$_3$ and lithium.
    D. Odds of beating the depression increase with every additional treatment strategy.

11. A 29-year-old female patient has severe depressive symptoms and functional impairment. She has not responded to multiple adequate trials of antidepressant medication. Which of the following additional features would be the *strongest* indication for ECT for this patient?

    A. Delusional belief that she has terminal cancer.
    B. Family member who received ECT.
    C. Lack of response to a 4-week trial of a monoamine oxidase inhibitor (MAOI).
    D. Normal β-human chorionic gonadotropin.
    E. Suicide attempt during a previous episode of illness.

12. Evaluation of the efficacy of St. John's wort as a treatment for major depressive episodes has been complicated by which of the following?

    A. The absence of randomized, double-blind trials of St. John's wort.
    B. Unblinding caused by distinctive side effects of St. John's wort.
    C. Lack of standardization regarding the contained ingredients of St. John's wort preparations.
    D. High cost of St. John's wort preparations.

13. During an initial evaluation for depression, a 39-year-old woman reports feelings of severe fatigue and describes a heavy sensation in her legs and arms, which she attributes to a recent 15-pound gain in weight. She says her depression "comes and goes," and she seems particularly sensitive to events around her. She feels easily slighted by friends and coworkers, and this adds to her sense of helplessness about her future. Of the following changes in sleep pattern, which is this patient most likely to report?

    A. Difficulty falling asleep.
    B. Early morning awakening.
    C. Frequent refreshing daytime naps.
    D. Hypersomnia.

14. Mr. S presents with insomnia, anorexia with a 10-pound weight loss per month, overwhelming sadness, daylong fatigue, marked indecisiveness, and hallucinations telling him he is to die because of past sexual misconduct. Which of the following treatment approaches is most appropriate?

    A. Bupropion alone.
    B. Citalopram alone.
    C. Quetiapine alone.
    D. Bupropion and fluoxetine.
    E. Citalopram and quetiapine.

15. Mr. J presents with a 5-month history of poor sleep with early morning awakening, anorexia with a 10-pound weight loss per month, anhedonia, daylong fatigue, marked indecisiveness, and delusions that he is being investigated by the FBI for financial errors at his job as a bank teller. He had no response to a 6-week trial of citalopram at adequate dosage. When taking risperidone with venlafaxine, he developed prominent akathisia and showed no improvement in mood. Of the following treatment approaches, which is the most appropriate next step?

    A. ECT alone.
    B. ECT and lithium.
    C. Lithium alone.
    D. Lithium and tranylcypromine.
    E. Tranylcypromine alone.

16. A patient with a diagnosis of major depressive disorder had a 5-week trial of citalopram without improving, followed by a 4-week trial of sertraline without improving. Of the following, which is the most appropriate next step in management?

    A. Adding fluoxetine to sertraline.
    B. Adding tranylcypromine to sertraline.
    C. Adding venlafaxine to sertraline.
    D. Prescribing fluoxetine alone.
    E. Prescribing venlafaxine alone.

17. A very sad, pessimistic, constantly fatigued, hyperphagic, hypersomnic patient with very low self-esteem is briefly cheered when his favorite football team wins. This patient would be most likely to benefit from which of the following?

    A. Clomipramine.
    B. Nortriptyline.
    C. Phenelzine.
    D. Risperidone.
    E. Trimipramine.

18. A patient diagnosed with major depressive disorder has strong risk factors for coronary artery disease, including hypertension, hypercholesterolemia, overweight, angina during exercise, and a history of heavy smoking. He acknowledges that he still occasionally smokes. His current medication regimen includes an angiotensin-converting enzyme (ACE) inhibitor, a statin, and aspirin. He also uses sildenafil for erectile dysfunction. Of the following antidepressants, which is the most appropriate to initiate treatment with?

    A. Bupropion.
    B. Fluoxetine.
    C. Nortriptyline.
    D. Phenelzine.
    E. Venlafaxine.

19. A patient started on bupropion for 1 week continues to experience symptoms of severe depression, reporting in therapy that he feels "essentially unchanged" from the day he attempted suicide. If he continues to have no symptomatic improvement, at what point after initiation of treatment should the treatment approach be changed?

    A. 1 week after treatment initiation (i.e., now).
    B. 2 weeks after treatment initiation.
    C. 4 weeks after treatment initiation.
    D. 6 weeks after treatment initiation.

20. After 8 weeks of treatment, a patient shows a moderate response to an antidepressant. He is sleeping better, he reports no suicidal thoughts, and he has begun working on a famous mathematics problem that carries a prize of $1 million. At a recent therapy session, the psychiatrist asked if working on this problem might be frustrating him and worsening his depression. He became enraged by the remark and threatened to drop out of treatment. He missed his following therapy appointment, and he has been arriving late for the past 2 weeks. Which of the following potential modifications in his treatment should be prioritized at this time?

    A. Add a second-generation antipsychotic.
    B. Improve the therapeutic alliance.
    C. Obtain medication blood levels.
    D. Switch to a different medication.

21. Mrs. Y is a 39-year-old woman with a 10-year history of mild to moderate depression. For the past year, her depressive symptoms have been well controlled by a treatment plan that includes 20 mg/day of paroxetine and monthly management sessions. She reports no side effects from the medication. Mrs. Y also receives acupuncture every 2 months and takes omega-3 fatty acid and folate supplements, at 1 g/day and 1 mg/day, respectively. She now states that some of her depressive symptoms have returned, including difficulty sleeping and lack of interest in usual activities. She says she is reluctant to increase her paroxetine dosage. She believes the acupuncture is helping and wonders if she should go more frequently, although it is expensive. She also asks if she should increase her dosage of omega-3 fatty acids or folate. Which of the following changes to her treatment regimen is most appropriate to recommend?

    A. Increase dosage of paroxetine to 40 mg/day.
    B. Increase frequency of acupuncture.
    C. Increase dosage of omega-3 fatty acids to 2 g/day.
    D. Increase dosage of folate to 2 mg/day.

22. Which of the following antidepressive agents would be LEAST appropriate to give as an initial therapy to a woman with significant depressive symptoms who is in her first trimester of pregnancy?

    A. Citalopram.
    B. Escitalopram.
    C. Fluoxetine.
    D. Paroxetine.
    E. Sertraline.

23. Which of the following is the primary risk associated with discontinuation of venlafaxine after long-term stability of euthymia?

    A. Return of depressive symptoms.
    B. Flu-like symptoms.
    C. Confusion of depressive relapse with medication discontinuation syndrome.
    D. Anorexia.
    E. Switch to hypomania.

24. A patient's venlafaxine is initially tapered from 150 to 75 mg/day. After 3 days, the patient calls the psychiatrist and says that he has been suffering intense headaches, insomnia, and an unpleasant sensation "like electrical shocks" in his back and neck. Which of the following approaches is most appropriate to treat his condition?

    A. Add fluoxetine at 20 mg/day, gradually taper the venlafaxine over several weeks, then discontinue the fluoxetine.
    B. Continue venlafaxine at 75 mg/day for 1 week, then discontinue the medication. Advise the patient that his discontinuation symptoms will soon pass.
    C. Immediately discontinue venlafaxine and substitute fluoxetine at 60 mg/day. Taper and discontinue the fluoxetine over several weeks.
    D. Add a benzodiazepine, continue the venlafaxine at 75 mg/day for 2 weeks, then discontinue both the venlafaxine and the benzodiazepine.
    E. Increase venlafaxine above 75 mg/day and then taper more gradually.

25. A 42-year-old man is being treated with cognitive-behavior therapy (CBT) for depression. He describes several mistakes he made at work, and he voices the belief that "no matter what I try, I always fail." This statement is an example of

    A. Automatic thought.
    B. Maladaptive schema.
    C. Full consciousness.
    D. Modified cognition.
    E. Unconscious conflict.

26. Which of the following has the strongest data supporting its use as an augmentation or combination agent in treatment-resistant depression?

    A. Lithium.
    B. Thyroid hormone (T_3).
    C. Buspirone.
    D. Bupropion.

27. Which cytochrome P450 enzyme is responsible for metabolizing 25% of medications?

    A. CYP2C19.
    B. CYP1A2.
    C. CYP2D6.
    D. CYP3A4.

28. A 46-year-old man takes citalopram 20 mg/day for a major depressive episode. After 4 weeks, he returns to his psychiatrist, citing little if any change in his symptoms. Which of the following would be the most appropriate next step in the patient's treatment?

    A. Increase the citalopram to 40 mg/day.
    B. Discontinue citalopram and begin venlafaxine.
    C. Continue citalopram but add lithium.
    D. Begin VNS.
    E. Continue citalopram and begin aripiprazole.

29. Which of the following antidepressants is an inhibitor of both dopamine and norepinephrine transporters?

    A. Bupropion.
    B. Tricyclic antidepressants (TCAs).
    C. Venlafaxine.
    D. MAOIs.
    E. Mirtazapine.

30. Which of the following describes the risk estimate for the genetic and environmental contributions to the development of depression?

    A. 2/3 genetic, 1/3 environmental.
    B. 2/3 environmental, 1/3 genetic.
    C. 1/2 environmental, 1/2 genetic.
    D. Not enough is known to estimate.

31. Which of the following types of psychotherapy emphasizes being a patient?

    A. Cognitive-behavior.
    B. Interpersonal.
    C. Psychodynamic.
    D. Dialectical behavior.
    E. Psychoeducation.

32. Mr. W is a 33-year-old man with HIV and mild to moderate depression. His antiretroviral therapy regimen includes tenofovir, lamivudine, and efavirenz. Which of the following should be avoided in treating his depression?

    A. Bupropion.
    B. Citalopram.
    C. Duloxetine.
    D. St. John's wort.

33. A 30-year-old graduate student has severe major depressive disorder and recently tried to kill himself. He has a long history of depression, especially during the winter season, but he has never previously received any treatment. He would prefer to try psychotherapy, but he is not absolutely opposed to taking medication. He is reluctant to try ECT because of the potential risk of memory loss. Which of the following modalities is appropriate to recommend as an initial treatment?

    A. Psychotherapy alone.
    B. Pharmacotherapy, either alone or in combination with psychotherapy.
    C. ECT alone.
    D. Bright light therapy alone.

34. A 3-day-postpartum mother with no prior psychiatric diagnosis is concerned about feeling depressed. She reports a decrease in energy, difficulty sleeping despite being tired, decreased appetite, and frequent mood swings, saying, "One minute I'm fine; the next minute, I'm crying." Which of the following is the most appropriate treatment?

    A. Psychoeducation.
    B. CBT.
    C. Pharmacotherapy.
    D. Hospitalization.
    E. Psychodynamic psychotherapy.

35. The diagnosis of a major depressive episode requires either a depressed mood or which of the following?

    A. Insomnia or hypersomnia.
    B. Recurrent thoughts of death.
    C. Feelings of worthlessness.
    D. Psychomotor agitation or retardation.
    E. Loss of interest or pleasure.

36. A 42-year-old man begins pharmacotherapy for treatment of major depressive disorder. Two weeks later he presents with complaints of dry mouth, impaired ability to focus at close range, constipation, urinary hesitation, tachycardia, and sexual dysfunction. Which of the following medications is most likely to have caused this presentation?

    A. Duloxetine.
    B. Fluoxetine.
    C. Imipramine.
    D. Mirtazapine.
    E. Venlafaxine.

37. A depressed 62-year-old man being treated with a selective serotonin reuptake inhibitor (SSRI) is admitted to the hospital with motoric immobility, posturing, grimacing, echolalia, and echopraxia. Intravenous administration of lorazepam and amobarbital with a concurrent antidepressant leads to no relief. Which of the following should be given or done next?

    A. Second antidepressant.
    B. Mood stabilizer.
    C. ECT.
    D. Dantrolene.
    E. Intravenous haloperidol.

38. A 48-year-old man has depression that has been resistant to treatment with a variety of antidepressants. The decision is made for him to try an MAOI. In order to avoid serotonin syndrome, a washout period of at least 5 weeks is MOST indicated if he has been taking which antidepressant?

    A. Bupropion.
    B. Clomipramine.
    C. Fluoxetine.
    D. Paroxetine.
    E. Venlafaxine.

39. A 65-year-old widower, accompanied by his daughter, presents to the clinic following the death of his wife 3 months ago. The daughter states that the couple had been married for 40 years, and that her father now feels utterly worthless without his wife. Since her death, he has stayed in the house, letting the newspapers pile up and not answering the phone. He stopped his weekly fishing trips with his neighbor, a pastime of his for 20 years. He denies suicidal ideation, but states that he wishes to join his wife. He has had a weight loss of 30 pounds over the past 3 months. He has stopped taking his hypertension medications. What is the most likely diagnosis?

    A. Bereavement.
    B. Adjustment disorder with depressed mood.
    C. Major depressive disorder.
    D. Depressive disorder not otherwise specified.
    E. Dysthymic disorder.

40. Which of the following SSRIs is most likely to be "self-tapering," thereby decreasing the chances of discontinuation effects?

    A. Citalopram.
    B. Escitalopram.
    C. Fluoxetine.
    D. Paroxetine.
    E. Sertraline.

41. Which of the following psychosocial treatments for depression has the most robust data supporting its use?

    A. Cognitive therapy.
    B. Dialectical behavior therapy.
    C. Group therapy.
    D. Psychodynamic psychotherapy.
    E. Supportive therapy.

42. Which of the following is a common symptom of seasonal affective disorder?

    A. Light sensitivity.
    B. Somatic complaints.
    C. Insomnia.
    D. Overeating.
    E. Impulsiveness.

43. Which of the following antidepressants has FDA approval for treating major depressive disorder in children and adolescents?

    A. Citalopram.
    B. Fluoxetine.
    C. Fluvoxamine.
    D. Sertraline.
    E. Paroxetine.

44. In the NIMH-sponsored clinical treatment trial STAR*D, level 1 remission rates after up to 14 weeks of treatment with the SSRI citalopram were

    A. 17%–23%.
    B. 27%–33%.
    C. 47%–53%.
    D. 67%–73%.

45. A psychiatrist is treating a 48-year-old man who has been diagnosed with major depressive disorder and who has functional impairments. Which of the following is the most appropriate course of action in therapy to assist in recovery?

    A. Assist the patient in modifying stressful responsibilities at home or at work.
    B. Encourage the patient to avoid procrastination and to make major life decisions as they arise.
    C. Have the patient take sole responsibility for scheduling time away from work if he is unable to function in the work environment.
    D. Recommend that the patient think positively and set goals beyond his usual level of function.

46. Which of the following is the best predictor of a recurrence of depression in someone with major depressive disorder?

    A. Family history of depression.
    B. Prior episodes of depression.
    C. Prior suicide attempt.
    D. Psychotic features.
    E. Severe functional impairments.

47. The available evidence on SSRI treatment of depression during pregnancy suggests that continuous SSRI use during pregnancy is associated with an increased risk of

    A. Minor physical anomalies.
    B. Maternal weight gain.
    C. Hypoglycemia.
    D. Preterm birth.
    E. Neonatal adaptation.

48. A patient has been free of major depressive symptoms for the last 12 months with a standard dose of an SSRI and biweekly CBT. This resolution of symptoms followed the patient's fourth episode of major depressive disorder. The patient asks how long treatment needs to continue. Which of the following is a recommended treatment strategy for maintaining the patient's functioning?

    A. Continue the current medication and taper CBT.
    B. Taper the medication and continue current CBT.
    C. Discontinue gradually both medication and CBT.
    D. Decrease medication level and CBT frequency.
    E. Continue current treatment indefinitely.

49. Standard of care guidelines recommend that patients with coronary heart disease be screened for depression because

    A. Depressed patients have a much higher cardiovascular morbidity.
    B. Becoming depressed is a normal response to having cardiovascular disease.
    C. The treatment for cardiovascular disease tends to cause depression.
    D. Depressed patients have different types of cardiovascular disease.
    E. Being depressed causes cardiovascular drugs to work differently.

50. A 35-year-old woman in her first trimester of pregnancy begins to experience frequent crying, mild insomnia, and increased sensitivity to rejection by her colleagues. She has no psychiatric history and no suicidal ideation, and continues to function close to her baseline. Which of the following treatment recommendations does the evidence base best support?

    A. Cognitive therapy.
    B. Group psychoeducation.
    C. ECT.
    D. An SSRI.
    E. Estrogen replacement therapy.

References

American Psychiatric Association: Diagnostic and Statistical Manual of Mental Disorders, 4th Edition, Text Revision. Washington, DC, American Psychiatric Association, 2000, p 356

American Psychiatric Association: Practice Guideline for the Treatment of Patients With Major Depressive Disorder, 3rd Edition. Arlington, VA, American Psychiatric Association, 2010. Available at: http://psychiatryonline.org/data/Books/prac/PG_Depression3rdEd.pdf. Accessed May 15, 2012.

Birmaher B, Brent D, Bernet W, et al: Practice parameter for the assessment and treatment of children and adolescents with depressive disorders. J Am Acad Child Adolesc Psychiatry 46:1503–1526, 2007. Reprinted with permission in FOCUS 6:379–400, 2008.

Clark DA, Hollifield M, Leahy R, et al: Theory of cognitive therapy, in Textbook of Psychotherapeutic Treatments. Edited by Gabbard GO. Washington, DC, American Psychiatric Publishing, 2009, pp 170–172

Cooper-Kazaz R, Lerer B: Efficacy and safety of triiodothyronine supplementation in patients with major depressive disorder treated with specific serotonin reuptake inhibitors. Int J Neuropsychopharmacol 11:685–699, 2008

de Leon J, Armstrong SC, Cozza KL: Clinical guidelines for psychiatrists for the use of pharmacogenetic testing for CYP450 2D6 and CYP450 2C19. Psychosomatics 47:75–85, 2006

Dey Pharma: Selegiline package insert. May 2009. Available at: http://packageinserts.bms.com/pi/pi_emsam.pdf. Accessed May 15, 2012.

Fitelson E, Kim S, Baker AS, et al: Treatment of postpartum depression: clinical, psychological and pharmacological options. Int J Womens Health 3:1–14, 2010

Gaynes BN, Warden D, Trivedi MH, et al: What did STAR*D teach us? Results from a large-scale, practical, clinical trial for patients with depression. Psychiatr Serv 60:1439–1445, 2009

George MS, Post RM: Daily left prefrontal repetitive transcranial magnetic stimulation for acute treatment of medication-resistant depression. Am J Psychiatry 168:356–364, 2011

Holtzheimer PE: Advances in the management of treatment-resistant depression. FOCUS 8:489–490, 2010

Iosifescu DV: "Supercharge" antidepressants by adding thyroid hormones. Why hormones help, and new data on SSRI augmentation. Curr Psychiatry 5:15–25, 2006

Joska JA, Stein DJ: Mood disorders, in The American Psychiatric Publishing Textbook of Psychiatry, 5th Edition. Edited by Hales RE, Yudofsky SC, Gabbard GO. Washington, DC, American Psychiatric Publishing, 2008, pp 479–485

Lichtman JH, Bigger JT, Blumenthal JA, et al: Depression and coronary heart disease: recommendations for screening, referral, and treatment: a science advisory from the American Heart Association Prevention Committee of the Council on Cardiovascular Nursing, Council on Clinical Cardiology, Council on Epidemiology and Prevention, and Interdisciplinary Council on Quality of Care and Outcomes Research: endorsed by the American Psychiatric Association. Circulation 118:1768–1775, 2008. Reprinted in FOCUS 7:406–413, 2009.

Markowitz JC: The clinical conduct of interpersonal psychotherapy. FOCUS 4:179–186, 2006

Myers AJ, Nemeroff CB: New vistas in the management of treatment refractory psychiatric disorders: genomics and personalized medicine. FOCUS 8:525–535, 2010

Nelson JC, Papakostas GI: Atypical antipsychotic augmentation in major depressive disorder: a meta-analysis of placebo-controlled randomized trials. Am J Psychiatry 166:980–991, 2009

Nemeroff CB: Recent findings in the pathophysiology of depression. FOCUS 6:3–14, 2008

Nierenberg AA, Fava M, Trivedi MH, et al: A comparison of lithium and T3 augmentation following two failed medication treatments for depression: a STAR*D report. Am J Psychiatry 163:1519–1530, 2006

Payne JL: Antidepressant use in the postpartum period: practical considerations. Am J Psychiatry 164:1329–1332, 2007

Robinson GE: Psychopharmacology in pregnancy and postpartum. FOCUS 10:3–14, 2012

Rush AJ, Warden D, Wisniewski SR, et al: STAR*D: revising conventional wisdom. CNS Drugs 23:627–647, 2009

Schatzberg AF, Cole JO, DeBattista C: Antidepressants: tricyclic and tetracyclic antidepressants, in Manual of Clinical Psychopharmacology, 7th Edition. Washington, DC, American Psychiatric Publishing, 2010, pp 105–121

Schatzberg AF, Cole JO, DeBattista C: Antidepressants: selective serotonin reuptake inhibitors, discontinuation, in Manual of Clinical Psychopharmacology, 7th Edition. Washington, DC, American Psychiatric Publishing, 2010, pp 72–74

Sindrup SH, Brøsen K: The pharmacogenetics of codeine hypoalgesia. Pharmacogenetics 5:335–346, 1995

Spina E, Santoro V, D'Arrigo C: Clinically relevant pharmacokinetic drug interactions with second-generation antidepressants: an update. Clin Ther 30:1206–1227, 2008

Sullivan PF, Neale MC, Kendler KS: Genetic epidemiology of major depression: review and meta-analysis. Am J Psychiatry 157:1552–1562, 2000

Suri R, Altshuler L: Postpartum depression: advances in recognition and treatment. FOCUS 10:15–21, 2012

Taurines R, Gerlach M, Warnke A, et al: Pharmacotherapy in depressed children and adolescents. World J Biol Psychiatry 12 (suppl 1):11–15, 2011

Thase ME, Friedman ES, Biggs MM, et al: Cognitive therapy versus medication in augmentation and switch strategies as second-step treatments: a STAR*D report. Am J Psychiatry 164:739–752, 2007

Udechuku A, Nguyen T, Hill R, et al: Antidepressants in pregnancy: a systematic review. Aust N Z J Psychiatry 44:978–996, 2010

U.S. Food and Drug Administration: Public Health Advisory: Paroxetine. December 18, 2005 (last updated January 27, 2010). Available at: http://www.fda.gov/Drugs/DrugSafety/PostmarketDrugSafetyInformationforPatientsandProviders/DrugSafetyInformationforHeathcareProfessionals/PublicHealthAdvisories/ucm051731.htm. Accessed October 1, 2011.

U.S. Food and Drug Administration: FDA Executive Summary Prepared for the January 27–28, 2011 meeting of the Neurological Devices Panel: Meeting to Discuss the Classification of Electroconvulsive Therapy Devices (ECT). Available at: http://www.fda.gov/downloads/AdvisoryCommittees/CommitteesMeetingMaterials/MedicalDevices/MedicalDevicesAdvisoryCommittee/NeurologicalDevicesPanel/UCM240933.pdf. Accessed March 27, 2012.

Wisner KL, Sit DK, Hanusa BH, et al: Major depression and antidepressant treatment: impact on pregnancy and neonatal outcomes. Am J Psychiatry 166:557–566, 2009. Reprinted in FOCUS 7:374–384, 2009.

Wright JH: Cognitive behavior therapy: basic principles and recent advances. FOCUS 4:173–178, 2006

Yonkers KA, Vigod S, Ross LE: Diagnosis, pathophysiology, and management of mood disorders in pregnant and postpartum women. Obstet Gynecol 117:961–977, 2011. Reprinted in FOCUS 10:51–66, 2012.

Zisook S: Ask the expert: psychopharmacology: major depressive disorder. FOCUS 4:484–486, 2006

MOC Part 4: Performance in Practice

Clinical Module for the Care of Patients With Major Depressive Disorder

Physician Practice Assessment
Retrospective Chart Review

STAGE A

Review of Five Patient Charts

STAGE A—Chart Review: In STAGE A, the physician compares his or her current practice (through a review of chart documentation) to guidelines and measures provided for the topic area. No patient or chart data need to be submitted, but the physician must evaluate the program online at www.apaeducation.org to earn continuing medical education (CME) credit and to document completion. When the evaluation is completed, STAGE A is recorded in the individual's CME transcript, and CME credit is awarded. Five credits are provided for STAGE A.

The evidence-based Performance in Practice: Clinical Module for the Care of Patients with Major Depressive Disorder presented here meets American Board of Psychiatry and Neurology Part 4 MOC requirements. In addition, this tool can facilitate implementation of a systematic approach to practice improvement for the assessment and treatment of patients with major depressive disorder.

PERFORMANCE IN PRACTICE:
Clinical Module for the Care of Patients with Major Depressive Disorder
Stage A: Physician Practice Assessment Retrospective Chart Review

Instructions: **Select charts for five patients** with a primary diagnosis of major depressive disorder. If the answer to a given question is "Yes," place a check mark in the appropriate box. If the answer to the question is "No" or "Unknown," leave the box unchecked. After reviewing the charts of all five patients, complete the penultimate column to determine the relative proportion of patients for whom the recommendation was followed. Any rows for which the total is less than 5 may be a useful focus for quality improvement efforts.

This activity is completed in the workbook on the form provided here for your use only. This form is *not* submitted to the American Psychiatric Association (APA) or to the ABPN. After the chart review step is complete, go to **www.apaeducation.org** to complete an evaluation for the program, document your participation, and receive a STAGE A certificate of credit.

Guideline recommendation being reviewed	Patient					Number of patients with checkmark in row	
Did the initial evaluation assess the following?	#1	#2	#3	#4	#5		Rationale and discussion
1 Signs/symptoms of major depression	❏	❏	❏	❏	❏	__/5	*Rationale:* Essential in establishing a diagnosis of major depressive disorder and determining response to treatment. *Discussion:* Before the clinician implements treatment of depression, a thorough diagnostic evaluation is needed, including assessment for the signs and symptoms of a major depressive episode. This evaluation will establish whether a diagnosis of major depressive disorder is warranted and provides baseline information against which to compare future changes in the patient's psychiatric status (sections A.II.A.2 and A.II.A.7 MDD PG). If self-assessment suggests that signs and symptoms of depression are inconsistently assessed, use of more formal rating scales such as the PHQ-9 may be considered.
2 Suicidal ideation/plans/intent	❏	❏	❏	❏	❏	__/5	*Rationale:* Essential in estimating suicide risk and determining appropriate treatment setting; public health importance of reducing suicide. *Discussion:* Assessing suicidal ideation, plans, and intent are essential elements of the initial evaluation. In addition to the relevance of suicidal ideation and plans to the diagnostic criteria for MDD (DSM-IV-TR), identifying the presence or absence of suicidal ideation, plans, and intent is important in assessing suicide risk and determining the most appropriate setting of treatment (sections A.II.A.3 MDD PG).

Guideline recommendation being reviewed	Patient					Number of patients with checkmark in row	
Did the initial evaluation assess the following?	#1	#2	#3	#4	#5		Rationale and discussion
3 Substance use/ abuse/dependence	❏	❏	❏	❏	❏		*Rationale:* Often unrecognized but common in individuals with MDD; essential in establishing the correct diagnosis (MDD vs. mood disorder due to substance intoxication or withdrawal), assessing suicide risk and planning treatment; public health importance of substance use disorders, including smoking. *Discussion:* Identifying past or current substance use disorders (including nicotine, alcohol, and other substances) is an important part of the initial evaluation of depressed patients (sections A.II.A.2 MDD PG) given the relevance of these disorders to risk assessment (sections A.II.A.3 MDD PG) and treatment planning.
Nicotine	❏	❏	❏	❏	❏	__/5	
Alcohol	❏	❏	❏	❏	❏	__/5	
Other substances	❏	❏	❏	❏	❏	__/5	
4 Presence/absence of other co-occurring psychiatric disorders	❏	❏	❏	❏	❏	__/5	*Rationale:* Other psychiatric disorders are common in individuals with MDD and may be unrecognized; essential in treatment planning and assessing suicide risk. *Discussion:* A crucial element of the initial evaluation is assessing for co-occurring psychiatric disorders (sections A.II.A.2, A.II.A.3, and A.II.B MDD PG). Anxiety disorders, dysthymic disorder, eating disorders, and personality disorders commonly co-occur with MDD and may increase suicide risk or require modifications in treatment (section A.III.A.3 MDD PG).
5 History of hypomanic or manic episodes	❏	❏	❏	❏	❏	__/5	*Rationale:* Often unrecognized but of relevance in distinguishing between MDD and bipolar disorder; essential in determining treatment. *Discussion:* Specific questioning about signs and symptoms of mania or hypomania is important in differentiating between MDD and bipolar disorder (sections A.II.A.2 MDD PG). This distinction has specific implications for treatment planning in order to minimize the risk of precipitating hypomania or mania with antidepressant treatment.

Guideline recommendation being reviewed		Patient					Number of patients with checkmark in row	
	Did the initial evaluation assess the following?	#1	#2	#3	#4	#5		Rationale and discussion
6	Presence/absence of general medical conditions	❑	❑	❑	❑	❑	__/5	*Rationale:* Essential in establishing the correct diagnosis (MDD vs. mood disorder due to general medical condition), planning treatment, interpreting potential side effects or interactions with prescribed medication, and avoiding worsening of preexisting conditions. *Discussion:* General medical conditions should be identified as part of the initial evaluation using information from the history, physical examination, and results of laboratory and other investigations, as they can be of relevance to diagnosis (DSM-IV-TR) and to the selection of treatments (sections A.II.B and A.III.C MDD PG) and treatment settings (section A.II.A.4 MDD PG).
Guideline recommendation being reviewed		Patient					Number of patients with checkmark in row	
	Was treatment concordant with Practice Guideline on MDD? (see Chart A)	#1	#2	#3	#4	#5		Rationale and discussion
								Rationale: Gaps in adhering to guideline-based recommendations are common, yet delivering recommended treatments can improve treatment outcomes. *Discussion:* Recommendations for treatment of MDD are presented in Chart A. If self-assessment identifies frequent divergences of care from guideline recommendations, further examination of practice patterns would help determine if deviations from guideline-recommended treatments are justified or if modifications in practice are needed to enhance patient outcomes.
7A	During the initial acute phase of treatment?	❑	❑	❑	❑	❑	__/5	
7B	At the time of the chart review (if the treatment plan differs from that in the initial phase of treatment)?	❑	❑	❑	❑	❑	__/5	

Guideline recommendation being reviewed	Patient					Number of patients with checkmark in row	
Has the treatment plan addressed the following?	#1	#2	#3	#4	#5		Rationale and discussion
8 Patient education about illness/ treatments	❏	❏	❏	❏	❏	__/5	*Rationale:* Increased provision of education can improve adherence and help patients make informed decisions about treatment. *Discussion:* Routinely providing patients and involved family members with education about MDD and its treatment can improve outcomes and enhance patients' involvement in decisions about their treatment (section A.II.A MDD PG).
9 Co-occurring substance use disorders	❏	❏	❏	❏	❏	__/__ (# applicable)	*Rationale:* Integrating treatment of MDD and co-occurring substance use disorders can improve outcomes yet is not always used. *Discussion:* If treatment of co-occurring substance use disorders is not addressed in individuals with MDD, the outcome of each disorder may be worse. Integrating MDD and co-occurring substance use disorders treatment is especially helpful in improving outcomes (A.III.A.3.d MDD PG). In addition, continued substance use may increase suicide risk.
10 Other co-occurring psychiatric disorders	❏	❏	❏	❏	❏	__/__ (# applicable)	*Rationale:* Integrating treatment of co-occurring psychiatric disorders can improve outcomes. *Discussion:* Other co-occurring psychiatric disorders (including dysthymic disorder, anxiety disorders, and personality disorders) are common among individuals with MDD, yet may be unidentified or undertreated. If these conditions are present, modifications in the treatment plan are often indicated (section A.III.A.3 MDD PG).

MDD=major depressive disorder; MDD PG=APA "Practice Guideline for the Treatment of Patients With Major Depressive Disorder," 3rd Edition (APA Practice Guidelines are available at: psychiatryonline.org); PHQ-9=nine-item depression scale of the Public Health Questionnaire.

Chart A

Recommendations for APA Practice Guideline–Concordant Treatment of Major Depressive Disorder (MDD)

If clinical presentation is characterized by:	Guideline concordant treatment will include:
Mild MDD (minor functional impairment, few symptoms beyond those required for diagnosis)	Antidepressant therapy alone OR Depression-focused psychotherapy alone[1] OR Combined treatment with depression-focused psychotherapy[1] and antidepressant medication[2] (if preferred by patient)
Moderate MDD (greater degree of functional impairment, some symptoms beyond those required for diagnosis)	Antidepressant therapy alone OR Depression-focused psychotherapy alone[1] OR Combined treatment with depression-focused psychotherapy[1] and antidepressant medication[2] OR Electroconvulsive therapy (ECT) (if preferred by the patient and depression is chronic)
Severe MDD (marked interference with social or occupational function; several symptoms in excess of those required for diagnosis)	Antidepressant therapy alone OR Combined treatment with depression-focused psychotherapy[1] and antidepressant medication[2] OR ECT (if preferred by the patient, if the patient has responded preferentially to ECT in the past, or if rapid treatment response is essential)
MDD with psychotic features	Combined treatment with an antidepressant and an antipsychotic medication (with or without depression-focused psychotherapy) OR ECT
MDD with catatonic features	Benzodiazepines OR ECT

[1]The presence of significant psychosocial stressors, interpersonal difficulties, co-occurring personality disorders, prior positive response to psychotherapy, or the stage, chronicity, and severity of the major depressive episode may add to the rationale for treating with psychotherapy. The availability of clinicians with appropriate training and expertise in specific therapeutic approaches can also be a factor in selecting among the depression-focused psychotherapies.

[2]In patients who have experienced only partial response to adequate trials of medications or psychotherapy alone, combination treatment may be considered.

Continuation Phase of Treatment
(focused on preserving symptom remission over the 4–9 months after full remission of symptoms is achieved)

If acute-phase treatment included:	Guideline-concordant treatment will include:
Depression-focused psychotherapy	Continued psychotherapy
Antidepressant medication	Antidepressant medication at a dose comparable to that used for acute treatment
Electroconvulsive therapy (ECT)	Pharmacotherapy or psychotherapy; continuation ECT is an acceptable alternative if pharmacotherapy or psychotherapy has not preserved remission in past

Maintenance Phase of Treatment
(focused on protecting against recurrence of major depressive episodes)

If treatment to prevent depressive recurrence is indicated[1] and acute treatment included:	Guideline-concordant treatment will include:
Depression-focused Psychotherapy	Continued depression-focused psychotherapy, with a decrease in visit frequency generally occurring
Antidepressant medication	Antidepressant medication, generally at a dose comparable to that used for acute treatment
Electroconvulsive therapy (ECT)	Pharmacotherapy or depression-focused psychotherapy; maintenance ECT may be considered if pharmacotherapy or psychotherapy has not preserved remission in past

[1]Indications for maintenance phase treatment are based on risk of recurrence (including consideration of number of prior episodes; presence of co-occurring conditions; interepisode residual symptoms, including sleep disturbance; family history of psychiatric illness, especially mood disorder; ongoing psychosocial stressors or impairment; negative cognitive style), severity of episodes (including consideration of suicidal ideas and behaviors, psychotic features, severe functional impairments), side effects experienced during continuation therapy, and patient preferences.

Performance in Practice

Clinical Module for the Care of Patients With Major Depressive Disorder

Physician Practice Assessment
Retrospective Chart Review

STAGE B

Improvement

In **STAGE B—Improvement,** based on the results of chart review, the physician identifies an area where improvement is needed and plans his or her strategy for improvement. This improvement plan is for the personal use of the physician and does not need to be submitted to the American Psychiatric Association (APA). Educational resources are provided in this workbook that can assist with an improvement plan; however, any activities relevant to the topic can be used for the improvement plan. During **STAGE B,** the physician implements the educational plan for as long as the doctor deems necessary, with a minimum of 30 days between STAGE A and STAGE C. This workbook includes some basic resources, such as the "Real-Time Assessment Tool for Patients with Depression," that guides the interviewer through a detailed assessment of one patient and can be copied and used with other patients or as a reference, and the Executive Summary from the APA "Practice Guideline on Treatment of Patients With Major Depressive Disorder, 3rd Edition." Key influential publications on aspects of depression and research into its treatment are also reprinted in the work-

book. Reading and studying these papers can be part of a STAGE B Improvement plan. Complete the continuing medical education (CME) evaluation for **STAGE B** at www.apaeducation.org.

After comparing the charted patient data to quality measures in STAGE A, the physician should initiate and document a plan for improvement, **STAGE B.** The physician may decide to access additional resources as part of the improvement plan. For example:

1. Use of specific recommendations and clinical resources outlined in STAGE A of the clinical module.
2. Completion of the "Real-Time Assessment Tool for Patients with Depression" (CME activity).
3. Review of the APA "Practice Guideline for Treatment of Patients With Major Depressive Disorders, 3rd Edition" (http://psychiatryonline.org/guidelines. aspx).
4. Review of Influential Publications on the topic of depression included in this workbook (see pages 43–156).
5. Individualized self-designed plan for improvement.

Five credits are awarded for completion of **Stage B.** In order to earn credit and document completion of **STAGE B,** log in to the course at apaeducation.org and document that you have completed a plan for improvement. Completion of Stage A provides automatic enrollment in **STAGE B.**

PERFORMANCE IN PRACTICE:
Clinical Module for the Care of Patients with Major Depressive Disorder
Stage B: Documentation of Your Improvement Plan

Record your improvement plan in the space below for your own use. Your improvement plan is not submitted to the American Board of Psychiatry and Neurology.

Use of PHQ-9 on admit and then weekly &
@ DC.

Performance in Practice

*Clinical Module for the Care of Patients
With Major Depressive Disorder*

**Physician Practice Assessment
Retrospective Chart Review**

STAGE C

Second Review of Five Patient Charts

Stage C—Second Chart Review: Following completion of STAGE B (education and improvement), the physician reassesses his or her performance with a second review of five patient charts and determines the results of his or her performance improvement effort. A minimum of 30 days is required between STAGE A and **STAGE C.** These can be a new group of patients seen since beginning the PIP activ-ities. Again, the physician retains all patient and chart data. After the physician completes the CME evaluation at www.apaeducation.org, credit and completion date for **STAGE C** will appear on his or her CME transcript. Ten credits are provided for **STAGE C.** Finishing the complete module, three stages in sequence within 24 months, earns the participant a total of 20 CME credits.

PERFORMANCE IN PRACTICE:
Clinical Module for the Care of Patients With Major Depressive Disorder
Stage C: Physician Practice Assessment Retrospective Chart Review

Instructions: **STAGE C,** a second retrospective chart review, must be completed within 24 months of STAGE A, the first retrospective chart review, and following completion of STAGE B, your plan for improvement and improvement action.

In **Stage C—Second Chart Review,** reassess your performance with review of five patient charts and determine the results of your performance improvement effort. These can be a new group of patients seen since beginning the PIP activities. Again, you retain all patient and chart data. After you complete the CME evaluation at www.apaeducation.org, credit and completion date for the entire PIP will appear on your CME transcript. The complete module, three stages in sequence within 24 months, earns the participant 20 CME credits total.

Select charts for five patients with a primary diagnosis of major depressive disorder. If the answer to a given question is "Yes," place a check mark in the appropriate box. If the answer to the question is "No" or "Unknown," leave the box unchecked. After reviewing the charts of all five patients, complete the penultimate column to determine the relative proportion of patients for whom the recommendation was followed and reflect on whether improvement objectives were accomplished within this set of charts.

Guideline recommendation being reviewed	Patient					Number of patients with checkmark in row	
Did the initial evaluation assess the following?	#1	#2	#3	#4	#5		Rationale and discussion
1 Signs/symptoms of major depression	❑	❑	❑	❑	❑	__/5	*Rationale:* Essential in establishing a diagnosis of major depressive disorder and determining response to treatment. *Discussion:* Before the clinician implements treatment of depression, a thorough diagnostic evaluation is needed, including assessment for the signs and symptoms of a major depressive episode. This evaluation will establish whether a diagnosis of major depressive disorder is warranted and provides baseline information against which to compare future changes in the patient's psychiatric status (sections A.II.A.2 and A.II.A.7 MDD PG). If self-assessment suggests that signs and symptoms of depression are inconsistently assessed, use of more formal rating scales such as the PHQ-9 may be considered.
2 Suicidal ideation/plans/intent	❑	❑	❑	❑	❑	__/5	*Rationale:* Essential in estimating suicide risk and determining appropriate treatment setting; public health importance of reducing suicide. *Discussion:* Assessing suicidal ideation, plans, and intent are essential elements of the initial evaluation. In addition to the relevance of suicidal ideation and plans to the diagnostic criteria for MDD (DSM-IV-TR), identifying the presence or absence of suicidal ideation, plans, and intent is important in assessing suicide risk and determining the most appropriate setting of treatment (sections A.II.A.3 MDD PG).

Guideline recommendation being reviewed	Patient					Number of patients with checkmark in row	
Did the initial evaluation assess the following?	#1	#2	#3	#4	#5		Rationale and discussion
3 Substance use/ abuse/dependence	❑	❑	❑	❑	❑		*Rationale:* Often unrecognized but common in individuals with MDD; essential in establishing the correct diagnosis (MDD vs. mood disorder due to substance intoxication or withdrawal), assessing suicide risk and planning treatment; public health importance of substance use disorders, including smoking. *Discussion:* Identifying past or current substance use disorders (including nicotine, alcohol, and other substances) is an important part of the initial evaluation of depressed patients (sections A.II.A.2 MDD PG) given the relevance of these disorders to risk assessment (sections A.II.A.3 MDD PG) and treatment planning.
Nicotine	❑	❑	❑	❑	❑	__/5	
Alcohol	❑	❑	❑	❑	❑	__/5	
Other substances	❑	❑	❑	❑	❑	__/5	
4 Presence/absence of other co-occurring psychiatric disorders	❑	❑	❑	❑	❑	__/5	*Rationale:* Other psychiatric disorders are common in individuals with MDD and may be unrecognized; essential in treatment planning and assessing suicide risk. *Discussion:* A crucial element of the initial evaluation is assessing for co-occurring psychiatric disorders (sections A.II.A.2, A.II.A.3, and A.II.B MDD PG). Anxiety disorders, dysthymic disorder, eating disorders, and personality disorders commonly co-occur with MDD and may increase suicide risk or require modifications in treatment (section A.III.A.3 MDD PG).
5 History of hypomanic or manic episodes	❑	❑	❑	❑	❑	__/5	*Rationale:* Often unrecognized but of relevance in distinguishing between MDD and bipolar disorder; essential in determining treatment. *Discussion:* Specific questioning about signs and symptoms of mania or hypomania is important in differentiating between MDD and bipolar disorder (sections A.II.A.2 MDD PG). This distinction has specific implications for treatment planning in order to minimize the risk of precipitating hypomania or mania with antidepressant treatment.

Guideline recommendation being reviewed	Patient					Number of patients with checkmark in row	
Did the initial evaluation assess the following?	#1	#2	#3	#4	#5		Rationale and discussion
6 — Presence/absence of general medical conditions	❏	❏	❏	❏	❏	__/5	*Rationale:* Essential in establishing the correct diagnosis (MDD vs. mood disorder due to general medical condition), planning treatment, interpreting potential side effects or interactions with prescribed medication, and avoiding worsening of preexisting conditions. *Discussion:* General medical conditions should be identified as part of the initial evaluation using information from the history, physical examination, and results of laboratory and other investigations, as they can be of relevance to diagnosis (DSM-IV-TR) and to the selection of treatments (sections A.II.B and A.III.C MDD PG) and treatment settings (section A.II.A.4 MDD PG).
Guideline recommendation being reviewed	Patient					Number of patients with checkmark in row	
Was treatment concordant with Practice Guideline on MDD? (see Chart A)	#1	#2	#3	#4	#5		Rationale and discussion
							Rationale: Gaps in adhering to guideline-based recommendations are common, yet delivering recommended treatments can improve treatment outcomes. *Discussion:* Recommendations for treatment of MDD are presented in Chart A. If self-assessment identifies frequent divergences of care from guideline recommendations, further examination of practice patterns would help determine if deviations from guideline-recommended treatments are justified or if modifications in practice are needed to enhance patient outcomes.
7A — During the initial acute phase of treatment?	❏	❏	❏	❏	❏	__/5	
7B — At the time of the chart review (if the treatment plan differs from that in the initial phase of treatment)?	❏	❏	❏	❏	❏	__/5	

Guideline recommendation being reviewed	Patient					Number of patients with checkmark in row	
Has the treatment plan addressed the following?	#1	#2	#3	#4	#5		Rationale and discussion
8 Patient education about illness/ treatments	❏	❏	❏	❏	❏	__/5	*Rationale:* Increased provision of education can improve adherence and help patients make informed decisions about treatment. *Discussion:* Routinely providing patients and involved family members with education about MDD and its treatment can improve outcomes and enhance patients' involvement in decisions about their treatment (section A.II.A MDD PG).
9 Co-occurring substance use disorders	❏	❏	❏	❏	❏	__/__ (# applicable)	*Rationale:* Integrating treatment of MDD and co-occurring substance use disorders can improve outcomes yet is not always used. *Discussion:* If treatment of co-occurring substance use disorders is not addressed in individuals with MDD, the outcome of each disorder may be worse. Integrating MDD and co-occurring substance use disorders treatment is especially helpful in improving outcomes (A.III.A.3.d MDD PG). In addition, continued substance use may increase suicide risk.
10 Other co-occurring psychiatric disorders	❏	❏	❏	❏	❏	__/__ (# applicable)	*Rationale:* Integrating treatment of co-occurring psychiatric disorders can improve outcomes. *Discussion:* Other co-occurring psychiatric disorders (including dysthymic disorder, anxiety disorders, and personality disorders) are common among individuals with MDD, yet may be unidentified or undertreated. If these conditions are present, modifications in the treatment plan are often indicated (section A.III.A.3 MDD PG).

MDD=major depressive disorder; MDD PG=APA "Practice Guideline for the Treatment of Patients With Major Depressive Disorder," 3rd Edition (APA Practice Guidelines are available at: psychiatryonline.org); PHQ-9=nine-item depression scale of the Public Health Questionnaire.

Improvement Activity: Real-Time Assessment Tool for Patients with Major Depressive Disorder

The Real-Time Assessment Tool for Patients with Major Depressive Disorder is a continuing medical education (CME) activity that may be used as a component of your self-determined improvement plan. The tool is provided as one resource you might use if after completing **STAGE A,** you determine that additional information about making an assessment of a patient with depression would provide information useful to you in improving practice.

After completing this assessment tool with one or more patients, go to **www.apaeducation.org** to docu-ment your CME credit (up to 5 AMA PRA Category 1 credits™) and evaluate the program. (Use of the unique purchaser number on the inside back cover of this work-book creates an enrollment for you in the activity.) Use the unique purchase number as described on p. xii. Once you have used the unique purchase number to enroll, click the **Launch Course** icon from your Student Home page to begin the course you choose.

Laura J. Fochtmann, M.D.
Farifteh F. Duffy, Ph.D.
Joyce C. West, Ph.D., M.P.P.
Robert Kunkle, M.A.
Robert M. Plovnick, M.D., M.S.

Performance in Practice:
Sample Tools for the Care of Patients with Major Depressive Disorder

Abstract: To facilitate continued clinical competence, the American Board of Medical Specialties and the American Board of Psychiatry and Neurology are implementing multi-faceted Maintenance of Certification programs, which include requirements for self-assessments of practice. Because psychiatrists may want to gain experience with self-assessment, two sample performance-in-practice tools are presented that are based on recommendations of the American Psychiatric Association's Practice Guideline for the Treatment of Patients with Major Depressive Disorder. One of these sample tools provides a traditional chart review approach to assessing care; the other sample tool presents a novel approach to real-time evaluation of practice. Both tools can be used as a foundation for subsequent performance improvement initiatives that are aimed at enhancing outcomes for patients with major depressive disorder.

Psychiatrists, like other medical professionals, are confronted by a need to maintain specialty specific knowledge despite an explosion in the amount of new information and the ongoing demands of clinical practice. Given these challenges, it is not surprising that researchers have consistently found gaps between actual care and recommended best-practices (1–10). In attempting to enhance the quality of delivered care, a number of approaches have been tried with varying degrees of success. Didactic approaches, including dissemination of written educational materials or practice guidelines, produce limited behavioral change (11–19). Embedding of patient-specific reminders into routine care can lead to benefits in specific quality measures (11, 13–16, 20–23) but these improvements may be narrow in scope, limited to the period of intervention or unassociated with improved patient outcomes (24–27). Receiving feedback after self or peer-review of practice patterns may also produce some enhancements in care (13–15, 23, 28–30). Given the limited effects of the above approaches when implemented alone, the diverse practice styles of physicians and the multiplicity of contexts in which care is delivered, a combination of quality improvement approaches may be needed to improve patient outcomes (14, 19, 28, 29, 31–34).

With these factors in mind, the American Board of Medical Specialties and the American Board of Psychiatry and Neurology are implementing multi-faceted Maintenance of Certification (MOC) Programs that include requirements for self-assessments of practice through reviewing the care of at least 5 patients (35). As with the original impetus to create specialty board certification, the MOC programs are intended to enhance quality of patient care in addition to assessing and verifying the competence of medical practitioners over time (36, 37). Although the MOC phase-in schedule will not require completion of a Performance in Practice (PIP) unit until 2014 (35), individuals may wish to begin assessing their own practice patterns before

---

CME Disclosure

Laura J. Fochtmann, M.D., Professor, Department of Psychiatry and Behavioral Science and Department of Pharmacological Sciences, State University of New York at Stony Brook, and Practice Guidelines Medical Editor, American Psychiatric Association

Robert Kunkle, M.A., and Robert M. Plovnick, M.D., M.S., Department of Quality Improvement and Psychiatric Services, American Psychiatric Association, 1000 Wilson Blvd., Ste. 1825, Arlington, VA 22209-3901

Farifteh F. Duffy, Ph.D., and Joyce C. West, Ph.D., M.P.P., American Psychiatric Institute for Research and Education, 1000 Wilson Blvd, Suite 1825, Arlington, Virginia, 22209

No relevant financial relationships to disclose.

Address correspondence to: Laura J. Fochtmann, M.D., Department of Psychiatry and Behavioral Science, Stony Brook University School of Medicine, HSC-T10, Stony Brook, NY 11794-8101, E-mail: laura.fochtmann@stonybrook.edu

Table 1. Aspects of Major Depressive Disorder Treatment Addressed by Sample Performance-In-Practice Tools

Recommendation	Source of Recommendation[1]	Performance Tool[2]
Identify signs and symptoms of depression	MDD PG	A, B, PCPI
Assess suicidal ideation, plans and intent	MDD PG; SB PG	A, B, PCPI
Identify past or current symptoms of mania or hypomania	MDD PG; BP PG	A, B
Identify past and current substance use disorders, including nicotine, alcohol and other substances	MDD PG; SUD PG; SB PG	A, B
Identify other past and current co-occurring psychiatric disorders	MDD PG	A, B
Identify past and current general medical conditions	MDD PG	A, B
Use treatments that are concordant with practice guideline recommendations (see Appendix A).	MDD PG	A, B, PCPI
Integrate treatment of any substance use disorders or other co-occurring psychiatric disorders with treatment for MDD	MDD PG; SUD PG; SB PG	A, B
Provide education to patients/families about depression and its treatment	MDD PG	A, B
Consider factors such as age, sex, ethnicity, cultural or religious beliefs in planning treatment	MDD PG	B
Assess the patient's level of functioning in social, occupational and other important realms	MDD PG	B
Determine whether cognitive impairment is present	MDD PG	B
Determine whether aggressive behavior is present	SB PG	B
Determine whether suicide attempts or other self-harming behaviors are present	MDD PG; SB PG	B
Determine the degree of adherence to treatment	MDD PG	B
Determine if side effects of treatment are present and, if so, which ones	MDD PG	B

[1] Source of Recommendation: MDD PG= Practice Guideline for the Treatment of Patients with Major Depressive Disorder (38); SUD PG= Practice Guideline for the Treatment of Patients with Substance Use Disorders (61); BP PG = Practice Guideline for the Treatment of Patients with Bipolar Disorder (42); SB PG = Practice Guideline for the Assessment and Treatment of Patients with Suicidal Behaviors (62)
[2] Performance Tool: A = Sample retrospective PIP tool of Appendix A; B = Sample prospective PIP tool of Appendix B; PCPI = Major depressive disorder measures of the American Medical Association Physician Consortium for Performance Improvement (63)

that time. To facilitate such self-assessment related to the treatment of depression, this paper will discuss several approaches to reviewing one's clinical practice and will provide sample PIP tools that are based on recommendations of the American Psychiatric Association's Practice Guideline for the Treatment of Patients with Major Depressive Disorder (38).

Traditionally, most quality improvement programs have focused on retrospective assessments of practice at the level of organizations or departments (39). The Healthcare Effectiveness Data and Information Set (HEDIS) measures of the National Committee for Quality Assurance (NCQA) (40) are a commonly used group of quality indicators that measure health organization performance.

When used under such circumstances, quality indicators are typically expressed as a percentage that reflects the extent of adherence to a particular indicator. For example, in the quality of care measures for bipolar disorder (41) derived from the American Psychiatric Association's 2002 Practice Guideline for the Treatment of Patients with Bipolar Disorder (42), one of the indicators is that "Patients in an acute depressive episode of bipolar disorder who are treated with antidepressants, [are] also receiving an antimanic agent such as valproate or lithium." In this example, to calculate the percentage of patients for whom the indicator is fulfilled, the numerator will be the "Number of patients in an acute depressive episode of bipolar disorder, who are receiving an antidepressant, and who are also receiving an anti-manic agent such as valproate or lithium." and the denominator will be the "Number of patients in an acute depressive episode of bipolar disorder who are receiving an antidepressant" (41).

As in the above example, most quality indicators are derived from evidence-based practice guidelines, which are intended to apply to typical patients in a population rather than being universally applicable to all patients with a particular disorder (43, 44). In addition, practice guideline recommendations are mainly informed by data from randomized controlled trials. Patients in such trials may have significant differences from those seen in routine clinical practice (45), including clinical presentation, preference for treatment, response to treatment, and presence of co-occurring psychiatric and general medical conditions (43, 46, 47). These differences may result in treatment decisions for individual patients that are clinically appropriate but not concordant with practice guideline recommendations.

When quality indicators are used to compare individual physicians' practice patterns, quality measures can be influenced by practice size, patients' sociodemographic factors and illness severity as well as other practice-level and patient-level factors. For example, when small groups of patients are receiving care from an individual physician, a small shift in the number of individuals receiving a recommended intervention could lead to large shifts in the resulting rates of concordance with evidence-based care. Without appropriate application of case-mix adjustments, across-practice comparisons may result in erroneous conclusions about the quality of care being delivered (48, 49). For patients with complex conditions or multiple disorders receiving simultaneous treatment, composite measures of overall treatment quality may yield more accurate appraisals than measurement of single quality indicators (50–52).

With the above caveats, however, use of retrospective quality indicators can be beneficial for individual physicians who wish to assess their own patterns of practice. If a physician's self-assessment identified aspects of care that frequently differed from key quality indicators, further examination of practice patterns would be helpful. Through self-assessment, the physician may determine that deviations from the quality indicators are justified, or he may acquire new knowledge and modify practice to improve quality. It is this sort of self-assessment and performance improvement efforts that the MOC PIP program is designed to foster.

Appendices A and B provide sample PIP tools, each of which is designed to be relevant across clinical settings (e.g., inpatient, outpatient), straight-forward to complete and usable in a pen-and-paper format to aid adoption. Although the MOC program requires review of at least 5 patients as part of each PIP unit, it is important to note that larger samples will provide more accurate estimates of quality within a practice. Appendix A provides a sample retrospective chart review PIP tool that assesses the care given to patients with major depressive disorder. Although it is designed as a self-assessment tool, this form could also be used for retrospective peer-review initiatives. As with other retrospective chart review tools, some questions on the form relate to the initial assessment and treatment of the patient whereas other questions relate to subsequent care. Appendix B provides a prospective review form that is intended to be a cross-sectional assessment and could be completed immediately following a patient visit. As currently formatted, Appendix B is designed to be folded in half to allow real-time feedback based upon answers to the initial practice-based questions. This approach is more typical of clinical decision support systems that provide real-time feedback on the concordance between guideline recommendations and the individual patient's care. In the future, the same data recording and feedback steps could be implemented via a web-based or electronic record system enhancing integration into clinical workflow (53). This will make it more likely that psychiatrists will see the feedback as interactive, targeted to their needs and clinically relevant. Rather than relying on more global changes in practice patterns to enhance individual patients' care, such feedback also provides the opportunity to adjust the treatment plan of an individual patient to improve patient-specific outcomes (54–56). However, data from this form could also be used in aggregate to plan and implement broader quality improvement initiatives. For example, if self-assessment using the sample tools suggests that signs and symptoms of depression are inconsistently assessed, consistent use of more formal rating scales such as the PHQ-9 (57–59) could be considered.

Each of the sample tools attempts to highlight aspects of care that have significant public health implications (e.g., suicide, obesity, use of tobacco and other substances) or for which gaps in guideline adherence are common. Examples include under-detection and undertreatment of co-occuring substance use disorders (5) and the relatively low concordance with practice guideline recommendations for use of psychosocial therapies and for treatment of psychotic features with MDD (4). Table 1 summarizes specific aspects of care that are measured by these sample PIP tools. Quality improvement suggestions that arise from completion of these sample tools are intended to be within the control of individual psychiatrists rather than dependent upon other health care system resources.

After using one of the sample PIP tools to assess the pattern of care given to a group of 5 or more patients with major depressive disorder, the psychiatrist should determine whether specific aspects of care need to be improved. For example, if the presence or absence of co-occurring psychiatric disorders has not been assessed or if these disorders are present but not addressed in the treatment plan, then a possible area for improvement would involve greater consideration of co-occurring psychiatric disorders, which are common in patients with MDD.

These sample PIP tools can also serve as a foundation for more elaborate approaches to improving psychiatric practice as part of the MOC program. If systems are developed so that practice-related data can be entered electronically (either as part of an electronic health record or as an independent web-based application), algorithms can suggest areas for possible improvement using specific, measurable, achievable, relevant and time-limited objectives (60). Such electronic systems could also provide links to journal or textbook materials, clinical practice guidelines, patient educational materials, drug-drug interaction checking, evidence based tool kits or other clinical materials. In addition, future work will focus on developing more standardized approaches to integrating patient and peer feedback with personal performance review, developing and implementing programs of performance improvements and reassessment of performance and patient outcomes.

REFERENCES

1. Institute of Medicine. Crossing the quality chasm: a new health system for the 21st century. Washington, D.C: National Academy Press; 2001.
2. Institute of Medicine. Improving the quality of health care for mental and substance-use conditions. Washington, DC: National Academies Press; 2006.
3. Colenda CC, Wagenaar DB, Mickus M, Marcus SC, Tanielian T, Pincus HA. Comparing clinical practice with guideline recommendations for the treatment of depression in geriatric patients: findings from the APA practice research network. Am J Geriatr Psychiatry 2003 Jul; 11(4):448–57.
4. West JC, Duffy FF, Wilk JE, Rae DS, Narrow WE, Pincus HA, et al. Patterns and quality of treatment for patients with major depressive disorder in routine psychiatric practice. Focus 2005; 3(1):43–50.
5. Wilk JE, West JC, Narrow WE, Marcus S, Rubio-Stipec M, Rae DS, et al. Comorbidity patterns in routine psychiatric practice: is there evidence of underdetection and underdiagnosis? Compr Psychiatry 2006 Jul; 47(4): 258–64.
6. Pincus HA, Page AE, Druss B, Appelbaum PS, Gottlieb G, England MJ. Can psychiatry cross the quality chasm? Improving the quality of health care for mental and substance use conditions. Am J Psychiatry 2007 May; 164(5):712–9.
7. Rost K, Dickinson LM, Fortney J, Westfall J, Hermann RC. Clinical improvement associated with conformance to HEDIS-based depression care. Ment Health Serv Res 2005 Jun; 7(2):103–12.
8. Cochrane LJ, Olson CA, Murray S, Dupuis M, Tooman T, Hayes S. Gaps between knowing and doing: understanding and assessing the barriers to optimal health care. J Contin Educ Health Prof 2007; 27(2):94–102.
9. Chen RS, Rosenheck R. Using a computerized patient database to evaluate guideline adherence and measure patterns of care for major depression. J Behav Health Serv Res 2001 Nov; 28(4):466–74.
10. Cabana MD, Rushton JL, Rush AJ. Implementing practice guidelines for depression: applying a new framework to an old problem. Gen Hosp Psychiatry 2002 Jan; 24(1):35–42.
11. Davis D. Does CME work? An analysis of the effect of educational activities on physician performance or health care outcomes. Int J Psychiatry Med 1998; 28(1):21–39.
12. Sohn W, Ismail AI, Tellez M. Efficacy of educational interventions targeting primary care providers' practice behaviors: an overview of published systematic reviews. J Public Health Dent 2004; 64(3):164–72.
13. Bloom BS. Effects of continuing medical education on improving physician clinical care and patient health: a review of systematic reviews. Int J Technol Assess Health Care 2005; 21(3):380–5.
14. Chaillet N, Dube E, Dugas M, Audibert F, Tourigny C, Fraser WD, et al. Evidence-based strategies for implementing guidelines in obstetrics: a systematic review. Obstet Gynecol 2006 Nov; 108(5):1234–45.
15. Grimshaw J, Eccles M, Thomas R, MacLennan G, Ramsay C, Fraser C, et al. Toward evidence-based quality improvement. Evidence (and its limitations) of the effectiveness of guideline dissemination and implementation strategies 1966–1998. J Gen Intern Med 2006 Feb; 21 Suppl 2:S14–S20.
16. Grimshaw JM, Shirran L, Thomas R, Mowatt G, Fraser C, Bero L, et al. Changing provider behavior: an overview of systematic reviews of interventions. Med Care 2001 Aug; 39(8 Suppl 2):II2–45.
17. Grol R. Changing physicians' competence and performance: finding the balance between the individual and the organization. J Contin Educ Health Prof 2002; 22(4):244–51.
18. Oxman TE. Effective educational techniques for primary care providers: application to the management of psychiatric disorders. Int J Psychiatry Med 1998; 28(1):3–9.
19. Green LA, Wyszewianski L, Lowery JC, Kowalski CP, Krein SL. An observational study of the effectiveness of practice guideline implementation strategies examined according to physicians' cognitive styles. Implement Sci 2007 Dec 1; 2(1):41.
20. Balas EA, Weingarten S, Garb CT, Blumenthal D, Boren SA, Brown GD. Improving preventive care by prompting physicians. Arch Intern Med 2000 Feb 14; 160(3):301–8.
21. Feldstein AC, Smith DH, Perrin N, Yang X, Rix M, Raebel MA, et al. Improved therapeutic monitoring with several interventions: a randomized trial. Arch Intern Med 2006 Sep 25; 166(17):1848–54.
22. Kucher N, Koo S, Quiroz R, Cooper JM, Paterno MD, Soukonnikov B, et al. Electronic alerts to prevent venous thromboembolism among hospitalized patients. N Engl J Med 2005 Mar 10; 352(10):969–77.
23. Weingarten SR, Henning JM, Badamgarav E, Knight K, Hasselblad V, Gano A, Jr., et al. Interventions used in disease management programmes for patients with chronic illness-which ones work? Meta-analysis of published reports. BMJ 2002 Oct 26; 325(7370):925.
24. O'Connor PJ, Crain AL, Rush WA, Sperl-Hillen JM, Gutenkauf JJ, Duncan JE. Impact of an electronic medical record on diabetes quality of care. Ann Fam Med 2005 Jul; 3(4):300–6.
25. Rollman BL, Hanusa BH, Lowe HJ, Gilbert T, Kapoor WN, Schulberg HC. A randomized trial using computerized decision support to improve treatment of major depression in primary care. J Gen Intern Med 2002 Jul; 17(7):493–503.
26. Sequist TD, Gandhi TK, Karson AS, Fiskio JM, Bugbee D, Sperling M, et al. A randomized trial of electronic clinical reminders to improve quality of care for diabetes and coronary artery disease. J Am Med Inform Assoc 2005 Jul; 12(4):431–7.
27. Tierney WM, Overhage JM, Murray MD, Harris LE, Zhou XH, Eckert GJ, et al. Can computer-generated evidence-based care suggestions enhance evidence-based management of asthma and chronic obstructive pulmonary disease? A randomized, controlled trial. Health Serv Res 2005 Apr; 40(2):477–97.
28. Arnold SR, Straus SE. Interventions to improve antibiotic prescribing practices in ambulatory care. Cochrane Database Syst Rev 2005; (4): CD003539.
29. Bradley EH, Holmboe ES, Mattera JA, Roumanis SA, Radford MJ, Krumholz HM. Data feedback efforts in quality improvement: lessons learned from US hospitals. Qual Saf Health Care 2004 Feb; 13(1):26–31.
30. Paukert JL, Chumley-Jones HS, Littlefield JH. Do peer chart audits improve residents' performance in providing preventive care? Acad Med 2003 Oct; 78(10 Suppl):S39–S41.
31. Roumie CL, Elasy TA, Greevy R, Griffin MR, Liu X, Stone WJ, et al. Improving blood pressure control through provider education, provider alerts, and patient education: a cluster randomized trial. Ann Intern Med 2006 Aug 1; 145(3):165–75.

32. Hysong SJ, Best RG, Pugh JA. Clinical practice guideline implementation strategy patterns in Veterans Affairs primary care clinics. Health Serv Res 2007 Feb; 42(1 Pt 1):84–103.

33. Dykes PC, Acevedo K, Boldrighini J, Boucher C, Frumento K, Gray P, et al. Clinical practice guideline adherence before and after implementation of the HEARTFELT (HEART Failure Effectiveness & Leadership Team) intervention. J Cardiovasc Nurs 2005 Sep; 20(5):306–14.

34. Greene RA, Beckman H, Chamberlain J, Partridge G, Miller M, Burden D, et al. Increasing adherence to a community-based guideline for acute sinusitis through education, physician profiling, and financial incentives. Am J Manag Care 2004 Oct; 10(10):670–8.

35. American Board of Psychiatry and Neurology. Maintenance of Certification for Psychiatry. 2007. Accessed on 11-23-0007. Available from: URL:http://www.abpn.com/moc_psychiatry.htm

36. Institute of Medicine. Health professions education: A bridge to quality. Washington, D.C: National Academies Press; 2003.

37. Miller SH. American Board of Medical Specialties and repositioning for excellence in lifelong learning: maintenance of certification. J Contin Educ Health Prof 2005; 25(3):151–6.

38. American Psychiatric Association. Practice guideline for the treatment of patients with major depressive disorder (revision). Am J Psychiatry 2000 Apr; 157(4 Suppl):1–45.

39. Hermann RC. Improving mental healthcare: A guide to measurement-based quality improvement. Washington, DC: American Psychiatric Pub; 2005.

40. National Committee for Quality Assurance. HEDIS and quality measurement. National Committee for Quality Assurance 2007. Accessed on 12-30-2007. Available from: URL: http://web.ncqa.org/tabid/59/Default.aspx

41. Duffy FF, Narrow W, West JC, Fochtmann LJ, Kahn DA, Suppes T, et al. Quality of care measures for the treatment of bipolar disorder. Psychiatr Q 2005; 76(3):213–30.

42. American Psychiatric Association. Practice guideline for the treatment of patients with bipolar disorder (revision). Am J Psychiatry 2002 Apr; 159(4 Suppl):1–50.

43. American Psychiatric Association. American Psychiatric Association practice guidelines for the treatment of psychiatric disorders. Arlington, Va: American Psychiatric Association; 2006.

44. Sachs GS, Printz DJ, Kahn DA, Carpenter D, Docherty JP. The Expert Consensus Guideline Series: Medication Treatment of Bipolar Disorder 2000. Postgrad Med 2000 Apr; Spec No:1–104.

45. Zarin DA, Young JL, West JC. Challenges to evidence-based medicine: a comparison of patients and treatments in randomized controlled trials with patients and treatments in a practice research network. Soc Psychiatry Psychiatr Epidemiol 2005 Jan; 40(1):27–35.

46. Eddy D. Reflections on science, judgment, and value in evidence-based decision making: a conversation with David Eddy by Sean R. Tunis. Health Aff (Millwood) 2007 Jul; 26(4):w500–w515.

47. Kobak KA, Taylor L, Katzelnick DJ, Olson N, Clagnaz P, Henk HJ. Antidepressant medication management and Health Plan Employer Data Information Set (HEDIS) criteria: reasons for nonadherence. J Clin Psychiatry 2002 Aug; 63(8):727–32.

48. Hofer TP, Hayward RA, Greenfield S, Wagner EH, Kaplan SH, Manning WG. The unreliability of individual physician "report cards" for assessing the costs and quality of care of a chronic disease. JAMA 1999 Jun 9; 281(22):2098–105.

49. Greenfield S, Kaplan SH, Kahn R, Ninomiya J, Griffith JL. Profiling care provided by different groups of physicians: effects of patient case-mix (bias) and physician-level clustering on quality assessment results. Ann Intern Med 2002 Jan 15; 136(2):111–21.

50. Parkerton PH, Smith DG, Belin TR, Feldbau GA. Physician performance assessment: nonequivalence of primary care measures. Med Care 2003 Sep; 41(9):1034–47.

51. Lipner RS, Weng W, Arnold GK, Duffy FD, Lynn LA, Holmboe ES. A three-part model for measuring diabetes care in physician practice. Acad Med 2007 Oct; 82(10 Suppl):S48–S52.

52. Nietert PJ, Wessell AM, Jenkins RG, Feifer C, Nemeth LS, Ornstein SM. Using a summary measure for multiple quality indicators in primary care: the Summary QUality InDex (SQUID). Implement Sci 2007; 2:11.

53. Rollman BL, Gilbert T, Lowe HJ, Kapoor WN, Schulberg HC. The electronic medical record: its role in disseminating depression guidelines in primary care practice. Int J Psychiatry Med 1999; 29(3):267–86.

54. Trivedi MH, Daly EJ. Measurement-based care for refractory depression: a clinical decision support model for clinical research and practice. Drug Alcohol Depend 2007 May;,88 Suppl 2:S61–S71.

55. Hepner KA, Rowe M, Rost K, Hickey SC, Sherbourne CD, Ford DE, et al. The effect of adherence to practice guidelines on depression outcomes. Ann Intern Med 2007 Sep 4; 147(5):320–9.

56. Dennehy EB, Suppes T, Rush AJ, Miller AL, Trivedi MH, Crismon ML, et al. Does provider adherence to a treatment guideline change clinical outcomes for patients with bipolar disorder? Results from the Texas Medication Algorithm Project. Psychol Med 2005 Dec; 35(12):1695–706.

57. Kroenke K, Spitzer RL, Williams JB. The PHQ-9: validity of a brief depression severity measure. J Gen Intern Med 2001 Sep; 16(9):606–13.

58. Lowe B, Kroenke K, Herzog W, Grafe K. Measuring depression outcome with a brief self-report instrument: sensitivity to change of the Patient Health Questionnaire (PHQ-9). J Affect Disord 2004 Jul; 81(1):61–6.

59. Lowe B, Schenkel I, Carney-Doebbeling C, Gobel C. Responsiveness of the PHQ-9 to Psychopharmacological Depression Treatment. Psychosomatics 2006 Jan; 47(1):62–7.

60. MacDonald G, Starr G, Schooley M, Yee SL, Klimowski K, Turner K. Introduction to program evaluation for comprehensive tobacco control programs. Centers for Disease Control and Prevention 2001 Accessed on 12-17-2007. Available from: URL: http://www.cdc.gov/tobacco/tobacco_control_programs/surveillance_evaluation/evaluation_manual/00_pdfs/Evaluation.pdf

61. American Psychiatric Association. Practice guideline for the treatment of patients with substance use disorders, second edition. Am J Psychiatry 2007 Apr; 164(4 Suppl):5–123.

62. American Psychiatric Association. Practice guideline for the assessment and treatment of patients with suicidal behaviors. Am J Psychiatry 2003 Nov; 160(11 Suppl):1–60.

63. American Medical Association Physician Consortium for Performance Improvement. AMA (CQI) Major depressive disorder. American Medical Association Physician Consortium for Performance Improvement Accessed on 12-17-2007. Available from: URL: http://www.ama-assn.org/ama/pub/category/16494.html

NOTES

"Real-Time" Assessment Tool for Patients with Depression

This "real time" tool is intended to be a prospective cross-sectional assessment that could be completed immediately following a patient visit. As currently formatted, the tool is designed to be folded in half to allow real-time feedback based upon answers to initial practice based questions.

Patient Characteristics: Age: ☐ Sex: ☐

Estimated duration of depressive illness:

Length of time in treatment for current depressive episode:

Which of the following is the patient experiencing?

	Yes	No	Unknown
Little interest or pleasure in doing things?	☐	☐	☐
Feeling down, depressed, or hopeless?	☐	☐	☐
Trouble falling or staying asleep, or sleeping too much?	☐	☐	☐
Feeling tired or having little energy?	☐	☐	☐
Poor appetite or overeating?	☐	☐	☐
Negative feelings about self?	☐	☐	☐
Trouble concentrating	☐	☐	☐
Psychomotor retardation or agitation?	☐	☐	☐
Thoughts of suicide, self-harm, or being better off dead?	☐	☐	☐

To establish a diagnosis of depression, at least 5 of these symptoms need to be experienced nearly every day over a 2 week period (with one of the symptoms being either depressed mood or loss of interest or pleasure). However, other symptom assessment intervals may be appropriate when monitoring the presence or absence of symptoms over time.

If associated symptoms of depression are not routinely assessed (as indicated by multiple boxes on the left that are checked as unassessed or unknown), consider using a standardized tool for assessing and recording depressive symptoms such as the PHQ-9.

If the patient has thoughts of suicide, self-harm, or being better off dead, was there a specific inquiry into:

Suicide plans	Yes ☐	No ☐
Suicide intent	Yes ☐	No ☐
Suicide methods	Yes ☐	No ☐

When patients are experiencing thoughts of suicide, self-harm, or of being better off dead, more detailed questioning is crucial. The presence of suicide plans or intent indicates a significant increase in suicide risk. An intention to use a highly lethal suicide method (e.g., guns, hanging, jumping) will also confer an increase in suicide risk. When a suicide method is identified, the accessibility of the method is an additional part of the inquiry.

	Yes	No	Unknown
Is the patient experiencing clinically significant distress or impairment in social, occupational, or other important areas of functioning that is a change from the baseline level of function?	☐	☐	☐

The presence of clinically significant distress or functional impairment is one of the criteria used in making a diagnosis of depression. In addition to being a primary focus of patients and their families, functional impairment is a major determinant of illness-related disability and should be routinely assessed.

Distress and impairment are equally important to assess in examining response to treatment. If clinically significant distress or functional impairment are present, consider whether a change in treatment plan is indicated. Depending on the duration of treatment and persistence of symptoms, consideration may be given to changing a medication dose, modifying or adding a psychosocial treatment, changing or adding a medication, or revising the primary diagnosis.

"Real-Time" Assessment Tool for Patients with Depression
(p. 2 of 6)

	Current	Past	Unknown
Current Depressive Diagnosis:			
Other Psychiatric Diagnoses:			
Anxiety disorder(s):	☐	☐	☐
Nicotine dependence	☐	☐	☐
Alcohol use disorder:	☐	☐	☐
Other substance use disorder:	☐	☐	☐
Personality disorder:	☐	☐	☐
Other:	☐	☐	☐

In establishing a diagnosis of depression, it is essential to determine whether the patient has had multiple depressive episodes or only a single episode of depression as this will have implications for treatment planning. It is also important to identify other co-occurring psychiatric disorders as part of the initial assessment. Such disorders are common in depressed patients and need to be considered in planning care.

Other psychiatric issues:	Current	Past	Unknown
Psychosis	☐	☐	☐
Impaired cognition	☐	☐	☐
Problematic use of alcohol or other substances (not meeting criteria for a substance use disorder diagnosis)	☐	☐	☐

The presence of psychotic symptoms in a depressed patient will generally necessitate treatment with an antipsychotic and an antidepressant medication or with ECT.

Cognitive impairment may be associated with depression, medication side effects, or other underlying causes. It can also influence adherence with treatment and patient safety.

Use of alcohol or other substances can be problematic in depressed patients and can influence treatment response and suicide risk even in the absence of a substance use disorder.

Additional psychiatric history:	Yes	No	Unknown
Hospitalizations	☐	☐	☐
Suicide attempts	☐	☐	☐
Other self-harming behaviors	☐	☐	☐
Aggressive behavior	☐	☐	☐
Mania/Hypomania	☐	☐	☐

A history of hospitalization, suicide attempts, or other self-harming behaviors is relevant in estimating suicide risk. The presence or absence of aggressive behaviors can also be important to risk assessment.

If not specifically assessed, manic or hypomanic episodes may not be reported. The treatment of a depressive episode may need to be modified if Bipolar I or Bipolar II disorder is identified, as use of an antidepressant in bipolar patients may be associated with occurrence of hypomanic or manic episodes.

If any of the aspects of psychiatric diagnosis, symptoms, or history on this page are not routinely assessed, increasing rates of assessment may be a useful goal for performance improvement.

"Real-Time" Assessment Tool for Patients with Depression (p. 3 of 6)

General Medical Conditions (including side effects of meds):	Yes	No	Unknown
Hypertension	☐	☐	☐
Cardiovascular disorders	☐	☐	☐
Asthma/COPD	☐	☐	☐
Renal disorders	☐	☐	☐
Hepatic disorders	☐	☐	☐
Infectious diseases (e.g., HIV, Hepatitis C)	☐	☐	☐
Thyroid disease	☐	☐	☐
Seizure disorder	☐	☐	☐
Sleep apnea	☐	☐	☐
Obesity	☐	☐	☐
Diabetes	☐	☐	☐
Hyperlipidemia	☐	☐	☐
Other:	☐	☐	☐

When present, general medical conditions and their treatments can contribute to depressive symptoms or require adjustments in medication doses. Medications prescribed for psychiatric disorders can interact with those for general medical conditions and can produce side effects in various organ systems (e.g., renal or thyroid difficulties with lithium, seizures with clozapine and other psychotropic medications, glucose dysregulation and hyperlipidemia with second generation antipsychotic medications). In addition, individuals with psychiatric illnesses may be at increased risk of acquiring general medical conditions (e.g., HIV and Hepatitis C acquired through intravenous substance use, cardiovascular and respiratory conditions through smoking). Weight gain is common with psychiatric medications and obesity contributes to morbidity and mortality. Sleep apnea can be an unrecognized complication of obesity that can be exacerbated by sedating medications.

If general medical conditions and medication-related side effects are not being routinely identified, this may be a useful focus of performance improvement efforts

If obesity is present, is the patient's weight being monitored?

Yes ☐   No ☐

Given the rise in obesity as a public health problem and the common occurrence of weight gain with psychotropic medications, monitoring of weight and recommendations about weight control strategies are increasingly relevant elements of treatment planning.

have nutrition and exercise been discussed?

Yes ☐   No ☐

If the patient has current general medical conditions, has contact been made with the patient's primary care physician?

Yes ☐   No ☐

Collaborating with other clinicians is an important part of psychiatric management. When a patient has a current general medical condition, communication with the patient's primary care physician may be indicated.

Current nonpsychiatric medication(s)	Dose	Frequency	Route

Knowledge of medications that patients are receiving for treatment of nonpsychiatric disorders is important in looking for potential drug-drug interactions and interpreting reported side effects of treatment. Such information can also alert the clinician to the presence of general medical conditions that may not have been reported by the patient (e.g., hypertension, hyperlipidemias) or to side effects of treatment that may require changes in medications or medication doses.

"Real-Time" Assessment Tool for Patients with Depression
(p. 4 of 6)

Current psychiatric medication(s)	Dose	Frequency	Route	
				Knowledge of medications that patients are receiving for treatment of psychiatric disorders is important in assessing the patient's response to treatment and interpreting reported side effects of treatment. In reviewing the list of the patient's current medications, infrequently administered medications (e.g., long-acting injectable antipsychotic medications) should not be overlooked. If the patient has residual symptoms, assess the adequacy of the medication dose and determine if changes in medication, medication dose, or concomitant psychosocial therapy are indicated.

Has the potential for drug-drug interactions been assessed for the patient's current medication regimen? Yes ☐ No ☐ N/A ☐	Many psychotropic medications are metabolized through the cytochrome P450 and uridine 5′-diphosphate glucuronosyl-transferase enzyme systems, have high degrees of binding to plasma proteins, or act on the P-glycoprotein transporter in the gastrointestinal tract. Consequently, there are many opportunities for clinically relevant drug-drug interactions to occur when patients are receiving psychotropic medications. If identification of potential drug-drug interactions is not routinely done, this may be a useful focus for performance improvement.
If any of the patient's medications require laboratory monitoring (e.g., medication blood levels, evaluation of side effects), has this been performed? Yes ☐ No ☐ N/A ☐	Specific medications may also require blood level monitoring or other follow-up laboratory testing to assess for the presence of side effects. If such monitoring is indicated but sometimes overlooked, this may also be a useful focus for performance improvement initiatives.
Is each medication essential? Yes ☐ No ☐	Continued use of nonessential medications increases costs as well as side effects and drug-drug interactions. With the fragmentation of health care, medications that were intended to be tapered may have been continued inadvertently. As a result, patients may be taking multiple medications of the same class without evidence in the literature that this improves outcomes. Regular review of patients' medication regimens may help determine which medications are essential (and should not be stopped) and which may be able to be tapered and discontinued.

Other somatic treatment approaches:

	Current	Past	Unknown	
Electroconvulsive therapy	☐	☐	☐	The current and past use of other somatic treatment approaches is relevant to treatment planning as well as to assessment of therapeutic responses and treatment-related side effects. Inquiring about past experiences with these treatments is sometimes overlooked as part of the evaluation of patients with depression.
Vagal nerve stimulation therapy	☐	☐	☐	
Other:	☐	☐	☐	

"Real-Time" Assessment Tool for Patients with Depression (p. 5 of 6)

Psychosocial treatments used (by psychiatrist or other clinicians):	Current	Past	Unknown
Psychodynamic psychotherapy	☐	☐	☐
Cognitive psychotherapy	☐	☐	☐
Behavioral psychotherapy	☐	☐	☐
Interpersonal psychotherapy	☐	☐	☐
Supportive psychotherapy	☐	☐	☐
Education about illness or treatment	☐	☐	☐
Medication management	☐	☐	☐
Self-management approaches	☐	☐	☐
Other:	☐	☐	☐

The current and past use of psychosocial treatment approaches is relevant to treatment planning as well as to assessment of therapeutic responses. Inquiring about past experiences with these treatments is sometimes overlooked as part of the evaluation of patients with depression. If the past and current use of psychosocial treatments is not routinely assessed, this may be a useful focus for performance improvement. If psychosocial treatments are being provided by other clinicians, it will be crucial to collaborate with these clinicians in the care of the patient.

In reviewing the psychosocial treatment approaches that are being used:

Does the treatment approach adequately target core symptoms?
Yes ☐   No ☐

Are modifications needed to address residual symptoms?
Yes ☐   No ☐

If psychosocial treatment approaches are infrequently utilized as part of the treatment of depressed patients, this might prompt a review of typical treatment planning approaches. If the psychosocial treatments being employed do not adequately address core symptoms or residual symptoms, modifications in the patient's plan of treatment may be indicated depending upon factors such as the type and duration of treatment.

Estimated degree of adherence to treatment:
Good ☐   Fair ☐   Poor ☐   Unknown ☐

Is additional education or discussion of the treatment plan needed to enhance the patient's understanding and adherence?
Yes ☐   No ☐

Difficulty adhering to treatment is a common cause of inadequate response. Treatment of depression can be enhanced by assessing adherence, providing additional education to patients and their involved family members and discussing barriers to adherence such as costs, concerns about medication use, complexity, and side effects of medication regimens, and obstacles to keeping appointments (e.g., transportation, childcare, schedule constraints).

Estimated magnitude of treatment-related side effects:
Severe ☐   Moderate ☐   Mild ☐   Unknown ☐

Side effects experienced:

Assessment of side effects of treatment is crucial in all patients and could be a focus for performance improvement if not routinely determined. Although side effects are less commonly considered in patients receiving psychosocial treatments, intensive insight-oriented treatments or exposure therapies may be associated with increases in anxiety for some patients. With antidepressant medication, common side effects include sleep-related effects (i.e., sedation, insomnia), gastrointestinal effects (e.g., diarrhea, constipation, nausea), restlessness/anxiety, sexual dysfunction, headache, and anticholinergic effects. Effects on cardiac conduction can be a particular problem with tricyclic antidepressants. For all antidepressants, the FDA has issued warnings that the potential for increased suicidal thoughts or behaviors with antidepressant therapy in individuals under the age of 25 must be balanced against the benefits of treatment.

"Real-Time" Assessment Tool for Patients with Depression
(p. 6 of 6)

Based on the severity of the patient's depressive disorder, is the overall treatment approach concordant with that recommended practice guideline on the preceding page? Yes ☐ No ☐ What patient specific factors (if any) have led to modifications in the approach to treating the patient's depression compared to that recommended by the practice guideline?	Although care is often noted to diverge from guideline based recommendations, other evidence suggests that providing guideline-concordant care is likely to improve patient outcomes. However, these data are based upon populations of patients and the samples in randomized trials (on which guidelines are typically based) have different characteristics than patients seen in actual practice. If a patient's plan of treatment does diverge from that recommended in the practice guideline, it is useful to consider the patient-specific factors relevant to the treatment plan as well as the rationale for the current plan of care. If patients' treatment plans infrequently follow guideline recommendations, this might serve as a focus for performance improvement.
If the patient has current or past co-occurring psychiatric disorders, are these being addressed in the treatment plan? Yes ☐ No ☐ N/A ☐	Co-occurring psychiatric disorders are common in depressed patients and need to be considered in planning care. Including treatment for each disorder in the treatment plan is likely to improve outcomes for each disorder. Substance use disorders, in particular, are often underrecognized and undertreated, despite the fact that integrated treatment is effective. Performance improvement efforts might be focused on increasing the rates of treatment for all co-occurring disorders or may focus on specific disorders with high rates of occurrence in individuals with depression (e.g., smoking cessation in individuals with nicotine dependence).
Has the treatment plan considered factors such as age, sex, ethnicity, culture, and religious/spiritual beliefs that may require a modified treatment approach? Yes ☐ No ☐ N/A ☐	In individualizing the patient's plan of treatment, factors such as age, sex, ethnicity, culture, and religious/spiritual beliefs are essential yet are often overlooked. If such factors are unassessed or infrequently incorporated into treatment planning, this might serve as a focus for performance improvement.
	Are any changes in this patient's treatment plan likely as a result of this review process?
	Are any performance improvement initiatives or further reviews of practice planned as a result of this review process?

Go to **www.apaeducation.org** to evaluate this activity and record your CME credit. Use the unique purchaser number printed on the inside back cover to enroll in the course (see p. xii).

Influential Publications: Major Depressive Disorder

Influential publications included in the workbook may also be used as a component of your self-determined improvement plan. These papers, selected by experts in the field, are provided as a resource available to you if after completing **STAGE A**, you determined as your **STAGE B** plan of improvement that additional information about the current clinical practice, research, and biology of depression would lead to improvement in your practice.

Influential Publications

Practice Guideline for the Treatment of Patients With Major Depressive Disorder, 3rd Edition: Executive Summary
The complete guideline is available at psychiatryonline.org.

Gartlehner G, Hansen RA, Morgan MA, et al: Comparative benefits and harms of second-generation antidepressants for treating major depressive disorder. Ann Intern Med 155:772–785, 2011
Published in 2011, this paper reports the findings of a comparative effectiveness analysis review of 234 studies of second-generation antidepressants. The primary funding source for this work was the Agency for Healthcare Research and Quality.

Nelson JC, Papakostas GI: Atypical antipsychotic augmentation in major depressive disorder: a meta-analysis of placebo-controlled randomized trials. Am J Psychiatry 166(9):980–991, 2009
Atypical antipsychotics are being increasingly used in nonpsychotic patients. Physicians should be aware of the pitfalls of using these agents for augmentation and be able to weigh the risk of adverse effects against the potential for benefit.

Rush AJ, Trivedi MH, Stewart JW, et al: Combining medications to enhance depression outcomes (CO-MED): acute and long-term outcomes of a single-blind randomized study. Am J Psychiatry 168(7):689–701, 2011
Although this study was single-blind, not double-blind, it emphasizes that it is best not to begin treatment of depressed patients on two antidepressants simultaneously.

Krishnan V, Nestler EJ: Linking molecules to mood: new insight into the biology of depression. Am J Psychiatry 167(11):1305–1320, 2010
An overview that summarizes the current knowledge of the neurobiology of depression by combining insights from human clinical studies and molecular explanations from animal models. The authors provide recommendations for future research, with a focus on translating today's discoveries into improved diagnostic tests and treatments.

Holtzheimer PE: Advances in the management of treatment-resistant depression. Focus 8:488–500, 2010
This paper discusses epidemiology and current approaches to management, an important topic useful to the clinician.

Gaynes BN, Warden D, Trivedi MH, et al: What did STAR*D teach us? Results from a large-scale, practical, clinical trial for patients with depression. Psychiatr Serv 60(11):1439–1445, 2009

*The authors provide an overview of the Sequenced Treatment Alternatives to Relieve Depression (STAR*D) study, a large-scale practical clinical trial to determine which of several treatments are the most effective "next-steps" for patients with major depressive disorder whose symptoms do not remit or who cannot tolerate an initial treatment and, if needed, ensuing treatments. This paper discusses the STAR*D trial as a whole and frames the study results in terms of implications for clinicians.*

Beck AT: The evolution of the cognitive model of depression and its neurobiological correlates. Am J Psychiatry 165(8):969–977, 2008

This paper gives an overview of cognitive theory as well as interconnections with biology. Molecular/neurobiological theory is likely to play an increasingly important role in the future, and most psychiatrists will need to prepare. The author discusses the pharmacology of depression and examines the neurobiological connections to psychotherapy.

Hansen R, Gaynes B, Thieda P, et al: Meta-analysis of major depressive disorder relapse and recurrence with second-generation antidepressants. Psychiatr Serv 59(10):1121–1130, 2008

This paper emphasizes the importance of using continuation/maintenance treatment rather than simply focusing on acute treatment.

Treatment of Patients With Major Depressive Disorder

Third Edition

WORK GROUP ON MAJOR DEPRESSIVE DISORDER

Alan J. Gelenberg, M.D., Chair

Marlene P. Freeman, M.D.

John C. Markowitz, M.D.

Jerrold F. Rosenbaum, M.D.

Michael E. Thase, M.D.

Madhukar H. Trivedi, M.D.

Richard S. Van Rhoads, M.D., Consultant

INDEPENDENT REVIEW PANEL

Victor I. Reus, M.D., Chair

J. Raymond DePaulo, Jr., M.D.

Jan A. Fawcett, M.D.

Christopher D. Schneck, M.D.

David A. Silbersweig, M.D.

This practice guideline was approved in May 2010 and published in October 2010. A guideline watch, summarizing significant developments in the scientific literature since publication of this guideline, may be available at http://www.psychiatryonline.com/pracGuide/pracGuideTopic_7.aspx.

AMERICAN PSYCHIATRIC ASSOCIATION STEERING COMMITTEE ON PRACTICE GUIDELINES

John S. McIntyre, M.D., Chair (1999–2009), Consultant (2009–2010)

Joel Yager, M.D., Vice-Chair (2008–2009), Chair (2009–2010)

Daniel J. Anzia, M.D.

Thomas J. Craig, M.D., M.P.H.

Molly T. Finnerty, M.D.

Bradley R. Johnson, M.D.

Francis G. Lu, M.D.

James E. Nininger, M.D., Vice-Chair (2009–2010)

Barbara Schneidman, M.D.

Paul Summergrad, M.D.

Sherwyn M. Woods, M.D., Ph.D.

Michael J. Vergare, M.D.

M. Justin Coffey, M.D. (fellow)

Kristen Ochoa, M.D. (fellow)

Jeremy Wilkinson, M.D. (fellow)

Sheila Hafter Gray, M.D. (liaison)

STAFF

Robert Kunkle, M.A., Director, Practice Guidelines Project

Robert M. Plovnick, M.D., M.S., Director, Dept. of Quality Improvement and Psychiatric Services

Darrel A. Regier, M.D., M.P.H., Director, Division of Research

MEDICAL EDITOR

Laura J. Fochtmann, M.D.

Part A
TREATMENT RECOMMENDATIONS

I. EXECUTIVE SUMMARY

A. CODING SYSTEM

Each recommendation is identified as falling into one of three categories of endorsement, indicated by a bracketed Roman numeral following the statement. The three categories represent varying levels of clinical confidence:

[I] Recommended with substantial clinical confidence
[II] Recommended with moderate clinical confidence
[III] May be recommended on the basis of individual circumstances

B. SUMMARY OF RECOMMENDATIONS

1. Psychiatric management

Psychiatric management consists of a broad array of interventions and activities that psychiatrists should initiate and continue to provide to patients with major depressive disorder through all phases of treatment [I].

a. Establish and maintain a therapeutic alliance

In establishing and maintaining a therapeutic alliance, it is important to collaborate with the patient in decision making and attend to the patient's preferences and concerns about treatment [I]. Management of the therapeutic alliance should include awareness of transference and countertransference issues, even if these are not directly addressed in treatment [II]. Severe or persistent problems of poor alliance or nonadherence to treatment may be caused by the depressive symptoms themselves or may represent psychological conflicts or psychopathology for which psychotherapy should be considered [II].

b. Complete the psychiatric assessment

Patients should receive a thorough diagnostic assessment in order to establish the diagnosis of major depressive disorder, identify other psychiatric or general medical conditions that may require attention, and develop a comprehensive plan for treatment [I]. This evaluation generally includes a history of the present illness and current symptoms; a psy-

chiatric history, including identification of past symptoms of mania, hypomania, or mixed episodes and responses to previous treatments; a general medical history; a personal history including information about psychological development and responses to life transitions and major life events; a social, occupational, and family history (including mood disorders and suicide); review of the patient's prescribed and over-the-counter medications; a review of systems; a mental status examination; a physical examination; and appropriate diagnostic tests as indicated to rule out possible general medical causes of depressive symptoms [I]. Assessment of substance use should evaluate past and current use of illicit drugs and other substances that may trigger or exacerbate depressive symptoms [I].

c. Evaluate the safety of the patient

A careful and ongoing evaluation of suicide risk is necessary for all patients with major depressive disorder [I]. Such an assessment includes specific inquiry about suicidal thoughts, intent, plans, means, and behaviors; identification of specific psychiatric symptoms (e.g., psychosis, severe anxiety, substance use) or general medical conditions that may increase the likelihood of acting on suicidal ideas; assessment of past and, particularly, recent suicidal behavior; delineation of current stressors and potential protective factors (e.g., positive reasons for living, strong social support); and identification of any family history of suicide or mental illness [I]. In addition to assessing suicide risk per se, it is important to assess the patient's level of self-care, hydration, and nutrition, each of which can be compromised by severe depressive symptoms [I]. As part of the assessment process, impulsivity and potential for risk to others should also be evaluated, including any history of violence or violent or homicidal ideas, plans, or intentions [I]. An evaluation of the impact of the depression on the patient's ability to care for dependents is an important component of the safety evaluation [I]. The patient's risk of harm to him- or herself and to others should also be monitored as treatment proceeds [I].

d. Establish the appropriate setting for treatment

The psychiatrist should determine the least restrictive setting for treatment that will be most likely not only to address the patient's safety, but also to promote improvement in the patient's condition [I]. The determination of an appropriate setting for treatment should include consideration of the patient's symptom severity, co-occurring psychiatric or general medical conditions, available support system, and level of functioning [I]. The determination of a treatment setting should also include consideration of the patient's ability to adequately care for him- or herself, to provide reliable feedback to the psychiatrist, and to cooperate with treatment of the major depressive disorder [I]. Measures such as hospitalization should be considered for patients who pose a serious threat of harm to themselves or others [I]. Patients who refuse inpatient treatment can be hospitalized involuntarily if their condition meets the criteria of the local jurisdiction for involuntary admission [I]. Admission to a hospital or, if available, an intensive day program, may also be indicated for severely ill patients who lack adequate social support outside of a hospital setting, who have complicating psychiatric or general medical conditions, or who have not responded adequately to outpatient treatment [I]. The optimal treatment setting and the patient's likelihood of benefit from a different level of care should be reevaluated on an ongoing basis throughout the course of treatment [I].

e. Evaluate functional impairment and quality of life

Major depressive disorder can alter functioning in numerous spheres of life including work, school, family, social relationships, leisure activities, or maintenance of health and hygiene. The psychiatrist should evaluate the patient's activity in each of these domains and determine the presence, type, severity, and chronicity of any dysfunction [I]. In developing a treatment plan, interventions should be aimed at maximizing the patient's level of functioning as well as helping the patient to set specific goals appropriate to his or her functional impairments and symptom severity [I].

f. Coordinate the patient's care with other clinicians

Many patients with major depressive disorder will be evaluated by or receive treatment from other health care professionals in addition to the psychiatrist. If more than one clinician is involved in providing the care, all treating clinicians should have sufficient ongoing contact with the patient and with each other to ensure that care is coordinated, relevant information is available to guide treatment decisions, and treatments are synchronized [I].

In ruling out general medical causes of depressive symptoms, it is important to ensure that a general medical evaluation has been done [I], either by the psychiatrist or by another health care professional. Extensive or specialized testing for general medical causes of depressive symptoms may be conducted based on individual characteristics of the patient [III].

g. Monitor the patient's psychiatric status

The patient's response to treatment should be carefully monitored [I]. Continued monitoring of co-occurring psychiatric and/or medical conditions is also essential to developing and refining a treatment plan for an individual patient [I].

h. Integrate measurements into psychiatric management

Tailoring the treatment plan to match the needs of the particular patient requires a careful and systematic assessment of the type, frequency, and magnitude of psychiatric symptoms as well as ongoing determination of the therapeutic benefits and side effects of treatment [I]. Such assessments can be facilitated by integrating clinician- and/or patient-administered rating scale measurements into initial and ongoing evaluation [II].

i. Enhance treatment adherence

The psychiatrist should assess and acknowledge potential barriers to treatment adherence (e.g., lack of motivation or excessive pessimism due to depression; side effects of treatment; problems in the therapeutic relationship; logistical, economic, or cultural barriers to treatment) and collaborate with the patient (and if possible, the family) to minimize the impact of these potential barriers [I]. In addition, the psychiatrist should encourage patients to articulate any fears or concerns about treatment or its side effects [I]. Patients should be given a realistic notion of what can be expected during the different phases of treatment, including the likely time course of symptom response and the importance of adherence for successful treatment and prophylaxis [I].

j. Provide education to the patient and the family

Education about the symptoms and treatment of major depressive disorder should be provided in language that is readily understandable to the patient [I]. With the patient's permission, family members and others involved in the patient's day-to-day life may also benefit from education about the illness, its effects on functioning (including family and other interpersonal relationships), and its treatment [I]. Common misperceptions about antidepressants (e.g., they are addictive) should be clarified [I]. In addition, education about major depressive disorder should address the need for a full acute course of treatment, the risk of relapse, the early recognition of recurrent symptoms, and the need to seek treatment as early as possible to reduce the risk of complications or a full-blown episode of major depression [I]. Patients should also be told about the need to taper antidepressants, rather than discontinuing them precipitously, to minimize the risk of withdrawal symptoms or symptom recurrence [I]. Patient education also includes general promotion of healthy behaviors such as exercise, good sleep hygiene, good nutrition, and decreased use of tobacco, alcohol, and other potentially deleterious substances [I]. Educational tools such as books, pamphlets, and trusted web sites can augment the face-to-face education provided by the clinician [I].

2. Acute phase

a. Choice of an initial treatment modality

Treatment in the acute phase should be aimed at inducing remission of the major depressive episode and achieving a full return to the patient's baseline level of functioning [I]. Acute phase treatment may include pharmacotherapy, depression-focused psychotherapy, the combination of medications and psychotherapy, or other somatic therapies such as electroconvulsive therapy (ECT), transcranial magnetic stimulation (TMS), or light therapy, as described in the sections that follow. Selection of an initial treatment modality should be influenced by clinical features (e.g., severity of symptoms, presence of co-occurring disorders or psychosocial stressors) as well as other factors (e.g., patient preference, prior treatment experiences) [I]. Any treatment should be integrated with psychiatric management and any other treatments being provided for other diagnoses [I].

1. Pharmacotherapy

An antidepressant medication is recommended as an initial treatment choice for patients with mild to moderate major depressive disorder [I] and definitely should be provided for those with severe major depressive disorder unless ECT is planned [I]. Because the effectiveness of antidepressant medications is generally comparable between classes and within classes of medications, the initial selection of an antidepressant medication will largely be based on the anticipated side effects, the safety or tolerability of these side effects for the individual patient, pharmacological properties of the medication (e.g., half-life, actions on cytochrome P450 enzymes, other drug interactions), and additional factors such as medication response in prior episodes, cost, and patient preference [I]. For most patients, a selective serotonin reuptake inhibitor (SSRI), serotonin norepinephrine reuptake inhibitor (SNRI), mirtazapine, or bupropion is optimal [I]. In general, the use of nonselective monoamine oxidase inhibitors (MAOIs) (e.g., phenelzine, tranylcypromine, isocarboxazid) should be restricted

to patients who do not respond to other treatments [I], given the necessity for dietary restrictions with these medications and the potential for deleterious drug-drug interactions. In patients who prefer complementary and alternative therapies, *S*-adenosyl methionine (SAMe) [III] or St. John's wort [III] might be considered, although evidence for their efficacy is modest at best, and careful attention to drug-drug interactions is needed with St. John's wort [I].

Once an antidepressant medication has been initiated, the rate at which it is titrated to a full therapeutic dose should depend upon the patient's age, the treatment setting, and the presence of co-occurring illnesses, concomitant pharmacotherapy, or medication side effects [I]. During the acute phase of treatment, patients should be carefully and systematically monitored on a regular basis to assess their response to pharmacotherapy, identify the emergence of side effects (e.g., gastrointestinal symptoms, sedation, insomnia, activation, changes in weight, and cardiovascular, neurological, anticholinergic, or sexual side effects), and assess patient safety [I]. The frequency of patient monitoring should be determined based upon the patient's symptom severity (including suicidal ideas), co-occurring disorders (including general medical conditions), cooperation with treatment, availability of social supports, and the frequency and severity of side effects with the chosen treatment [II]. If antidepressant side effects do occur, an initial strategy is to lower the dose of the antidepressant or to change to an antidepressant that is not associated with that side effect [I].

2. Other somatic therapies

ECT is recommended as a treatment of choice for patients with severe major depressive disorder that is not responsive to psychotherapeutic and/or pharmacological interventions, particularly in those who have significant functional impairment or have not responded to numerous medication trials [I]. ECT is also recommended for individuals with major depressive disorder who have associated psychotic or catatonic features [I], for those with an urgent need for response (e.g., patients who are suicidal or nutritionally compromised due to refusal of food or fluids) [I], and for those who prefer ECT or have had a previous positive response to ECT [II].

Bright light therapy might be used to treat seasonal affective disorder as well as nonseasonal depression [III].

3. Psychotherapy

Use of a depression-focused psychotherapy alone is recommended as an initial treatment choice for patients with mild to moderate major depressive disorder [I], with clinical evidence supporting the use of cognitive-behavioral therapy (CBT) [I], interpersonal psychotherapy [I], psychodynamic therapy [II], and problem-solving therapy [III] in individual [I] and in group [III] formats. Factors that may suggest the use of psychotherapeutic interventions include the presence of significant psychosocial stressors, intrapsychic conflict, interpersonal difficulties, a co-occurring axis II disorder, treatment availability, or—most important—patient preference [II]. In women who are pregnant, wish to become pregnant, or are breast-feeding, a depression-focused psychotherapy alone is recommended [II] and depending on the severity of symptoms, should be considered as an initial option [I]. Considerations in the choice of a specific type of psychotherapy include the goals of treatment (in addition to resolving major depressive symptoms), prior positive response to a specific type of psychotherapy, patient preference, and the availability of clinicians skilled in the specific psychotherapeutic approach [II]. As with patients who are receiving pharmacotherapy, patients receiving psychotherapy should be carefully and systematically monitored on a regular basis to assess their response to treatment and assess patient safety [I]. When determining the frequency of psychotherapy sessions for an individual patient, the psychiatrist should consider multiple factors, including the specific type and goals of psychotherapy, symptom severity (including suicidal ideas), co-occurring disorders, cooperation with treatment, availability of social supports, and the frequency of visits necessary to create and maintain a therapeutic relationship, ensure treatment adherence, and monitor and address depressive symptoms and suicide risk [II]. Marital and family problems are common in the course of major depressive disorder, and such problems should be identified and addressed, using marital or family therapy when indicated [II].

4. *Psychotherapy plus antidepressant medication*

The combination of psychotherapy and antidepressant medication may be used as an initial treatment for patients with moderate to severe major depressive disorder [I]. In addition, combining psychotherapy and medication may be a useful initial treatment even in milder cases for patients with psychosocial or interpersonal problems, intrapsychic conflict, or co-occurring Axis II disorder [III]. In general, when choosing an antidepressant or psychotherapeutic approach for combination treatment, the same issues should be considered as when selecting a medication or psychotherapy for use alone [I].

b. Assessing the adequacy of treatment response

In assessing the adequacy of a therapeutic intervention, it is important to establish that treatment has been administered for a sufficient duration and at a sufficient frequency or, in the case of medication, dose [I]. Onset of benefit from

psychotherapy tends to be a bit more gradual than that from medication, but no treatment should continue unmodified if there has been no symptomatic improvement after 1 month [I]. Generally, 4–8 weeks of treatment are needed before concluding that a patient is partially responsive or unresponsive to a specific intervention [II].

c. Strategies to address nonresponse

For individuals who have not responded fully to treatment, the acute phase of treatment should not be concluded prematurely [I], as an incomplete response to treatment is often associated with poor functional outcomes. If at least a moderate improvement in symptoms is not observed within 4–8 weeks of treatment initiation, the diagnosis should be reappraised, side effects assessed, complicating co-occurring conditions and psychosocial factors reviewed, and the treatment plan adjusted [I]. It is also important to assess the quality of the therapeutic alliance and treatment adherence [I]. For patients in psychotherapy, additional factors to be assessed include the frequency of sessions and whether the specific approach to psychotherapy is adequately addressing the patient's needs [I]. If medications are prescribed, the psychiatrist should determine whether pharmacokinetic [I] or pharmacodynamic [III] factors suggest a need to adjust medication doses. With some TCAs, a drug blood level can help determine if additional dose adjustments are required [I].

After an additional 4–8 weeks of treatment, if the patient continues to show minimal or no improvement in symptoms, the psychiatrist should conduct another thorough review of possible contributory factors and make additional changes in the treatment plan [I]. Consultation should also be considered [II].

A number of strategies are available when a change in the treatment plan seems necessary. For patients treated with an antidepressant, optimizing the medication dose is a reasonable first step if the side effect burden is tolerable and the upper limit of a medication dose has not been reached [II]. Particularly for those who have shown minimal improvement or experienced significant medication side effects, other options include augmenting the antidepressant with a depression-focused psychotherapy [I] or with other agents [II] or changing to another non-MAOI antidepressant [I]. Patients may be changed to an antidepressant from the same pharmacological class (e.g., from one SSRI to another SSRI) or to one from a different class (e.g., from an SSRI to a tricyclic antidepressant [TCA]) [II]. For patients who have not responded to trials of SSRIs, a trial of an SNRI may be helpful [II]. Augmentation of antidepressant medications can utilize another non-MAOI antidepressant [II], generally from a different pharmacological class, or a non-antidepressant medication such as lithium [II], thyroid hormone [II], or a second-generation antipsychotic [II]. Additional strategies with less evidence for efficacy include augmentation using an anticonvulsant [III], omega-3 fatty acids [III], folate [III], or a psychostimulant medication [III], including modafinil [III]. If anxiety or insomnia are prominent features, consideration can be given to anxiolytic and sedative-hypnotic medications [III], including buspirone, benzodiazepines, and selective γ-aminobutyric acid (GABA) agonist hypnotics (e.g., zolpidem, eszopiclone). For patients whose symptoms have not responded adequately to medication, ECT remains the most effective form of therapy and should be considered [I]. In patients capable of adhering to dietary and medication restrictions, an additional option is changing to a non-selective MAOI [II] after allowing sufficient time between medications to avoid deleterious interactions [I]. Transdermal selegiline, a relatively selective MAO B inhibitor with fewer dietary and medication restrictions, or transcranial magnetic stimulation could also be considered [II]. Vagus nerve stimulation (VNS) may be an additional option for individuals who have not responded to at least four adequate trials of antidepressant treatment, including ECT [III].

For patients treated with psychotherapy, consideration should be given to increasing the intensity of treatment or changing the type of therapy [II]. If psychotherapy is used alone, the possible need for medications in addition to or in lieu of psychotherapy should be assessed [I]. Patients who have a history of poor treatment adherence or incomplete response to adequate trials of single treatment modalities may benefit from combined treatment with medication and a depression-focused psychotherapy [II].

3. Continuation phase

During the continuation phase of treatment, the patient should be carefully monitored for signs of possible relapse [I]. Systematic assessment of symptoms, side effects, adherence, and functional status is essential [I] and may be facilitated through the use of clinician- and/or patient-administered rating scales [II]. To reduce the risk of relapse, patients who have been treated successfully with antidepressant medications in the acute phase should continue treatment with these agents for 4–9 months [I]. In general, the dose used in the acute phase should be used in the continuation phase [II]. To prevent a relapse of depression in the continuation phase, depression-focused psychotherapy is recommended [I], with the best evidence available for CBT.

Patients who respond to an acute course of ECT should receive continuation pharmacotherapy [I], with the best evidence available for the combination of lithium and nortriptyline. Alternatively, patients who have responded to an acute course of ECT may be given continuation ECT, particularly if medication or psychotherapy has been ineffective in maintaining remission [II].

4. Maintenance phase

In order to reduce the risk of a recurrent depressive episode, patients who have had three or more prior major depressive episodes or who have chronic major depressive disorder should proceed to the maintenance phase of treatment after completing the continuation phase [I]. Maintenance therapy should also be considered for patients with additional risk factors for recurrence, such as the presence of residual symptoms, ongoing psychosocial stressors, early age at onset, and family history of mood disorders [II]. Additional considerations that may play a role in the decision to use maintenance therapy include patient preference, the type of treatment received, the presence of side effects during continuation therapy, the probability of recurrence, the frequency and severity of prior depressive episodes (including factors such as psychosis or suicide risk), the persistence of depressive symptoms after recovery, and the presence of co-occurring disorders [II]. Such factors also contribute to decisions about the duration of the maintenance phase [II]. For many patients, particularly for those with chronic and recurrent major depressive disorder or co-occurring medical and/or psychiatric disorders, some form of maintenance treatment will be required indefinitely [I].

During the maintenance phase, an antidepressant medication that produced symptom remission during the acute phase and maintained remission during the continuation phase should be continued at a full therapeutic dose [II]. If a depression-focused psychotherapy has been used during the acute and continuation phases of treatment, maintenance treatment should be considered, with a reduced frequency of sessions [II]. For patients whose depressive episodes have not previously responded to acute or continuation treatment with medications or a depression-focused psychotherapy but who have shown a response to ECT, maintenance ECT may be considered [III]. Maintenance treatment with VNS is also appropriate for individuals whose symptoms have responded to this treatment modality [III].

Due to the risk of recurrence, patients should be monitored systematically and at regular intervals during the maintenance phase [I]. Use of standardized measurement aids in the early detection of recurrent symptoms [II].

5. Discontinuation of treatment

When pharmacotherapy is being discontinued, it is best to taper the medication over the course of at least several weeks [I]. To minimize the likelihood of discontinuation symptoms, patients should be advised not to stop medications abruptly and to take medications with them when they travel or are away from home [I]. A slow taper or temporary change to a longer half-life antidepressant may reduce the risk of discontinuation syndrome [II] when discontinuing antidepressants or reducing antidepressant doses. Before the discontinuation of active treatment, patients should be informed of the potential for a depressive relapse and a plan should be established for seeking treatment in the event of recurrent symptoms [I]. After discontinuation of medications, patients should continue to be monitored over the next several months and should receive another course of adequate acute phase treatment if symptoms recur [I].

For patients receiving psychotherapy, it is important to raise the issue of treatment discontinuation well in advance of the final session [I], although the exact process by which this occurs will vary with the type of therapy.

6. Clinical factors influencing treatment

a. Psychiatric factors

For suicidal patients, psychiatrists should consider an increased intensity of treatment, including hospitalization when warranted [I] and/or combined treatment with pharmacotherapy and psychotherapy [II]. Factors to consider in determining the nature and intensity of treatment include (but are not limited to) the nature of the doctor-patient alliance, the availability and adequacy of social supports, access to and lethality of suicide means, the presence of a co-occurring substance use disorder, and past and family history of suicidal behavior [I].

For patients who exhibit psychotic symptoms during an episode of major depressive disorder, treatment should include a combination of antipsychotic and antidepressant medications or ECT [I]. When patients exhibit cognitive dysfunction during a major depressive episode, they may have an increased likelihood of future dementia, making it important to assess cognition in a systematic fashion over the course of treatment [I].

Catatonic features that occur as part of a major depressive episode should be treated with a benzodiazepine [I] or barbiturate [II], typically in conjunction with an antidepressant [II]. If catatonic symptoms persist, ECT is recommended [I]. To reduce the likelihood of general medical complications, patients with catatonia may also require supportive medical interventions, such as hydration, nutritional support, prophylaxis against deep vein thrombo-

sis, turning to reduce risks of decubitus ulcers, and passive range of motion to reduce risk of contractures [I]. If antipsychotic medication is needed, it is important to monitor for signs of neuroleptic malignant syndrome, to which patients with catatonia may have a heightened sensitivity [II].

When patients with a major depressive disorder also have a co-occurring psychiatric illness, the clinician should address each disorder as part of the treatment plan [I]. Benzodiazepines may be used adjunctively in individuals with major depressive disorder and co-occurring anxiety [II], although these agents do not treat depressive symptoms, and careful selection and monitoring is needed in individuals with co-occurring substance use disorders [I].

In patients who smoke, bupropion [I] or nortriptyline [II] may be options to simultaneously treat depression and assist with smoking cessation. When possible, a period of substance abstinence can help determine whether the depressive episode is related to substance intoxication or withdrawal [II]. Factors that suggest a need for antidepressant treatment soon after cessation of substance use include a family history of major depressive disorder and a history of major depressive disorder preceding the onset of the substance use disorder or during periods of sobriety [II].

For patients who have a personality disorder as well as major depressive disorder, psychiatrists should institute treatment for the major depressive disorder [I] and consider psychotherapeutic and adjunctive pharmacotherapeutic treatment for personality disorder symptoms [II].

b. Demographic and psychosocial factors

Several aspects of assessment and treatment differ between women and men. Because the symptoms of some women may fluctuate with gonadal hormone levels, the evaluation should include a detailed assessment of mood changes across the reproductive life history (e.g., menstruation, pregnancy, birth control including oral contraception use, abortions, menopause) [I]. When prescribing medications to women who are taking oral contraceptives, the potential effects of drug-drug interactions must be considered [I]. For women in the perimenopausal period, SSRI and SNRI antidepressants are useful in ameliorating depression as well as in reducing somatic symptoms such as hot flashes [II]. Both men and women who are taking antidepressants should be asked whether sexual side effects are occurring with these medications [I]. Men for whom trazodone is prescribed should be warned of the risk of priapism [I].

The treatment of major depressive disorder in women who are pregnant or planning to become pregnant requires a careful consideration of the benefits and risks of available treatment options for the patient and the fetus [I]. For women who are currently receiving treatment for depression, a pregnancy should be planned, whenever possible, in consultation with the treating psychiatrist, who may wish to consult with a specialist in perinatal psychiatry [I]. In women who are pregnant, planning to become pregnant, or breast-feeding, depression-focused psychotherapy alone is recommended [II] and should always be considered as an initial option, particularly for mild to moderate depression, for patients who prefer psychotherapy, or for those with a prior positive response to psychotherapy [I]. Antidepressant medication should be considered for pregnant women who have moderate to severe major depressive disorder as well as for those who are in remission from major depressive disorder, are receiving maintenance medication, and are deemed to be at high risk for a recurrence if the medication is discontinued [II]. When antidepressants are prescribed to a pregnant woman, changes in pharmacokinetics during pregnancy may require adjustments in medication doses [I]. Electroconvulsive therapy may be considered for the treatment of depression during pregnancy in patients who have psychotic or catatonic features, whose symptoms are severe or have not responded to medications, or who prefer treatment with ECT [II]. When a woman decides to nurse, the potential benefits of antidepressant medications for the mother should be balanced against the potential risks to the newborn from receiving antidepressant in the mother's milk [I]. For women who are depressed during the postpartum period, it is important to evaluate for the presence of suicidal ideas, homicidal ideas, and psychotic symptoms [I]. The evaluation should also assess parenting skills for the newborn and for other children in the patient's care [I].

In individuals with late-life depression, identification of co-occurring general medical conditions is essential, as these disorders may mimic depression or affect choice or dosing of medications [I]. Older individuals may also be particularly sensitive to medication side effects (e.g., hypotension, anticholinergic effects) and require adjustment of medication doses for hepatic or renal dysfunction [I]. In other respects, treatment for depression should parallel that used in younger age groups [I].

The assessment and treatment of major depressive disorder should consider the impact of language barriers, as well as cultural variables that may influence symptom presentation, treatment preferences, and the degree to which psychiatric illness is stigmatized [I]. When antidepressants are prescribed, the psychiatrist should recognize that ethnic groups may differ in their metabolism and response to medications [II].

Issues relating to the family situation and family history, including mood disorders and suicide, can also affect treatment planning and are an important element of the initial evaluation [I]. A family history of bipolar disorder or acute psychosis suggests a need for increased attention to possible signs of bipolar illness in the patient (e.g., with antidepressant treatment) [I]. A family history of recurrent major depressive disorder increases the likelihood of recurrent episodes in the patient and supports a need for maintenance treatment [II]. Family history of a response to a particular antidepressant may sometimes help in choosing a specific antidepressant for the patient [III]. Because problems within the family may become an ongoing stressor that hampers the patient's response to treatment, and because depression in a family is a major stress in itself, such factors should be identified and strong consideration given to educating the family about the nature of the illness, enlisting the family's support, and providing family therapy, when indicated [II].

For patients who have experienced a recent bereavement, psychotherapy or antidepressant treatment should be used when the reaction to a loss is particularly prolonged or accompanied by significant psychopathology and functional impairment [I]. Support groups may be helpful for some bereaved individuals [III].

c. Co-occurring general medical conditions

In patients with major depressive disorder, it is important to recognize and address the potential interplay between major depressive disorder and any co-occurring general medical conditions [I]. Communication with other clinicians who are providing treatment for general medical conditions is recommended [I]. The clinical assessment should include identifying any potential interactions between medications used to treat depression and those used to treat general medical conditions [I]. Assessment of pain is also important as it can contribute to and co-occur with depression [I]. In addition, the psychiatrist should consider the effects of prescribed psychotropic medications on the patient's general medical conditions, as well as the effects of interventions for such disorders on the patient's psychiatric condition [I].

In patients with preexisting hypertension or cardiac conditions, treatment with specific antidepressant agents may suggest a need for monitoring of vital signs or cardiac rhythm (e.g., electrocardiogram [ECG] with TCA treatment; heart rate and blood pressure assessment with SNRIs and TCAs) [I]. When using antidepressant medications with anticholinergic side effects, it is important to consider the potential for increases in heart rate in individuals with cardiac disease, worsening cognition in individuals with dementia, development of bladder outlet obstruction in men with prostatic hypertrophy, and precipitation or worsening of narrow angle glaucoma [I]. Some antidepressant drugs (e.g., bupropion, clomipramine, maprotiline) reduce the seizure threshold and should be used with caution in individuals with preexisting seizure disorders [II]. In individuals with Parkinson's disease, the choice of an antidepressant should consider that serotonergic agents may worsen symptoms of the disease [II], that bupropion has potential dopamine agonist effects (benefitting symptoms of Parkinson's disease but potentially worsening psychosis) [II], and that selegiline has antiparkinsonian and antidepressant effects but may interact with L-dopa and with other antidepressant agents [I]. In treating the depressive syndrome that commonly occurs following a stroke, consideration should be given to the potential for interactions between antidepressants and anticoagulating (including antiplatelet) medications [I]. Given the health risks associated with obesity and the tendency of some antidepressant medications to contribute to weight gain, longitudinal monitoring of weight (either by direct measurement or patient report) is recommended [I], as well as calculation of body mass index (BMI) [II]. If significant increases are noted in the patient's weight or BMI, the clinician and patient should discuss potential approaches to weight control such as diet, exercise, change in medication, nutrition consultation, or collaboration with the patient's primary care physician [I]. In patients who have undergone bariatric surgery to treat obesity, adjustment of medication formulations or doses may be required because of altered medication absorption [I]. For diabetic patients, it is useful to collaborate with the patient's primary care physician in monitoring diabetic control when initiating antidepressant therapy or making significant dosing adjustments [II]. Clinicians should be alert to the possibility of sleep apnea in patients with depression, particularly those who present with daytime sleepiness, fatigue, or treatment-resistant symptoms [II]. In patients with known sleep apnea, treatment choice should consider the sedative side effects of medication, with minimally sedating options chosen whenever possible [I]. Given the significant numbers of individuals with unrecognized human immunodeficiency virus (HIV) infection and the availability of effective treatment, consideration should be given to HIV risk assessment and screening [I]. For patients with HIV infection who are receiving antiretroviral therapy, the potential for drug-drug interactions needs to be assessed before initiating any psychotropic medications [I]. Patients who are being treated with antiretroviral medications should be cautioned about drug-drug interactions with St. John's wort that can reduce the effectiveness of HIV treatments [I]. In patients with hepatitis C infection, interferon can exacerbate depressive symptoms, making it important to monitor patients carefully for worsening depressive symptoms during the course of interferon treatment [I]. Because tamoxifen requires active 2D6 enzyme function to be clinically efficacious, patients who receive tamoxifen for breast cancer or other indications should generally be treated with an antidepressant (e.g., citalopram, escitalopram, venlafaxine, desvenlafaxine) that has minimal effect on metabolism through the cytochrome P450 2D6 isoenzyme [I]. When depression occurs in the context of chronic pain, SNRIs and TCAs may be preferable to other antidepressive agents [II]. When ECT is used to treat major depressive disorder in an individual with a co-occurring general medical condition, the evaluation should identify conditions that could require modifications in ECT technique (e.g., cardiac conditions, hypertension, central nervous system lesions) [I]; these should be addressed insofar as possible and discussed with the patient as part of the informed consent process [I].

Comparative Benefits and Harms of Second-Generation Antidepressants for Treating Major Depressive Disorder
An Updated Meta-analysis

Gerald Gartlehner, MD, MPH; Richard A. Hansen, PhD, RPh; Laura C. Morgan, MA; Kylie Thaler, MD, MPH; Linda Lux, MPA; Megan Van Noord, MSIS; Ursula Mager, PhD, MPH; Patricia Thieda, MA; Bradley N. Gaynes, MD, MPH; Tania Wilkins, MSc; Michaela Strobelberger, MA; Stacey Lloyd, MPH; Ursula Reichenpfader, MD, MPH; and Kathleen N. Lohr, PhD

Background: Second-generation antidepressants dominate the management of major depressive disorder (MDD), but evidence on the comparative benefits and harms of these agents is contradictory.

Purpose: To compare the benefits and harms of second-generation antidepressants for treating MDD in adults.

Data Sources: English-language studies from PubMed, Embase, the Cochrane Library, PsycINFO, and International Pharmaceutical Abstracts from 1980 to August 2011 and reference lists of pertinent review articles and gray literature.

Study Selection: 2 independent reviewers identified randomized trials of at least 6 weeks' duration to evaluate efficacy and observational studies with at least 1000 participants to assess harm.

Data Extraction: Reviewers abstracted data about study design and conduct, participants, and interventions and outcomes and rated study quality. A senior reviewer checked and confirmed extracted data and quality ratings.

Data Synthesis: Meta-analyses and mixed-treatment comparisons of response to treatment and weighted mean differences were conducted on specific scales to rate depression. On the basis of 234 studies, no clinically relevant differences in efficacy or effectiveness were detected for the treatment of acute, continuation, and maintenance phases of MDD. No differences in efficacy were seen in patients with accompanying symptoms or in subgroups based on age, sex, ethnicity, or comorbid conditions. Individual drugs differed in onset of action, adverse events, and some measures of health-related quality of life.

Limitations: Most trials were conducted in highly selected populations. Publication bias might affect the estimates of some comparisons. Mixed-treatment comparisons cannot conclusively exclude differences in efficacy. Evidence within subgroups was limited.

Conclusion: Current evidence does not warrant recommending a particular second-generation antidepressant on the basis of differences in efficacy. Differences in onset of action and adverse events may be considered when choosing a medication.

Primary Funding Source: Agency for Healthcare Research and Quality.

Ann Intern Med. 2011;155:772-785.   www.annals.org
For author affiliations, see end of text.

Major depressive disorder (MDD) affects more than 16% of adults at some point during their lifetime (1). The estimated U.S. economic burden of depressive disorders is approximately $83 billion annually (2), and projected workforce productivity losses related to depression are $24 billion annually (3).

Pharmacotherapy is the primary choice for medical management of MDD. As of 2005, approximately 27 million persons in the United States had received antidepressant therapy (4). Second-generation antidepressants now comprise most antidepressant prescriptions. These drugs include selective serotonin reuptake inhibitors (SSRIs), serotonin and norepinephrine reuptake inhibitors, and other drugs with related mechanisms of action that selectively target neurotransmitters (**Table 1**). In 2009, these drugs accounted for $9.9 billion in U.S. sales and were the fourth top-selling therapeutic class of prescription drugs (5).

Several systematic reviews have assessed the comparative efficacy and safety of second-generation antidepressants (6–14). Two recent comparative effectiveness reviews provide the most comprehensive, albeit contradictory, assessments to date (15, 16). One review, conducted by some of the authors of this article, concluded that efficacy does not differ substantially among second-generation antidepressants (16); conversely, the MANGA (Multiple Meta-Analyses of New Generation Antidepressants) study group reported that escitalopram and sertraline have the best efficacy–acceptability ratio compared with other second-generation antidepressants (15).

This article updates a previous systematic review funded by the Agency for Healthcare Research and Quality (AHRQ) (16) and uses the same statistical approach as the MANGA study group did. We assessed evidence on comparative benefits and harms of second-generation antidepressants for acute, continuation, and maintenance phases of MDD, including variations of effects in patients with accompanying symptoms and among patient subgroups.

METHODS

An open process involving the public (described at www .effectivehealthcare.ahrq.gov/index.cfm/what-is-comparative -effectiveness-research1/what-is-the-research-process), the Scientific Resource Center for the Effective Health Care Program of the AHRQ, and various stakeholder groups produced key questions. We followed a standardized protocol for all review steps (17).

Data Soures and Searches

We searched PubMed, Embase, PsycINFO, the Cochrane Library, and International Pharmaceutical Abstracts from 1980 to August 2011. We used Medical Subject Heading terms as search terms when available or keywords when appropriate. We combined terms for MDD with a list of 13 second-generation antidepressants (bupropion, citalopram, desvenlafaxine, duloxetine, escitalopram, fluoxetine, fluvoxamine, mirtazapine, nefazodone, paroxetine, sertraline, trazodone, and venlafaxine) and their trade names. We limited electronic searches to "adult 19 + years," "human," and "English language." We also performed semiautomated manual searches of reference lists of pertinent review articles and letters to the editor by using Scopus (18).

Context

Multiple second-generation antidepressants with different pharmacologic actions are available for treating major depressive disorder in adults.

Contribution

This comparative effectiveness review of 234 studies found no clinically important differences in treatment response among second-generation antidepressants. Differences among agents did exist in onset of action, dosing regimens, and adverse effects.

Caution

Most studies were efficacy trials conducted in selected populations.

Implication

Possible side effects, convenience of dosing regimens, and costs may best guide the choice of a second-generation antidepressant for treating major depression in adults, because these agents probably have similar efficacy.

—The Editors

Table 1. **Second-Generation Antidepressants Approved for Use in the United States**

Generic Name	U.S. Trade Name*	Dosage Forms	Therapeutic Classification	Labeled Uses	Cost, $†	
					Generic	Brand Name
Bupropion‡	Wellbutrin, Wellbutrin SR, Wellbutrin XL	75- or 100-mg tablets; 100-, 150-, or 200- mg SR tablets; 150- or 300-mg XL tablets	Other	MDD, seasonal affective disorder	53–166	235–499
Citalopram‡	Celexa	10-, 20-, or 40-mg tablets; 2-mg/mL solution	SSRI	MDD	31–38	127–143
Desvenlafaxine	Pristiq	50- or 100-mg tablets	SNRI	MDD	–	157
Duloxetine	Cymbalta	20-, 30-, or 60-mg capsules	SNRI	MDD, GAD, neuropathic pain, fibromyalgia	–	166–181
Escitalopram	Lexapro	5-, 10-, or 20-mg tablets; 1-mg/mL solution	SSRI	MDD, GAD	–	121–125
Fluoxetine‡	Prozac, Prozac Weekly	10-, 20-, 40-, or 90-mg capsules; 4-mg/mL solution	SSRI	MDD, OCD, PMDD, panic disorder, bulimia nervosa	22–136	176–449
Fluvoxamine‡	Luvox	25-, 50-, or 100-mg tablets	SSRI	OCD	99–106	213–234
Mirtazapine‡	Remeron, Remeron SolTab	15-, 30-, or 45-mg tablets; 15-, 30-, or 45-mg orally disintegrating tablets	Other	MDD	44–77	124–190
Nefazodone‡	Serzone	50-, 100-, 150-, 200-, or 250-mg tablets	Other	MDD	–	65–70
Paroxetine‡	Paxil, Paxil CR	10-, 20-, 30-, or 40-mg tablets; 2-mg/mL solution; 12.5-, 25-, or 37.5-mg CR tablets	SSRI	MDD, OCD, panic disorder, social anxiety disorder, GAD, PTSD, PMDD§	20–115	130–163
Sertraline‡	Zoloft	25-, 50-, or 100-mg tablets; 20-mg/mL solution	SSRI	MDD, OCD, panic disorder, PTSD, PMDD, social anxiety disorder	28–29	146–152
Trazodone‡	Desyrel	50-, 100-, 150-, or 300-mg tablets	Other	MDD	NR	NR
Venlafaxine‡	Effexor, Effexor XR	25-, 37.5-, 50-, 75-, or 100-mg tablets; 37.5-, 75-, or 150-mg XR capsules	SNRI	MDD, GAD, panic disorder, social anxiety disorder‖	88–129	168–193

CR = controlled release; GAD = generalized anxiety disorder; MDD = major depressive disorder; NR = not reported; OCD = obsessive-compulsive disorder; PMDD = premenstrual dysphoric disorder; PTSD = posttraumatic stress disorder; SNRI = serotonin and norepinephrine reuptake inhibitor; SR = sustained release; SSRI = selective serotonin reuptake inhibitor; XL = extended release; XR = extended release.
* Wellbutrin, Wellbutrin SR, Wellbutrin XL, Paxil, and Paxil CR (GlaxoSmithKline, Middlesex, United Kingdom); Celexa and Lexapro (Forest Laboratories, New York, New York); Pristiq, Zoloft, Effexor, and Effexor XR (Pfizer, New York, New York); Cymbalta, Prozac, and Prozac Weekly (Eli Lilly, Indianapolis, Indiana); Luvox (Jazz Pharmaceuticals, Palo Alto, California); Remeron and Remeron SolTab (Merck, Whitehouse Station, New Jersey); and Serzone and Desyrel (Bristol-Myers Squibb, Princeton, New Jersey).
† Cost estimates are ranges for various formulations and dosages of the same drug. From Consumer Reports Best Buy Drugs. The Antidepressants: Treating Depression. Comparing Effectiveness, Safety, and Price. April 2011. Accessed at www.consumerreports.org/health/resources/pdf/best-buy-drugs/Antidepressants_update.pdf.
‡ Generic available for some dosage forms.
§ Only Paxil CR (not Paxil) is approved for the treatment of PMDD.
‖ Only Effexor XR (not Effexor) is approved for the treatment of GAD and social anxiety disorder.

The Scientific Resource Center searched the following sources for potentially relevant unpublished literature: the U.S. Food and Drug Administration (FDA) Web site, Health Canada, Authorized Medicines for the European Union, ClinicalTrials.gov, Current Controlled Trials, Clinical Study Results, the World Health Organization International Clinical Trials Registry Platform, Conference Papers Index, the National Institutes of Health Research Portfolio Online Reporting Tools, the U.S. National Library of Medicine Health Services Research Projects in Process, the Hayes Health Technology Assessment, and the New York Academy of Medicine's gray literature index. The Scientific Resource Center also invited pharmaceutical manufacturers to submit dossiers on completed research for each drug. We received dossiers from AstraZeneca (London, United Kingdom) and Warner Chilcott (Dublin, Ireland).

Study Selection

Two persons independently reviewed abstracts and full-text articles. Studies reported only in abstract form were excluded. To assess efficacy or effectiveness, we included head-to-head randomized, controlled trials (RCTs) of at least 6 weeks' duration that compared 2 drugs. Because many comparisons lacked head-to-head evidence, we included placebo-controlled trials for indirect comparisons. All outcomes of interest were health-related (for example, response, remission and quality of life).

To specifically assess harms, we examined RCTs as well as data from observational studies with 1000 participants or more and a follow-up of 12 weeks or more. To determine the differences of benefits and harms in subgroups and participants with accompanying symptoms, we reviewed head-to-head and placebo-controlled trials. We included meta-analyses if we believed them to be relevant for a key question and of good or fair methodological quality (19).

We excluded studies that both reviewers agreed did not meet eligibility criteria. Investigators resolved disagreements about inclusion or exclusion by consensus or by involving a third reviewer.

Data Extraction and Quality Assessment

Trained reviewers abstracted data from each study and assigned an initial quality rating by using the Web-based data abstraction form SRSNexus, version 4.0 (Mobius Analytics, Ottawa, Ontario, Canada). A senior reviewer evaluated completeness of data abstraction and confirmed the quality rating.

To assess trial quality (risk for bias), we used predefined criteria based on those developed by the U.S. Preventive Services Task Force (ratings of good, fair, or poor) (20) and the National Health Service Centre for Reviews and Dissemination (21). To assess the quality of observational studies, we used criteria outlined by Deeks and colleagues (22). We rated studies with a high risk for bias in 1 or more categories as "poor" quality and excluded them from the analyses.

To identify effectiveness studies, we used a tool that distinguishes them from efficacy trials on the basis of certain elements of study design (23). To evaluate the comparability of drug doses, we considered a large range of doses within and across studies. Because no reference standard exists for comparing doses among drugs, we had previously created a comparative dose classification system to identify gross inequities in comparisons of drug doses (24). We used this roster, which does not indicate dosing equivalence, to detect inequalities in dosing that could affect comparative efficacy and effectiveness.

Data Synthesis and Analysis

We conducted meta-analyses of head-to-head comparisons if 3 or more studies provided data to calculate either the odds ratio (OR) of achieving response (defined as >50% improvement from baseline) or the weighted mean difference of changes on the Hamilton Rating Scale for Depression (HAM-D) or the Montgomery-Asberg Depression Rating Scale (MADRS).

For each meta-analysis, we tested for heterogeneity by using the Cochran Q test and estimated the extent of heterogeneity by using the I^2 statistic. If heterogeneity was high (>60%), we explored differences in clinical and methodological characteristics among studies considered for meta-analyses. We assessed publication bias by using funnel plots and Kendall τ rank correlation.

Lacking head-to-head evidence for many drug comparisons, we conducted mixed-treatment comparisons of head-to-head and placebo-controlled trials by using Bayesian methods (25, 26). Because of clinical heterogeneity, we did not include studies conducted in patients older than 65 years. Our outcome measure of choice was the rate of response on the HAM-D. We recalculated response rates for each study by using the number of all randomly assigned patients as the denominator.

We gave all drug effect parameters flat normal (0, 1000) priors and gave the between-study SD flat, uniform distributions with a large range. We discarded a burn-in of 20 000 simulations. All results are based on a further sample of 80 000 simulations. We calculated the OR and 95% credible interval (CrI) for all possible comparisons among our drugs of interest.

All statistical analyses were performed by using StatsDirect Statistical Software, version 2.7.7 (StatsDirect, Cheshire, United Kingdom). We computed Bayesian inferences by using a Markov-chain Monte Carlo simulation with WinBUGS, version 1.4.3 (Medical Research Council Biostatistical Unit, Cambridge, United Kingdom). We evaluated the strength of evidence for major comparisons and outcomes by using a modified Grading of Recommendations Assessment, Development and Evaluation approach (27).

Role of the Funding Source

The AHRQ participated in formulating the key questions and reviewed planned methods and data analyses, as well as interim and final evidence reports. The AHRQ had no role in study selection, quality ratings, and interpretation in or synthesis of the evidence.

RESULTS

Our searches identified 3927 citations (**Appendix Figure 1**, available at www.annals.org). We included 234 studies of good or fair quality, of which 118 were head-to-head RCTs presented in report form at www.effectivehealthcare.ahrq.gov. Pharmaceutical companies financially supported most of the studies (77%), governmental agencies or independent funds supported 7%, and undetermined sources funded 16%. Funnel plots of head-to-head trials did not indicate publication bias.

Overall, comparative efficacy and effectiveness of second-generation antidepressants did not differ substantially for treating patients with MDD. These findings pertain to patients in the acute, continuation, and maintenance phases of this condition; those with accompanying symptom clusters; and subgroups defined by age, sex, ethnicity, or comorbid conditions, although only sparse evidence for these findings exists for subgroups. Overall, 37% of patients with acute-phase MDD who received first-line treatment did not achieve response within 6 to 12 weeks, and 53% did not achieve remission.

Comparative Efficacy for Acute-Phase Treatment of MDD

Ninety-three good- or fair-quality head-to-head trials that included more than 20 000 patients compared the efficacy or effectiveness of the treatment of acute-phase MDD. These studies provided direct evidence for 40 of 78 possible comparisons among these drugs. Direct evidence from head-to-head trials was sufficient to conduct meta-analyses for 6 drug–drug comparisons. In addition, we conducted mixed-treatment comparisons of response rates for all comparisons, incorporating 64 placebo-controlled or head-to-head trials.

Overall, treatment effects were similar among second-generation antidepressants (**Table 2**). Some analyses yielded statistically significant differences among treatments, but the magnitudes of differences were modest and probably not clinically relevant.

Meta-analyses of head-to-head trials showed statistically significantly greater response rates for escitalopram than citalopram (1 unpublished study [28] and 5 published studies [29–33] involving 1802 patients [OR, 1.49 {95% CI, 1.07 to 2.01}]), sertraline than fluoxetine (4 studies [34–37] involving 960 patients [OR, 1.42 {CI, 1.08 to 1.85}]) (**Figure 1**), and venlafaxine than fluoxetine (6 studies [38–43] involving 1197 patients [OR, 1.47 {CI, 1.16 to 1.86}]) (**Figure 2**).

The 2 largest relative differences in response rates were between escitalopram and citalopram and fluoxetine and venlafaxine, but absolute differences were modest. On average, 62% of patients receiving escitalopram and 56% receiving citalopram achieved a response. The pooled difference of the reduction of points on the MADRS scale was 1.52 in favor of escitalopram (CI, 0.59 to 2.45 points), which is approximately one sixth of the average SD of change on the MADRS scale in trials.

The additional benefit of venlafaxine versus fluoxetine was similarly modest. On average, 65% of patients receiving venlafaxine and 60% receiving fluoxetine achieved a response. Pooled results of reductions of points on the HAM-D showed a non–statistically significant 1.30-point greater reduction for patients receiving venlafaxine versus fluoxetine (CI, 0.32 lower reduction to 2.92 greater reduction).

Mixed-treatment comparisons of drugs (**Figures 1 to 3** and **Appendix Figure 2**, available at www.annals.org) did not show statistically significant differences in response rates except for escitalopram over duloxetine (OR, 0.74 [95% CrI, 0.56 to 0.98]) and escitalopram over fluoxetine (OR, 0.66 [CrI, 0.49 to 0.89]).

Seventeen studies (*n* = 3960) indicated no differences in health-related quality of life (**Table 2**) (30, 37, 41, 44–47, 49–58) Seven studies, all funded by the maker of mirtazapine, reported that this agent has a significantly faster onset of action than some comparators (49, 50, 55, 59–62). After 4 weeks of treatment, most response rates among the drugs studied were similar. In 1 trial, mirtazapine and venlafaxine did not differ in speed of action (52).

Achieving Response in Unresponsive or Recurrent Disease

Overall, 37% of patients did not achieve a treatment response during 6 to 12 weeks of treatment with second-generation antidepressants, and 53% did not achieve remission. The STAR*D (Sequenced Treatment Alternatives to Relieve Depression) trial (63) provides the best evidence for assessing alternative medications among patients in whom initial therapy has failed. Approximately 1 in 4 of the 727 participants who switched medications after initial treatment failure became symptom-free; however, no statistically significant difference was seen in patients who switched to sustained-release bupropion, sertraline, or extended-release venlafaxine. In 3 additional head-to-head trials involving patients with treatment-resistant depression, response and remission rates were numerically better with venlafaxine than with comparators (64–67), but differences generally were not statistically significant.

Maintaining Response or Remission After Successful Treatment

In several head-to-head trials (68–75), overall efficacy in maintaining remission did not significantly differ between escitalopram and desvenlafaxine (74), escitalopram and paroxetine (72), fluoxetine and sertraline (68), fluox-

Table 2. Comparative Efficacy and Effectiveness of Second-Generation Antidepressants: Findings and Strength of Evidence

Outcome	Strength of Evidence*	Findings
Treating acute-phase MDD		
Comparative efficacy	Moderate	Results from direct and indirect comparisons indicate that clinical response and remission rates are similar among second-generation antidepressants.
Comparative effectiveness	Moderate	One good-quality and 2 fair-quality effectiveness studies indicate that no substantial differences in effectiveness exist among second-generation antidepressants.
Quality of life	Moderate	Consistent results from 17 mostly fair-quality studies indicate that the efficacy of second-generation antidepressants regarding quality of life does not differ among drugs.
Onset of action	Moderate	Consistent results from 7 fair-quality trials suggest that mirtazapine has a statistically significantly faster onset of action than citalopram, fluoxetine, paroxetine, and sertraline. Whether this difference favoring mirtazapine can be extrapolated to other second-generation antidepressants is unclear. Most other trials do not indicate a faster onset of action of a particular second-generation antidepressant compared with another.
Maintaining response or remission†		
Comparative efficacy	Moderate	Findings from 5 efficacy trials and 1 naturalistic study show no statistically significant differences in preventing relapse or recurrence between escitalopram and paroxetine, fluoxetine and sertraline, fluoxetine and venlafaxine, fluvoxamine and sertraline, and trazodone and venlafaxine.
Managing treatment-resistant depression		
Comparative efficacy	Low	Results from 3 trials support modestly better efficacy for venlafaxine compared with citalopram, fluoxetine, and paroxetine.
Comparative effectiveness	Low	Results from 2 effectiveness studies are conflicting. One good-quality trial showed no statistically significant differences in effectiveness among sustained-release bupropion, sertraline, and extended-release venlafaxine. One fair-quality effectiveness trial found venlafaxine to be modestly superior to citalopram, fluoxetine, mirtazapine, paroxetine, and sertraline; however, differences may not be clinically relevant.
Treating depression in patients with accompanying symptom clusters		
Anxiety		
Comparative efficacy for depression	Moderate	Results from 5 fair-quality head-to-head trials suggest that efficacy does not differ substantially for treatment of depression in patients with accompanying anxiety.
Comparative efficacy for anxiety	Moderate	Results from 8 fair-quality head-to-head trials and 3 fair-quality placebo-controlled trials suggest that no substantial differences in efficacy exist among second-generation antidepressants for treatment of accompanying anxiety.
Insomnia		
Comparative efficacy for depression	Insufficient	Evidence from 1 fair-quality head-to-head study is insufficient to draw conclusions about the comparative efficacy for treating depression in patients with coexisting insomnia.
Comparative efficacy for insomnia	Low	Evidence from 5 fair-quality head-to-head trials suggests that no substantial differences in efficacy exist among second-generation antidepressants for treatment of accompanying insomnia. Results are limited by study design; differences in outcomes are of unknown clinical significance.
Low energy		
Comparative efficacy for depression	Insufficient	Evidence from 1 placebo-controlled trial of bupropion XL is insufficient to draw conclusions about treating depression in patients with coexisting low energy.
Comparative efficacy for low energy	Insufficient	Evidence from 1 placebo-controlled trial of bupropion XL is insufficient to draw conclusions about treating low energy in patients with depression.
Melancholia		
Comparative efficacy for depression	Insufficient	Evidence from 2 fair-quality head-to-head studies is insufficient to draw conclusions about treating depression in patients with coexisting melancholia. Results are inconsistent across studies.
Comparative efficacy for melancholia	No evidence	–
Pain		
Comparative efficacy for depression	Insufficient	Evidence from 2 fair-quality placebo-controlled studies is conflicting about the superiority of duloxetine over placebo. Results from head-to-head trials are not available.
Comparative efficacy for pain	Moderate	Evidence from 1 systematic review, 2 head-to-head trials (1 fair-quality trial and 1 poor-quality trial), and 5 placebo-controlled trials indicate no difference in efficacy between paroxetine and duloxetine.
Psychomotor changes		
Comparative efficacy for depression	Insufficient	Evidence from 1 fair-quality head-to-head trial is insufficient to draw conclusions about the comparative efficacy for treating depression in patients with coexisting psychomotor change. Results indicate that comparative outcomes for psychomotor retardation and psychomotor change may differ.
Comparative efficacy for psychomotor change	No evidence	–
Somatization		
Comparative efficacy for depression	No evidence	–
Comparative efficacy for somatization	Insufficient	Evidence from 1 randomized, head-to-head trial is insufficient to draw conclusions about the comparative efficacy for treating somatization in patients with depression. Results indicate similar improvement in somatization.

MDD = major depressive disorder; XL = extended release.
* High strength of evidence indicates high confidence that the evidence reflects the true effect. Further research is very unlikely to change our confidence in the estimate of effect. Moderate strength of evidence indicates that the evidence reflects the true effect. Further research may change our confidence in the estimate of effect and may change the estimate. Low strength of evidence indicates that the evidence reflects the true effect. Further research is likely to change both the confidence in the estimate of effect and the estimate. Insufficient strength of evidence indicates that evidence is either unavailable or does not permit a conclusion.
† Preventing relapse or recurrence.

Figure 1. Odds ratios of response rates comparing selective serotonin reuptake inhibitors.

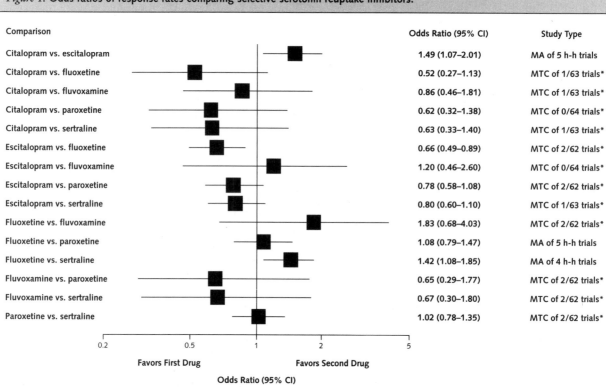

h-h = head-to-head; MA = meta-analysis; MTC = mixed-treatment comparison.
* The first number indicates the number of trials comparing 2 drugs; the second indicates the number of additional studies used to perform MTCs.

etine and venlafaxine (73, 75), fluvoxamine and sertraline (69, 70), and trazodone and venlafaxine (71). One of these studies reported a significantly shorter time to recurrence with fluoxetine than with venlafaxine during 2 years of maintenance treatment (75). In one naturalistic study, re-hospitalization rates did not differ between patients continuing therapy with fluoxetine versus venlafaxine (76).

Efficacy or Effectiveness in Treating Depression or Accompanying Symptoms

Clinicians may use symptom clusters that accompany depression (for example, anxiety and insomnia) to guide antidepressant selection. We identified studies addressing 7 symptom clusters: anxiety, insomnia, low energy, pain, psychomotor change (retardation or agitation), melancholia (a subtype of depression that is a severe form of MDD with characteristic somatic symptoms), and somatization (physical symptoms that are manifestations of depression rather than of an underlying physical illness). **Table 2** summarizes these findings.

Treatment of Depression in Patients With Accompanying Symptom Clusters

For patients with MDD and accompanying anxiety, 4 head-to-head trials (45, 77–79) suggested that antide-

pressants have similar antidepressive efficacy. Two of these studies compared SSRIs (fluoxetine, paroxetine, and sertraline) (77, 78), 1 compared sertraline and sustained-release bupropion (79), and 1 compared sertraline and extended-release venlafaxine (45). One study reported a greater decrease in severity of depression and higher response rates with venlafaxine than with fluoxetine (75% vs. 49%) (39).

For other symptom clusters, such as insomnia (35), melancholia (78, 80), or psychomotor changes (78), most studies indicated similar treatment effects for depression among compared drugs. Because these studies were small or had conflicting results, the strength of the evidence is low.

Treatment of Accompanying Symptom Clusters in Patients With Depression

Results from 8 head-to-head trials suggested that antidepressant medications do not differ in efficacy for treating anxiety associated with MDD. Among these studies, 4 compared SSRIs (including escitalopram, fluoxetine, sertraline, and paroxetine) (77, 81–83); 3 compared paroxetine and nefazodone (84), citalopram and mirtazapine (50), and sertraline and sustained-release

Figure 2. Odds ratios of response rates comparing SSRIs with SNRIs and comparing SNRIs with one another.

Comparison		Odds Ratio (95% CI)	Study Type
SSRIs vs. SNRIs			
Citalopram vs. desvenlafaxine		0.64 (0.32–1.48)	MTC of 0/64 trials*
Citalopram vs. duloxetine		0.58 (0.30–1.27)	MTC of 0/64 trials*
Citalopram vs. venlafaxine		0.74 (0.38–1.65)	MTC of 1/63 trials*
Escitalopram vs. desvenlafaxine		0.81 (0.56–1.23)	MTC of 0/64 trials*
Escitalopram vs. duloxetine		0.74 (0.56–0.98)	MTC of 3/61 trials*
Escitalopram vs. venlafaxine		0.93 (0.67–1.33)	MTC of 2/62 trials*
Fluoxetine vs. desvenlafaxine		1.27 (0.89–1.76)	MTC of 0/64 trials*
Fluoxetine vs. duloxetine		1.13 (0.87–1.46)	MTC of 1/63 trials*
Fluoxetine vs. venlafaxine		1.47 (1.16–1.86)	MA of 5 h-h trials
Fluvoxamine vs. desvenlafaxine		0.68 (0.30–1.89)	MTC of 0/64 trials*
Fluvoxamine vs. duloxetine		0.62 (0.28–1.64)	MTC of 0/64 trials*
Fluvoxamine vs. venlafaxine		0.78 (0.35–2.13)	MTC of 0/64 trials*
Paroxetine vs. desvenlafaxine		1.07 (0.73–1.51)	MTC of 0/64 trials*
Paroxetine vs. duloxetine		0.93 (0.72–1.22)	MA of 5 h-h trials
Paroxetine vs. venlafaxine		1.07 (0.73–1.50)	MTC of 3/61 trials*
Sertraline vs. desvenlafaxine		1.04 (0.72–1.44)	MTC of 0/64 trials*
Sertraline vs. duloxetine		0.93 (0.70–1.20)	MTC of 0/64 trials*
Sertraline vs. venlafaxine		1.17 (0.89–1.53)	MTC of 3/61 trials*
SNRIs vs. SNRIs			
Duloxetine vs. desvenlafaxine		1.13 (0.80–1.55)	MTC of 1/63 trials*
Duloxetine vs. venlafaxine		1.25 (0.92–1.74)	MTC of 0/64 trials*
Desvenlafaxine vs. venlafaxine		1.12 (0.78–1.68)	MTC of 0/64 trials*

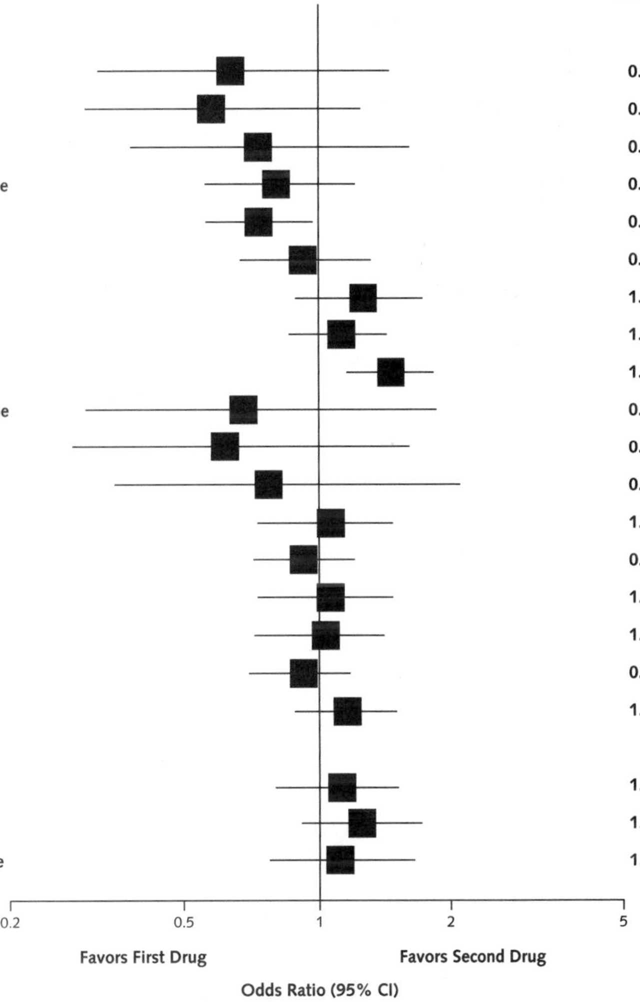

0.2   0.5   1   2   5

Favors First Drug   Favors Second Drug

Odds Ratio (95% CI)

h-h = head-to-head; MA = meta-analysis; MTC = mixed-treatment comparison; SNRI = serotonin and norepinephrine reuptake inhibitor; SSRI = serotonin reuptake inhibitor.
* The first number indicates the number of trials directly comparing 2 drugs; the second indicates the number of additional studies used to perform MTCs.

bupropion (79); and 1 compared extended-release venlafaxine and sertraline (45). Only 1 trial (146 participants) reported that patients receiving venlafaxine had statistically significantly greater reductions in Covi Anxiety Scale scores (5.7 vs. 3.9) than those receiving fluoxetine (39).

For insomnia, 2 studies suggested greater improvement in sleep scores with trazodone than with fluoxetine (47) and venlafaxine (71). In 3 other studies, rates of insomnia did not significantly differ in patients receiving escitalopram or fluoxetine (83); fluoxetine, paroxetine, or sertaline (35); or fluoxetine or mirtazapine (55). A well-conducted meta-analysis (85) of 3 fair-quality head-to-head trials (86–88) and 1 poor-quality

trial (89) (1466 participants) found no substantial difference between duloxetine and paroxetine in the relief of accompanying pain.

Risk for Harms

We analyzed 93 head-to-head studies and 48 additional studies of both experimental and observational design to assess the comparative risk for harm. We distinguished adverse events from serious adverse events on the basis of an FDA classification. A serious adverse event is any medical occurrence that results in death, is life-threatening, requires hospitalization, results in persistent or substantial disability or incapacity, or is a congenital birth defect (90). **Table 3** summarizes these findings.

Adverse Events and Discontinuation of Therapy

In efficacy trials, an average of 63% of patients experienced at least 1 adverse event during treatment. Diarrhea, dizziness, dry mouth, fatigue, headache, nausea, sexual dysfunction, sweating, tremor, and weight gain were commonly reported. Overall, second-generation antidepressants caused similar adverse events; however, the frequency of specific events differed among some drugs (**Appendix Table 1**, available at www.annals.org).

Overall discontinuation rates were similar between SSRIs and other second-generation antidepressants (range of means, 15% to 25%). Duloxetine had a 67% (CI, 17% to 139%) and venlafaxine had a 40% (CI, 16% to 73%) higher risk for discontinuation of therapy because of adverse events than SSRIs as a class did. Discontinuation rates due to lack of efficacy were similar between SSRIs and other second-generation antidepressants except for venlafaxine. Venlafaxine had a 34% (CI, 47 to 93) lower risk for discontinuation of therapy because of lack of efficacy than SSRIs did.

Serious Adverse Events

Except for sexual dysfunction, trials and observational studies were too small and than durations were too short to

Figure 3. Odds ratios of response rates comparing SSRIs with other second-generation antidepressants.

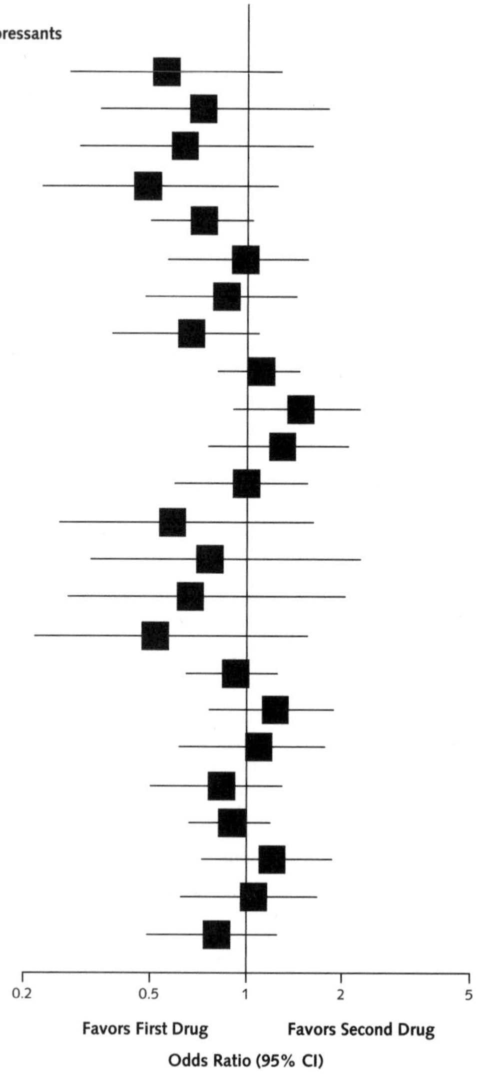

Comparison	Odds Ratio (95% CI)	Study Type
SSRIs vs. other second-generation antidepressants		
Citalopram vs. bupropion	0.56 (0.28–1.29)	MTC of 0/64 trials*
Citalopram vs. mirtazapine	0.73 (0.35–1.83)	MTC of 1/63 trials*
Citalopram vs. nefazodone	0.64 (0.30–1.63)	MTC of 0/64 trials*
Citalopram vs. trazodone	0.49 (0.23–1.26)	MTC of 0/64 trials*
Escitalopram vs. bupropion	0.74 (0.50–1.06)	MTC of 0/64 trials*
Escitalopram vs. mirtazapine	0.99 (0.57–1.59)	MTC of 0/64 trials*
Escitalopram vs. nefazodone	0.87 (0.48–1.45)	MTC of 0/64 trials*
Escitalopram vs. trazodone	0.67 (0.38–1.10)	MTC of 0/64 trials*
Fluoxetine vs. bupropion	1.11 (0.81–1.48)	MTC of 2/62 trials*
Fluoxetine vs. mirtazapine	1.48 (0.91–2.28)	MTC of 3/61 trials*
Fluoxetine vs. nefazodone	1.30 (0.76–2.10)	MTC of 1/63 trials*
Fluoxetine vs. trazodone	1.00 (0.60–1.57)	MTC of 2/62 trials*
Fluvoxamine vs. bupropion	0.59 (0.26–1.65)	MTC of 0/64 trials*
Fluvoxamine vs. mirtazapine	0.77 (0.33–2.32)	MTC of 0/64 trials*
Fluvoxamine vs. nefazodone	0.67 (0.28–2.05)	MTC of 0/64 trials*
Fluvoxamine vs. trazodone	0.52 (0.22–1.58)	MTC of 0/64 trials*
Paroxetine vs. bupropion	0.93 (0.65–1.28)	MTC of 2/62 trials*
Paroxetine vs. mirtazapine	1.24 (0.77–1.89)	MTC of 3/61 trials*
Paroxetine vs. nefazodone	1.09 (0.62–1.78)	MTC of 2/62 trials*
Paroxetine vs. trazodone	0.84 (0.50–1.32)	MTC of 1/63 trials*
Sertraline vs. bupropion	0.90 (0.67–1.20)	MTC of 3/61 trials*
Sertraline vs. mirtazapine	1.21 (0.73–1.88)	MTC of 1/63 trials*
Sertraline vs. nefazodone	1.06 (0.63–1.69)	MTC of 1/63 trials*
Sertraline vs. trazodone	0.82 (0.49–1.28)	MTC of 1/63 trials*

Favors First Drug   Favors Second Drug
Odds Ratio (95% CI)

MTC = mixed-treatment comparison; SSRI = selective serotonin reuptake inhibitor.
* The first number indicates the number of trials directly comparing 2 drugs; the second indicates the number of additional studies used to perform MTCs.

Table 3. Comparative Adverse Events: Findings and Strength of Evidence

Outcome	Strength of Evidence*	Comparative Risk for Harms
General tolerability		
Adverse events profiles	High	Adverse events profiles are similar among second-generation antidepressants. Differences exist in the incidence of specific adverse events.
Nausea and vomiting	High	Meta-analysis of 15 fair-quality studies indicates that venlafaxine has a higher rate of nausea and vomiting than SSRIs as a class.
Diarrhea	Moderate	Evidence from multiple fair-quality studies indicates that sertraline has a higher incidence of diarrhea than bupropion, citalopram, fluoxetine, fluvoxamine, mirtazapine, nefazodone, paroxetine, and venlafaxine.
Weight change	Moderate	Seven fair-quality trials indicate that mirtazapine causes greater weight gain than citalopram, fluoxetine, paroxetine, and sertraline.
Somnolence	Moderate	Six fair-quality studies provide evidence that trazodone has a higher rate of somnolence than bupropion, fluoxetine, mirtazapine, paroxetine, and venlafaxine.
The discontinuation syndrome	Moderate	A good-quality systematic review provides evidence that paroxetine and venlafaxine have the highest rates of the discontinuation syndrome; fluoxetine has the lowest.
Discontinuation rates	High	Meta-analyses of efficacy trials indicate that overall discontinuation rates are similar among second-generation antidepressants. Venlafaxine has a higher rate of discontinuation due to and a lower rate of discontinuation due to lack of efficacy than SSRIs as a class.
Serious adverse events		
Suicidality	Insufficient	Evidence from existing studies is insufficient to draw conclusions about the comparative risk for suicidality.
Sexual adverse events	High	Five fair-quality trials and a pooled analysis of 2 identical randomized, controlled trials provide evidence that bupropion causes significantly less sexual dysfunction than escitalopram, fluoxetine, paroxetine, and sertraline.
Cardiovascular adverse events	Insufficient	Evidence from existing studies is insufficient to draw conclusions about the comparative risk for cardiovascular adverse events. Insufficient evidence indicates that venlafaxine might cause an increased risk for cardiovascular adverse events.
Hyponatremia	Insufficient	Evidence from existing studies is insufficient to draw conclusions about the comparative risk for hyponatremia.
Seizures	Insufficient	Evidence from existing studies is insufficient to draw conclusions about the comparative risk for seizures. Insufficient evidence indicates that bupropion might increase risk for seizures.
Hepatotoxicity	Insufficient	Evidence from existing studies is insufficient to draw conclusions about the comparative risk for hepatotoxicity. Insufficient evidence indicates that nefazodone might have an increased risk for hepatotoxicity.
The serotonin syndrome	Insufficient	Evidence from existing studies is insufficient to draw conclusions about the comparative risk for the serotonin syndrome. Observational studies indicate no differences in risk among second-generation antidepressants.

SSRI = selective serotonin reuptake inhibitor.

* High strength of evidence indicates high confidence that the evidence reflects the true effect. Further research is very unlikely to change our confidence in the estimate of effect. Moderate strength of evidence indicates that the evidence reflects the true effect. Further research may change our confidence in the estimate of effect and may change the estimate. Low strength of evidence indicates that the evidence reflects the true effect. Further research is likely to change both the confidence in the estimate of effect and the estimate. Insufficient strength of evidence indicates that evidence is either unavailable or does not permit a conclusion.

assess the comparative risks for rare but serious adverse events, such as suicidality, seizures, cardiovascular events, the serotonin syndrome, hyponatremia, or hepatotoxicity.

Sexual Dysfunction. Five trials and a pooled analysis (2399 participants) of 2 identical RCTs provided evidence that bupropion causes lower rates of sexual dysfunction than escitalopram (91), fluoxetine (92), paroxetine (93), and sertraline (94–96). Compared with other second-generation antidepressants, paroxetine frequently caused higher rates of sexual dysfunction, particularly ejaculatory dysfunction. These differences, however, did not always reach statistical significance (35, 44, 60, 81, 97–101).

Underreporting of sexual dysfunction in efficacy studies is likely. A fair-quality Spanish prospective, observational study (1022 participants) reported that 59% of patients treated with second-generation antidepressants experienced sexual dysfunction (102).

Suicidality. Although suicide is relatively rare and affects approximately 1 in 8000 psychiatric patients treated with second-generation antidepressants, 1 in 166 patients reported suicidal feelings while receiving treatment with a second-generation antidepressant (103).

Thirteen studies assessed the risk for suicidality (defined as suicidal thinking or behavior) in patients treated with second-generation antidepressants (104–116). Data on the comparative risk for suicidality among second-generation antidepressants were sparse. Results from existing studies did not indicate that any particular drug of interest had an excess risk compared with other second-generation antidepressants (106–109, 113, 116).

Several large observational studies determined that second-generation antidepressants cause a general increase in the risk for suicidality (106, 107, 116). A recent meta-analysis of observational studies in a combined population of more than 200 000 patients indicated that SSRIs decreased the risk for attempted or completed suicide among adults (OR, 0.57 [CI, 0.47 to 0.70]) (116). These findings are consistent with an FDA data analysis of more than 99 000 participants of 372 trials (103). The FDA identified that the risk of suicidality is increased in children and patients aged 18 to 24 years but not in other adult patients.

Other Serious Adverse Events. Evidence on the comparative risk for rare but severe adverse events, such as seizures, cardiovascular events, hyponatremia, hepatotoxicity, and the serotonin syndrome, is insufficient to draw firm conclusions.

Treatment of Major Depressive Disorder in Subgroups

No study directly compared efficacy, effectiveness, and harms of second-generation antidepressants between subgroups and the general population for treatment of MDD. However, numerous studies conducted subgroup analyses or used subgroups as the study population (**Appendix Table 2**, available at www.annals.org).

Multiple head-to-head trials (36, 58, 117–125) indicated that the efficacy of second-generation antidepressants did not differ in participants aged 55 years or older. Efficacy trials usually did not address differences in efficacy or effectiveness between men and women. Two head-to-head RCTs provided limited evidence on adverse sexual effects of these agents; 1 reported a higher risk for sexual dysfunction in men than in women receiving paroxetine (93), and the other reported greater sexual dysfunction in women receiving paroxetine than in those receiving sertraline (44).

No head-to head trials or other studies directly compared differences in efficacy, effectiveness, and harms among groups identified by race or ethnicity or between patients with depression and comorbid conditions and the general population. One recent RCT reported no differences between citalopram and fluoxetine in participants with type 2 diabetes and MDD (126).

DISCUSSION

In this systematic review of data from 234 studies, direct and indirect comparisons of second-generation antidepressants showed no substantial differences in efficacy for the treatment of MDD. Statistically significant results were small and are unlikely to have clinical relevance. No differences in efficacy were seen in patients with accompanying symptoms or in subgroups based on age, sex, ethnicity, or comorbid conditions.

Although second-generation antidepressants are similar in efficacy, they cannot be considered identical drugs. Differences with respect to onset of action, adverse events, and some measures of health-related quality of life may be clinically relevant and influence the choice of a medication for a specific patient. For example, mirtazapine has a faster onset of action than citalopram, fluoxetine, paroxetine, and sertraline (49, 55, 60–62), whereas bupropion has fewer

sexual side effects than escitalopram, fluoxetine, paroxetine, and sertraline (91, 92, 94, 96, 127).

Our findings are consistent with results of most other systematic reviews assessing the comparative efficacy and safety of second-generation antidepressants (8–14). Our conclusions contradict some findings of the 2009 MANGA study, which indicated that escitalopram and sertraline have the best efficacy–acceptability ratio compared with that of other agents (15). The MANGA study, however, has been criticized for methodological shortcomings (128–132). Specifically, the authors included studies with a high risk for bias and open-label designs, assumed that a response on the HAM-D equals a response on MADRS or the Clinical Global Inventory, excluded placebo-controlled trials in their network meta-analysis, and overstated the importance of statistically significant findings without considering clinical relevance. In particular, the assumption that responses on different scales are comparable is not evidence-based (133) and thus might introduce substantial bias in a mixed-treatment comparison model.

For the current update of our review, we used the same statistical methods as the authors of the MANGA study, although we retained more rigid systematic review methods. We specifically excluded studies with high risk for bias or open-label designs and limited mixed-treatment comparisons to ORs of response on a single diagnostic scale (HAM-D). Furthermore, whenever possible, we used meta-analyses of head-to-head trials to determine the relative efficacy.

Our study has several limitations. Most important, we primarily derived our conclusions from efficacy trials with highly selected populations. For example, for data on acute-phase MDD, we found only 3 effectiveness studies (37, 120, 134) out of 93 head-to-head RCTs. Two of these effectiveness studies were conducted in Europe, and their applicability to the U.S. health care system might be limited. Although findings from effectiveness studies are generally consistent with those from efficacy trials, the evidence is limited to a few comparisons.

Indirect comparisons have methodological limitations, most prominently the assumption that prognostic factors for a specific outcome (for example, response to treatment) are similar across study populations in the network meta-analyses. Nevertheless, they are a valuable additional analytic tool when available head-to-head evidence is insufficient.

Publication bias is a concern for all systematic reviews and has been empirically proven to be problematic for placebo-controlled trials of second-generation antidepressants (135, 136). Selective availability of studies with positive results can seriously bias conclusions, particularly when a pharmaceutical company compares 2 of its own drugs (as in the case of citalopram and escitalopram). The small number of studies for individual comparisons limits the validity of statistical methods to explore publication bias, such as funnel plots.

How do these findings that pharmacologic differences among second-generation antidepressants do not translate into substantial clinical differences, although tolerability may differ, inform the practicing clinician? Given the difficulty in predicting what medication will be both efficacious for and tolerated by an individual patient, familiarity with a broad spectrum of antidepressants is prudent. Existing evidence of efficacy, however, does not warrant choosing a particular second-generation antidepressant as first-line therapy for acute-phase MDD or as a subsequent treatment in patients who do not respond to therapy or experience remission. Because of differences in adverse events and dosing regimens, engaging in informed decision making can help physicians to take patient preferences into consideration.

From Danube University, Krems, Austria; Auburn University, Auburn, Alabama; RTI International, Research Triangle Park, North Carolina; the University of North Carolina at Chapel Hill, Chapel Hill, North Carolina; and the Ludwig Boltzmann Institute for Health Promotion Research, Vienna, Austria.

Disclaimer: This manuscript and the work it is derived from was commissioned by the Agency of Healthcare Research and Quality (AHRQ), through a contract to the xyz Evidence-based Practice Center (contract 290200710056l#2). While AHRQ has approved the assertion of copyright by the authors, as noted in the attached letter from the AHRQ Contracting Officer, the government retains rights to the use of the manuscript according to the contract and the Federal Acquisition Regulations (FAR). In order to facilitate and meet the need of public access to research works and findings funded by the government, AHRQ will publish the full report from which this manuscript is derived. The original report from which this manuscript was derived has undergone rigorous peer and public review through the Effective Health Care Program.

Acknowledgment: The authors thank Shrikant Bangdiwala, Visali Peravali, Loraine Monroe, Irene Wild, and Evelyn Auer.

Financial Support: By contract 290200710056I#2 from the AHRQ to RTI International.

Potential Conflicts of Interest: Dr. Gartlehner: *Grant (money to institution):* AHRQ. Dr. Hansen: *Grant (money to institution):* AHRQ; *Consultancy:* Novartis and Takeda Pharmaceutical Company; *Grants/grants pending (money to institution):* AHRQ, North Carolina Department of Health and Human Services, and the Foundation for the National Institutes of Health; *Payment for development of educational presentations:* WebMD. Ms. Morgan: *Grant (money to institution):* AHRQ. Dr. Thaler: *Grant (money to institution):* AHRQ. Ms. Lux: *Grant (money to institution):* AHRQ. Dr. Mager and Ms. Strobelberger: *Grant (money to institution):* Danube University. Ms. Thieda: Grant *(money to institution):* AHRQ. Dr. Gaynes: *Grant (money to institution):* AHRQ; *Grants/grants pending (money to institution):* National Institute of Mental Health. Ms. Lloyd: *Grant (money to institution):* AHRQ. Disclosures can also be viewed at www.acponline.org/authors/icmje/ConflictOfInterestForms.do?msNum=M11-1590.

Current author addresses and author contributions are available at www.annals.org.

References

1. Kessler RC, Berglund P, Demler O, Jin R, Merikangas KR, Walters EE. Lifetime prevalence and age-of-onset distributions of DSM-IV disorders in the National Comorbidity Survey Replication. Arch Gen Psychiatry. 2005;62:593-602. [PMID: 15939837]

2. Wu E, Greenberg P, Yang E, Yu A, Ben-Hamadi R, Erder MH. Comparison of treatment persistence, hospital utilization and costs among major depressive disorder geriatric patients treated with escitalopram versus other SSRI/SNRI antidepressants. Curr Med Res Opin. 2008;24:2805-13. [PMID: 18755054]

3. Birnbaum HG, Ben-Hamadi R, Greenberg PE, Hsieh M, Tang J, Reygrobellet C. Determinants of direct cost differences among US employees with major depressive disorders using antidepressants. Pharmacoeconomics. 2009;27:507-17. [PMID: 19640013]

4. Olfson M, Marcus SC. National patterns in antidepressant medication treatment. Arch Gen Psychiatry. 2009;66:848-56. [PMID: 19652124]

5. Berkrot B. U.S. prescription drug sales hit $300 bln in 2009. Thomson Reuters. 1 April 2010. Accessed at www.reuters.com/article/2010/04/01/us-drug-sales-idUSTRE6303CU20100401 on 10 April 2010.

6. Hansen RA, Gartlehner G, Lohr KN, Gaynes BN, Carey TS. Efficacy and safety of second-generation antidepressants in the treatment of major depressive disorder. Ann Intern Med. 2005;143:415-26. [PMID: 16172440]

7. Williams JW Jr, Mulrow CD, Chiquette E, Noël PH, Aguilar C, Cornell J. A systematic review of newer pharmacotherapies for depression in adults: evidence report summary. Ann Intern Med. 2000;132:743-56. [PMID: 10787370]

8. Cipriani A, Furukawa TA, Geddes JR, Malvini L, Signoretti A, McGuire H, et al; MANGA Study Group. Does randomized evidence support sertraline as first-line antidepressant for adults with acute major depression? A systematic review and meta-analysis. J Clin Psychiatry. 2008;69:1732-42. [PMID: 19026250]

9. Omori IM, Watanabe N, Nakagawa A, Akechi T, Cipriani A, Barbui C, et al; Meta-Analysis of New Generation Antidepressants (MANGA) Study Group. Efficacy, tolerability and side-effect profile of fluvoxamine for major depression: meta-analysis. J Psychopharmacol. 2009;23:539-50. [PMID: 18562407]

10. Watanabe N, Omori IM, Nakagawa A, Cipriani A, Barbui C, McGuire H, et al; Multiple Meta-Analyses of New Generation Antidepressants (MANGA) Study Group. Mirtazapine versus other antidepressants in the acute-phase treatment of adults with major depression: systematic review and meta-analysis. J Clin Psychiatry. 2008;69:1404-15. [PMID: 19193341]

11. Weinmann S, Becker T, Koesters M. Re-evaluation of the efficacy and tolerability of venlafaxine vs SSRI: meta-analysis. Psychopharmacology (Berl). 2008;196:511-20; discussion 521-2. [PMID: 17955213]

12. Girardi P, Pompili M, Innamorati M, Mancini M, Serafini G, Mazzarini L, et al. Duloxetine in acute major depression: review of comparisons to placebo and standard antidepressants using dissimilar methods. Hum Psychopharmacol. 2009;24:177-90. [PMID: 19229839]

13. Eckert L, Falissard B. Using meta-regression in performing indirect-comparisons: comparing escitalopram with venlafaxine XR. Curr Med Res Opin. 2006;22:2313-21. [PMID: 17076991]

14. Eckert L, Lançon C. Duloxetine compared with fluoxetine and venlafaxine: use of meta-regression analysis for indirect comparisons. BMC Psychiatry. 2006;6:30. [PMID: 16867188]

15. Cipriani A, Furukawa TA, Salanti G, Geddes JR, Higgins JP, Churchill R, et al. Comparative efficacy and acceptability of 12 new-generation antidepressants: a multiple-treatments meta-analysis. Lancet. 2009;373:746-58. [PMID: 19185342]

16. Gartlehner G, Hansen RA, Thieda P, DeVeaugh-Geiss AM, Gaynes BN, Krebs EE, et al. Comparative Effectiveness of Second-Generation Antidepressants in the Pharmacologic Treatment of Adult Depression. Rockville, MD: Agency for Healthcare Research and Quality; 2007.

17. Gartlehner G, Hansen RA, Morgan LC, Thaler K, Lux LJ, Van Noord M, et al. Comparative Effectiveness of Second Generation Antidepressants in the Pharmacologic Treatment of Adult Depression: An Update to a 2007 Report. Research Protocol. 13 July 2011. Rockville, MD: Agency for Healthcare Research and Quality; 2011. Accessed at www.effectivehealthcare.ahrq.gov/index.cfm/search-for-guides-reviews-and-reports/?pageaction=displayproduct&productID

=59 on 21 October 2011.

18. **Chapman AL, Morgan LC, Gartlehner G.** Semi-automating the manual literature search for systematic reviews increases efficiency. Health Info Libr J. 2010;27:22-7. [PMID: 20402801]

19. **Balk EM, Lau J, Bonis PA.** Reading and critically appraising systematic reviews and meta-analyses: a short primer with a focus on hepatology. J Hepatol. 2005;43:729-36. [PMID: 16120472]

20. **Harris RP, Helfand M, Woolf SH, Lohr KN, Mulrow CD, Teutsch SM, et al; Methods Work Group, Third US Preventive Services Task Force.** Current methods of the US Preventive Services Task Force: a review of the process. Am J Prev Med. 2001;20:21-35 [PMID: 11306229]

21. **National Health Service Centre for Reviews and Dissemination.** Undertaking systematic reviews of research on effectiveness: CRD's guidance for those carrying out or commissioning reviews. Report no. 4, 2nd ed. March 2001. York, United Kingdom: Centre for Reviews and Dissemination, Univ York; 2001.

22. **Deeks JJ, Dinnes J, D'Amico R, Sowden AJ, Sakarovitch C, Song F, et al; International Stroke Trial Collaborative Group.** Evaluating non-randomised intervention studies. Health Technol Assess. 2003;7:iii-x, 1-173. [PMID: 14499048]

23. **Gartlehner G, Hansen RA, Nissman D, Lohr KN, Carey TS.** A simple and valid tool distinguished efficacy from effectiveness studies. J Clin Epidemiol. 2006;59:1040-8. [PMID: 16980143]

24. **Hansen RA, Moore CG, Dusetzina SB, Leinwand BI, Gartlehner G, Gaynes BN.** Controlling for drug dose in systematic review and meta-analysis: a case study of the effect of antidepressant dose. Med Decis Making. 2009;29:91-103. [PMID: 19141788]

25. **Jansen JP, Crawford B, Bergman G, Stam W.** Bayesian meta-analysis of multiple treatment comparisons: an introduction to mixed treatment comparisons. Value Health. 2008;11:956-64. [PMID: 18489499]

26. **Lu G, Ades AE.** Combination of direct and indirect evidence in mixed treatment comparisons. Stat Med. 2004;23:3105-24 [PMID: 15449338]

27. **Owens DK, Lohr KN, Atkins D, Treadwell JR, Reston JT, Bass EB, et al.** AHRQ series paper 5: grading the strength of a body of evidence when comparing medical interventions—AHRQ and the effective health-care program. J Clin Epidemiol. 2010;63:513-23 [PMID: 19595577]

28. **U.S. Food and Drug Administration.** FDA Center for Drug Evaluation and Research. Stastical review of NDA 21-323 (escitalopram oxalate). 2001. Accessed at www.fda.gov/downloads/Drugs/DevelopmentApprovalProcess/Development Resources/UCM226546.pdf on 22 October 2011.

29. **Yevtushenko VY, Belous AI, Yevtushenko YG, Gusinin SE, Buzik OJ, Agibalova TV.** Efficacy and tolerability of escitalopram versus citalopram in major depressive disorder: a 6-week, multicenter, prospective, randomized, double-blind, active-controlled study in adult outpatients. Clin Ther. 2007;29:2319-32. [PMID: 18158074]

30. **Burke WJ, Gergel I, Bose A.** Fixed-dose trial of the single isomer SSRI escitalopram in depressed outpatients. J Clin Psychiatry. 2002;63:331-6. [PMID: 12000207]

31. **Colonna L, Andersen HF, Reines EH.** A randomized, double-blind, 24-week study of escitalopram (10 mg/day) versus citalopram (20 mg/day) in primary care patients with major depressive disorder. Curr Med Res Opin. 2005; 21:1659-68. [PMID: 16238906]

32. **Lepola UM, Loft H, Reines EH.** Escitalopram (10-20 mg/day) is effective and well tolerated in a placebo-controlled study in depression in primary care. Int Clin Psychopharmacol. 2003;18:211-7. [PMID: 12817155]

33. **Moore N, Verdoux H, Fantino B.** Prospective, multicentre, randomized, double-blind study of the efficacy of escitalopram versus citalopram in outpatient treatment of major depressive disorder. Int Clin Psychopharmacol 2005;20: 131-7. [PMID: 15812262]

34. **Bennie EH, Mullin JM, Martindale JJ.** A double-blind multicenter trial comparing sertraline and fluoxetine in outpatients with major depression. J Clin Psychiatry. 1995;56:229-37. [PMID: 7775364]

35. **Fava M, Hoog SL, Judge RA, Kopp JB, Nilsson ME, Gonzales JS.** Acute efficacy of fluoxetine versus sertraline and paroxetine in major depressive disorder including effects of baseline insomnia. J Clin Psychopharmacol. 2002;22:137-47. [PMID: 11910258]

36. **Newhouse PA, Krishnan KR, Doraiswamy PM, Richter EM, Batzar ED, Clary CM.** A double-blind comparison of sertraline and fluoxetine in depressed elderly outpatients. J Clin Psychiatry. 2000;61:559-68. [PMID: 10982198]

37. **Sechter D, Troy S, Paternetti S, Boyer P.** A double-blind comparison of sertraline and fluoxetine in the treatment of major depressive episode in outpa-

tients. Eur Psychiatry. 1999;14:41-8. [PMID: 10572324]

38. **Alves C, Cachola I, Brandao J.** Efficacy and tolerability of venlafaxine and fluoxetine in outpatients with major depression. Primary Care Psychiatry. 1999; 5:57-63

39. **De Nayer A, Geerts S, Ruelens L, Schittecatte M, De Bleeker E, Van Eeckhoutte I, et al.** Venlafaxine compared with fluoxetine in outpatients with depression and concomitant anxiety. Int J Neuropsychopharmacol. 2002;5:115-20. [PMID: 12135535]

40. **Dierick M, Ravizza L, Realini R, Martin A.** A double-blind comparison of venlafaxine and fluoxetine for treatment of major depression in outpatients Prog Neuropsychopharmacol Biol Psychiatry. 1996;20:57-71. [PMID: 8861177]

41. **Nemeroff CB, Thase ME; EPIC 014 Study Group.** A double-blind, placebo-controlled comparison of venlafaxine and fluoxetine treatment in depressed outpatients. J Psychiatr Res. 2007;41:351-9. [PMID: 16165158]

42. **Rudolph RL, Feiger AD.** A double-blind, randomized, placebo-controlled trial of once-daily venlafaxine extended release (XR) and fluoxetine for the treatment of depression. J Affect Disord. 1999;56:171-81. [PMID: 10701474]

43. **Silverstone PH, Ravindran A.** Once-daily venlafaxine extended release (XR) compared with fluoxetine in outpatients with depression and anxiety. Venlafaxine XR 360 Study Group. J Clin Psychiatry. 1999;60:22-8. [PMID: 10074873]

44. **Aberg-Wistedt A, Agren H, Ekselius L, Bengtsson F, Akerblad AC.** Sertraline versus paroxetine in major depression: clinical outcome after six months of continuous therapy. J Clin Psychopharmacol. 2000;20:645-52. [PMID: 11106136]

45. **Sir A, D'Souza RF, Uguz S, George T, Vahip S, Hopwood M, et al.** Randomized trial of sertraline versus venlafaxine XR in major depression: efficacy and discontinuation symptoms. J Clin Psychiatry. 2005;66:1312-20. [PMID: 16259546]

46. **Ravindran AV, Guelfi JD, Lane RM, Cassano GB.** Treatment of dysthymia with sertraline: a double-blind, placebo-controlled trial in dysthymic patients without major depression. J Clin Psychiatry. 2000;61:821-7. [PMID: 11105734]

47. **Beasley CM Jr, Dornseif BE, Pultz JA, Bosomworth JC, Sayler ME.** Fluoxetine versus trazodone: efficacy and activating-sedating effects. J Clin Psychiatry. 1991;52:294-9. [PMID: 2071559]

48. **Devanand DP, Nobler MS, Cheng J, Turret N, Pelton GH, Roose SP, et al.** Randomized, double-blind, placebo-controlled trial of fluoxetine treatment for elderly patients with dysthymic disorder. Am J Geriatr Psychiatry. 2005;13: 59-68. [PMID: 15653941]

49. **Wheatley DP, van Moffaert M, Timmerman L, Kremer CM.** Mirtazapine: efficacy and tolerability in comparison with fluoxetine in patients with moderate to severe major depressive disorder. Mirtazapine-Fluoxetine Study Group. J Clin Psychiatry. 1998;59:306-12. [PMID: 9671343]

50. **Leinonen E, Skarstein J, Behnke K, Agren H, Helsdingen JT.** Efficacy and tolerability of mirtazapine versus citalopram: a double-blind, randomized study in patients with major depressive disorder. Nordic Antidepressant Study Group. Int Clin Psychopharmacol. 1999;14:329-37. [PMID: 10565799]

51. **McPartlin GM, Reynolds A, Anderson C, Casoy J.** A comparison of once-daily venlafaxine XR and paroxetine in depressed outpatients treated in general practice. Primary Care Psychiatry. 1998;4:127-32.

52. **Guelfi JD, Ansseau M, Timmerman L, Kørsgaard S; Mirtazapine-Venlafaxine Study Group.** Mirtazapine versus venlafaxine in hospitalized severely depressed patients with melancholic features. J Clin Psychopharmacol. 2001;21: 425-31. [PMID: 11476127]

53. **Vanelle JM, Attar-Levy D, Poirier MF, Bouhassira M, Blin P, Olié JP.** Controlled efficacy study of fluoxetine in dysthymia. Br J Psychiatry. 1997;170: 345-50. [PMID: 9246253]

54. **Weihs KL, Settle EC Jr, Batey SR, Houser TL, Donahue RM, Ascher JA.** Bupropion sustained release versus paroxetine for the treatment of depression in the elderly. J Clin Psychiatry. 2000;61:196-202. [PMID: 10817105]

55. **Versiani M, Moreno R, Ramakers-van Moorsel CJ, Schutte AJ; Comparative Efficacy Antidepressants Study Group.** Comparison of the effects of mirtazapine and fluoxetine in severely depressed patients. CNS Drugs. 2005;19:137-46. [PMID: 15697327]

56. **Boyer P, Danion JM, Bisserbe JC, Hotton JM, Troy S.** Clinical and economic comparison of sertraline and fluoxetine in the treatment of depression. A 6-month double-blind study in a primary-care setting in France. Pharmacoeconomics. 1998;13:157-69. [PMID: 10184835]

57. **Bielski RJ, Ventura D, Chang CC.** A double-blind comparison of escitalopram and venlafaxine extended release in the treatment of major depressive disorder. J Clin Psychiatry. 2004;65:1190-6. [PMID: 15367045]

58. Finkel SI, Richter EM, Clary CM, Batzar E. Comparative efficacy of sertraline vs. fluoxetine in patients age 70 or over with major depression. Am J Geriatr Psychiatry. 1999;7:221-7. [PMID: 10438693]

59. Hong CJ, Hu WH, Chen CC, Hsiao CC, Tsai SJ, Ruwe FJ. A double-blind, randomized, group-comparative study of the tolerability and efficacy of 6 weeks' treatment with mirtazapine or fluoxetine in depressed Chinese patients. J Clin Psychiatry. 2003;64:921-6. [PMID: 12927007]

60. Benkert O, Szegedi A, Kohnen R. Mirtazapine compared with paroxetine in major depression. J Clin Psychiatry. 2000;61:656-63. [PMID: 11030486]

61. Schatzberg AF, Kremer C, Rodrigues HE, Murphy GM Jr; Mirtazapine vs. Paroxetine Study Group. Double-blind, randomized comparison of mirtazapine and paroxetine in elderly depressed patients. Am J Geriatr Psychiatry. 2002;10: 541-50. [PMID: 12213688]

62. Behnke K, Søgaard J, Martin S, Bäuml J, Ravindran AV, Agren H, et al. Mirtazapine orally disintegrating tablet versus sertraline: a prospective onset of action study. J Clin Psychopharmacol. 2003;23:358-64. [PMID: 12920411]

63. Rush AJ, Trivedi MH, Wisniewski SR, Stewart JW, Nierenberg AA, Thase ME, et al; STAR*D Study Team. Bupropion-SR, sertraline, or venlafaxine-XR after failure of SSRIs for depression. N Engl J Med. 2006;354:1231-42. [PMID: 16554525]

64. Poirier MF, Boyer P. Venlafaxine and paroxetine in treatment-resistant depression. Double-blind, randomised comparison. Br J Psychiatry. 1999;175:12-6. [PMID: 10621762]

65. Lenox-Smith AJ, Jiang Q. Venlafaxine extended release versus citalopram in patients with depression unresponsive to a selective serotonin reuptake inhibitor. Int Clin Psychopharmacol. 2008;23:113-9. [PMID: 18408525]

66. Corya SA, Williamson D, Sanger TM, Briggs SD, Case M, Tollefson G. A randomized, double-blind comparison of olanzapine/fluoxetine combination, olanzapine, fluoxetine, and venlafaxine in treatment-resistant depression. Depress Anxiety. 2006;23:364-72. [PMID: 16710853]

67. Baldomero EB, Ubago JG, Cercós CL, Ruiloba JV, Calvo CG, López RP. Venlafaxine extended release versus conventional antidepressants in the remission of depressive disorders after previous antidepressant failure: ARGOS study. Depress Anxiety. 2005;22:68-76. [PMID: 16094658]

68. Van Moffaert M, Bartholome F, Cosyns P, De Nayer AR. A controlled comparison of sertraline and fluoxetine in acute and continuation treatment of major depression. Hum Psychopharmacol. 1995;10:393-405.

69. Franchini L, Gasperini M, Perez J, Smeraldi E, Zanardi R. A double-blind study of long-term treatment with sertraline or fluvoxamine for prevention of highly recurrent unipolar depression. J Clin Psychiatry. 1997;58:104-7. [PMID: 9108811]

70. Franchini L, Gasperini M, Zanardi R, Smeraldi E. Four-year follow-up study of sertraline and fluvoxamine in long-term treatment of unipolar subjects with high recurrence rate. J Affect Disord. 2000;58:233-6. [PMID: 10802132]

71. Cunningham LA, Borison RL, Carman JS, Chouinard G, Crowder JE, Diamond BI, et al. A comparison of venlafaxine, trazodone, and placebo in major depression. J Clin Psychopharmacol. 1994;14:99-106. [PMID: 8195464]

72. Baldwin DS, Cooper JA, Huusom AK, Hindmarch I. A double-blind, randomized, parallel-group, flexible-dose study to evaluate the tolerability, efficacy and effects of treatment discontinuation with escitalopram and paroxetine in patients with major depressive disorder. Int Clin Psychopharmacol. 2006;21:159-69. [PMID: 16528138]

73. Keller MB, Trivedi MH, Thase ME, Shelton RC, Kornstein SG, Nemeroff CB, et al. The Prevention of Recurrent Episodes of Depression with Venlafaxine for Two Years (PREVENT) study: outcomes from the acute and continuation phases. Biol Psychiatry. 2007;62:1371-9. [PMID: 17825800]

74. Soares CN, Thase ME, Clayton A, Guico-Pabia CJ, Focht K, Jiang Q, et al. Desvenlafaxine and escitalopram for the treatment of postmenopausal women with major depressive disorder. Menopause. 2010;17:700-11. [PMID: 20539246]

75. Thase ME, Gelenberg A, Kornstein SG, Kocsis JH, Trivedi MH, Ninan P, et al. Comparing venlafaxine extended release and fluoxetine for preventing the recurrence of major depression: results from the PREVENT study. J Psychiatr Res. 2011;45:412-20. [PMID: 20801464]

76. Lin CH, Lin KS, Lin CY, Chen MC, Lane HY. Time to rehospitalization in patients with major depressive disorder taking venlafaxine or fluoxetine. J Clin Psychiatry. 2008;69:54-9. [PMID: 18312038]

77. Fava M, Rosenbaum JF, Hoog SL, Tepner RG, Kopp JB, Nilsson ME. Fluoxetine versus sertraline and paroxetine in major depression: tolerability and efficacy in anxious depression. J Affect Disord. 2000;59:119-26. [PMID: 10837880]

78. Flament MF, Lane RM, Zhu R, Ying Z. Predictors of an acute antidepressant response to fluoxetine and sertraline. Int Clin Psychopharmacol. 1999;14: 259-75. [PMID: 10529069]

79. Rush AJ, Trivedi MH, Carmody TJ, Donahue RM, Houser TL, Bolden-Watson C, et al. Response in relation to baseline anxiety levels in major depressive disorder treated with bupropion sustained release or sertraline. Neuropsychopharmacology. 2001;25:131-8. [PMID: 11377926]

80. Tzanakaki M, Guazzelli M, Nimatoudis I, Zissis NP, Smeraldi E, Rizzo F. Increased remission rates with venlafaxine compared with fluoxetine in hospitalized patients with major depression and melancholia. Int Clin Psychopharmacol. 2000;15:29-34. [PMID: 10836283]

81. Chouinard G, Saxena B, Bélanger MC, Ravindran A, Bakish D, Beauclair L, et al. A Canadian multicenter, double-blind study of paroxetine and fluoxetine in major depressive disorder. J Affect Disord. 1999;54:39-48. [PMID: 10403145]

82. Gagiano CA. A double blind comparison of paroxetine and fluoxetine in patients with major depression. Br J Clin Res. 1993;4:145-52.

83. Mao PX, Tang YL, Jiang F, Shu L, Gu X, Li M, et al. Escitalopram in major depressive disorder: a multicenter, randomized, double-blind, fixed-dose, parallel trial in a Chinese population. Depress Anxiety. 2008;25:46-54. [PMID: 17149753]

84. Baldwin DS, Hawley CJ, Abed RT, Maragakis BP, Cox J, Buckingham SA, et al. A multicenter double-blind comparison of nefazodone and paroxetine in the treatment of outpatients with moderate-to-severe depression. J Clin Psychiatry. 1996;57 Suppl 2:46-52. [PMID: 8626363]

85. Krebs EE, Gaynes BN, Gartlehner G, Hansen RA, Thieda P, Morgan LC, et al. Treating the physical symptoms of depression with second-generation antidepressants: a systematic review and metaanalysis. Psychosomatics. 2008;49: 191-8. [PMID: 18448772]

86. Detke MJ, Wiltse CG, Mallinckrodt CH, McNamara RK, Demitrack MA, Bitter I. Duloxetine in the acute and long-term treatment of major depressive disorder: a placebo- and paroxetine-controlled trial. Eur Neuropsychopharmacol. 2004;14:457-70. [PMID: 15589385]

87. Perahia DG, Wang F, Mallinckrodt CH, Walker DJ, Detke MJ. Duloxetine in the treatment of major depressive disorder: a placebo- and paroxetine-controlled trial. Eur Psychiatry. 2006;21:367-78. [PMID: 16697153]

88. Eli Lilly. Duloxetine Versus Placebo and Paroxetine in the Acute Treatment of Major Depression, Study Group A. CT Registry ID #4091. Clinical Study Summary: Study F1J-MC-HMAT. 2004. Acessed at www.clinicalstudyresults.org/documents/company-study_170_0.pdf on 24 August 2006.

89. Goldstein DJ, Lu Y, Detke MJ, Wiltse C, Mallinckrodt C, Demitrack MA. Duloxetine in the treatment of depression: a double-blind placebo-controlled comparison with paroxetine. J Clin Psychopharmacol. 2004;24:389-99. [PMID: 15232330]

90. U.S. Food and Drug Administration. Guidance for Industry and Investigators. Safety Reporting Requirements for INDs and BA/BE Studies. Draft Guidance. Rockville, MD: U.S. Department of Health and Human Services; 2010.

91. Clayton AH, Croft HA, Horrigan JP, Wightman DS, Krishen A, Richard NE, et al. Bupropion extended release compared with escitalopram: effects on sexual functioning and antidepressant efficacy in 2 randomized, double-blind, placebo-controlled studies. J Clin Psychiatry. 2006;67:736-46. [PMID: 16841623]

92. Coleman CC, King BR, Bolden-Watson C, Book MJ, Segraves RT, Richard N, et al. A placebo-controlled comparison of the effects on sexual functioning of bupropion sustained release and fluoxetine. Clin Ther. 2001;23:1040-58. [PMID: 11519769]

93. Kennedy SH, Fulton KA, Bagby RM, Greene AL, Cohen NL, Rafi-Tari S. Sexual function during bupropion or paroxetine treatment of major depressive disorder. Can J Psychiatry. 2006;51:234-42. [PMID: 16629348]

94. Croft H, Settle E Jr, Houser T, Batey SR, Donahue RM, Ascher JA. A placebo-controlled comparison of the antidepressant efficacy and effects on sexual functioning of sustained-release bupropion and sertraline. Clin Ther. 1999;21: 643-58. [PMID: 10363731]

95. Segraves RT, Kavoussi R, Hughes AR, Batey SR, Johnston JA, Donahue R, et al. Evaluation of sexual functioning in depressed outpatients: a double-blind comparison of sustained-release bupropion and sertraline treatment. J Clin Psychopharmacol. 2000;20:122-8. [PMID: 10770448]

96. Coleman CC, Cunningham LA, Foster VJ, Batey SR, Donahue RM, Houser TL, et al. Sexual dysfunction associated with the treatment of depression:

a placebo-controlled comparison of bupropion sustained release and sertraline treatment. Ann Clin Psychiatry. 1999;11:205-15. [PMID: 10596735]

97. Fava M, Amsterdam JD, Deltito JA, Salzman C, Schwaller M, Dunner DL. A double-blind study of paroxetine, fluoxetine, and placebo in outpatients with major depression. Ann Clin Psychiatry. 1998;10:145-50. [PMID: 9988054]

98. Hicks JA, Argyropoulos SV, Rich AS, Nash JR, Bell CJ, Edwards C, et al. Randomised controlled study of sleep after nefazodone or paroxetine treatment in out-patients with depression. Br J Psychiatry. 2002;180:528-35. [PMID: 12042232]

99. Kiev A, Feiger A. A double-blind comparison of fluvoxamine and paroxetine in the treatment of depressed outpatients. J Clin Psychiatry. 1997;58:146-52. [PMID: 9164424]

100. Delgado PL, Brannan SK, Mallinckrodt CH, Tran PV, McNamara RK, Wang F, et al. Sexual functioning assessed in 4 double-blind placebo- and paroxetine-controlled trials of duloxetine for major depressive disorder. J Clin Psychiatry 2005;66:686-92. [PMID: 15960560]

101. Boulenger JP, Huusom AK, Florea I, Baekdal T, Sarchiapone M. A comparative study of the efficacy of long-term treatment with escitalopram and paroxetine in severely depressed patients. Curr Med Res Opin. 2006;22:1331-41. [PMID: 16834832]

102. Montejo AL, Llorca G, Izquierdo JA, Rico-Villademoros F. Incidence of sexual dysfunction associated with antidepressant agents: a prospective multicenter study of 1022 outpatients. Spanish Working Group for the Study of Psychotropic-Related Sexual Dysfunction. J Clin Psychiatry. 2001;62 Suppl 3:10-21. [PMID: 11229449]

103. Friedman RA, Leon AC. Expanding the black box - depression, antidepressants, and the risk of suicide. N Engl J Med. 2007;356:2343-6. [PMID: 17485726]

104. Report of the CSM expert working group on the safety of selective serotonin reuptake inhibitor antidepressants. 2004. Accessed at www.mhra.gov.uk/home/groups/pl-p/documents/drugsafetymessage/con019472.pdf on 22 October 2011.

105. Fergusson D, Doucette S, Glass KC, Shapiro S, Healy D, Hebert P, et al. Association between suicide attempts and selective serotonin reuptake inhibitors: systematic review of randomised controlled trials. BMJ. 2005;330:396. [PMID: 15718539]

106. Martinez C, Rietbrock S, Wise L, Ashby D, Chick J, Moseley J, et al. Antidepressant treatment and the risk of fatal and non-fatal self harm in first episode depression: nested case-control study. BMJ. 2005;330:389. [PMID: 15718538]

107. Gunnell D, Saperia J, Ashby D. Selective serotonin reuptake inhibitors (SSRIs) and suicide in adults: meta-analysis of drug company data from placebo controlled, randomised controlled trials submitted to the MHRA's safety review. BMJ. 2005;330:385. [PMID: 15718537]

108. Didham RC, McConnell DW, Blair HJ, Reith DM. Suicide and self-harm following prescription of SSRIs and other antidepressants: confounding by indication. Br J Clin Pharmacol. 2005;60:519-25. [PMID: 16236042]

109. Jick H, Kaye JA, Jick SS. Antidepressants and the risk of suicidal behaviors. JAMA. 2004;292:338-43. [PMID: 15265848]

110. Jick SS, Dean AD, Jick H. Antidepressants and suicide. BMJ. 1995;310:215-8. [PMID: 7677826]

111. Jick H, Ulcickas M, Dean A. Comparison of frequencies of suicidal tendencies among patients receiving fluoxetine, lofepramine, mianserin, or trazodone. Pharmacotherapy. 1992;12:451-4. [PMID: 1492009]

112. Aursnes I, Tvete IF, Gaasemyr J, Natvig B. Suicide attempts in clinical trials with paroxetine randomised against placebo. BMC Med. 2005;3:14. [PMID: 16115311]

113. Khan A, Khan S, Kolts R, Brown WA. Suicide rates in clinical trials of SSRIs, other antidepressants, and placebo: analysis of FDA reports. Am J Psychiatry. 2003;160:790-2. [PMID: 12668373]

114. López-Iibor JJ. Reduced suicidality with paroxetine. Eur Psychiatry. 1993;8(Suppl 1):17S-9S.

115. Olfson M, Marcus SC. A case-control study of antidepressants and attempted suicide during early phase treatment of major depressive episodes. J Clin Psychiatry. 2008;69:425-32. [PMID: 18294025]

116. Barbui C, Esposito E, Cipriani A. Selective serotonin reuptake inhibitors and risk of suicide: a systematic review of observational studies. CMAJ. 2009; 180:291-7. [PMID: 19188627]

117. Rocca P, Calvarese P, Faggiano F, Marchiaro L, Mathis F, Rivoira E, et al. Citalopram versus sertraline in late-life nonmajor clinically significant depression: a 1-year follow-up clinical trial. J Clin Psychiatry. 2005;66:360-9. [PMID: 15766303]

118. Schöne W, Ludwig M. A double-blind study of paroxetine compared with fluoxetine in geriatric patients with major depression. J Clin Psychopharmacol. 1993;13:34S-39S. [PMID: 8106654]

119. Geretsegger C, Böhmer F, Ludwig M. Paroxetine in the elderly depressed patient: randomized comparison with fluoxetine of efficacy, cognitive and behavioural effects. Int Clin Psychopharmacol. 1994;9:25-9. [PMID: 8195578]

120. Kroenke K, West SL, Swindle R, Gilsenan A, Eckert GJ, Dolor R, et al. Similar effectiveness of paroxetine, fluoxetine, and sertraline in primary care: a randomized trial. JAMA. 2001;286:2947-55. [PMID: 11743835]

121. Cassano GB, Puca F, Scapicchio PL, Trabucchi M; Italian Study Group on Depression in Elderly Patients. Paroxetine and fluoxetine effects on mood and cognitive functions in depressed nondemented elderly patients. J Clin Psychiatry. 2002;63:396-402. [PMID: 12019663]

122. Rossini D, Serretti A, Franchini L, Mandelli L, Smeraldi E, De Ronchi D, et al. Sertraline versus fluvoxamine in the treatment of elderly patients with major depression: a double-blind, randomized trial. J Clin Psychopharmacol. 2005;25:471-5. [PMID: 16160624]

123. Allard P, Gram L, Timdahl K, Behnke K, Hanson M, Søgaard J. Efficacy and tolerability of venlafaxine in geriatric outpatients with major depression: a double-blind, randomised 6-month comparative trial with citalopram. Int J Geriatr Psychiatry. 2004;19:1123-30. [PMID: 15526307]

124. Schatzberg A, Roose S. A double-blind, placebo-controlled study of venlafaxine and fluoxetine in geriatric outpatients with major depression. Am J Geriatr Psychiatry. 2006;14:361-70. [PMID: 16582045]

125. Halikas JA. Org 3770 (mirtazapine) versus trazodone: A placebo controlled trial in depressed elderly patients. Hum Psychopharmacol. 1995;10(Suppl 2):S125-33.

126. Khazaie H, Rahimi M, Tatari F, Rezaei M, Najafi F, Tahmasian M. Treatment of depression in type 2 diabetes with fluoxetine or citalopram? Neurosciences (Riyadh). 2011;16:42-5. [PMID: 21206443]

127. Feighner JP, Gardner EA, Johnston JA, Batey SR, Khayrallah MA, Ascher JA, et al. Double-blind comparison of bupropion and fluoxetine in depressed outpatients. J Clin Psychiatry. 1991;52:329-35. [PMID: 1907963]

128. Gartlehner G, Gaynes BN, Hansen RA, Lohr KN. Ranking antidepressants [Letter]. Lancet. 2009;373:1761. [PMID: 19465225]

129. Ioannidis JP. Ranking antidepressants [Letter]. Lancet. 2009;373:1759-60. [PMID: 19465221]

130. Turner E, Moreno SG, Sutton AJ. Ranking antidepressants [Letter]. Lancet. 2009;373:1760. [PMID: 19465223]

131. Seyringer ME, Kasper S. Ranking antidepressants [Letter]. Lancet. 2009; 373:1760-1; author reply 1761-2. [PMID: 19465224]

132. Schwan S, Hallberg P. Ranking antidepressants [Letter]. Lancet. 2009;373:1761. [PMID: 19465226]

133. Bagby RM, Ryder AG, Schuller DR, Marshall MB. The Hamilton Depression Rating Scale: has the gold standard become a lead weight? Am J Psychiatry. 2004;161:2163-77. [PMID: 15569884]

134. Ekselius L, von Knorring L, Eberhard G. A double-blind multicenter trial comparing sertraline and citalopram in patients with major depression treated in general practice. Int Clin Psychopharmacol. 1997;12:323-31. [PMID: 9547134]

135. Melander H, Ahlqvist-Rastad J, Meijer G, Beermann B. Evidence b(i)ased medicine—selective reporting from studies sponsored by pharmaceutical industry: review of studies in new drug applications. BMJ. 2003;326:1171-3. [PMID: 12775615]

136. Turner EH, Matthews AM, Linardatos E, Tell RA, Rosenthal R. Selective publication of antidepressant trials and its influence on apparent efficacy. N Engl J Med. 2008;358:252-60. [PMID: 18199864]

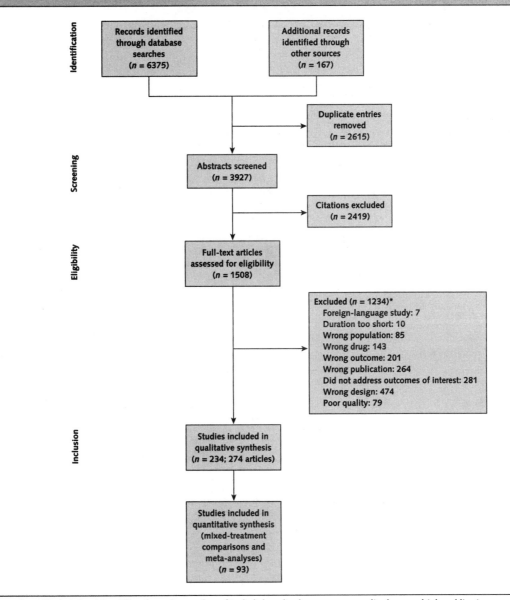

Appendix Figure 1. Summary of evidence search and selection.

* The number of included articles differs from the number of included studies because some studies have multiple publications.

Appendix Figure 2. Odds ratios of response rates comparing SNRIs with other second-generation antidepressants and comparing second-generation antidepressants with one another.

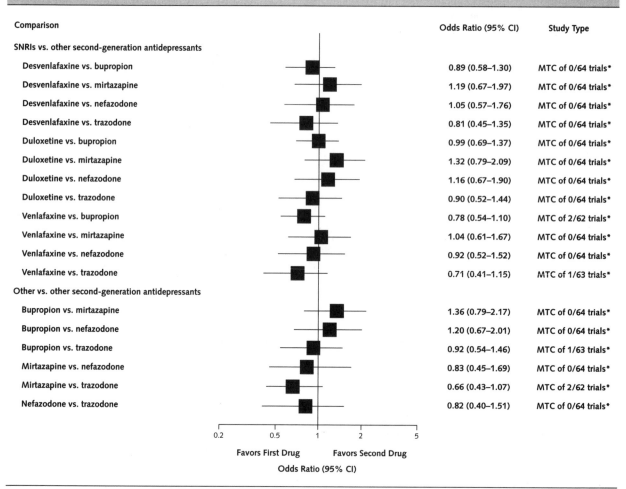

MTC = mixed-treatment comparison; SNRI = serotonin and norepinephrine reuptake inhibitor.
* The first number indicates the number of trials directly comparing 2 drugs; the second indicates the number of additional studies used to perform MTCs.

Appendix Table 1. Main Differences in Specific Adverse Events

Drug	Comparators	Differences in Adverse Events
Bupropion	Escitalopram, fluoxetine, paroxetine, sertraline	Lower incidence of sexual dysfunction than comparator drugs (6% vs. 16%)
Mirtazapine	Fluoxetine, paroxetine, trazodone, venlafaxine	Greater weight gain than comparator drugs (mean, 0.8–3.0 kg after 6–8 wk)
Paroxetine	Escitalopram, duloxetine, fluoxetine, mirtazapine, nefazodone, and sertraline	Higher incidence of sexual dysfunction, particularly ejaculatory dysfunction, than comparator drugs
Sertraline	Bupropion, citalopram, fluoxetine, fluvoxamine, mirtazapine, nefazodone, paroxetine, venlafaxine	Higher incidence of diarrhea than comparator drugs (mean, 16% [95% CI, 13%–20%] vs. 8% [CI, 4%–13%])
Trazodone	Bupropion, fluoxetine, mirtazapine, paroxetine, venlafaxine	Higher incidence of somnolence than comparator drugs (mean, 42% [CI, 19%–64% vs. 25% [CI, 3%–46%])
Venlafaxine	SSRIs as a class	Higher incidence of nausea and vomiting than SSRIs as a class (mean, 33% [CI, 23%–43%] vs. 22% [CI, 16%–29%])

SSRI = selective serotonin reuptake inhibitor.

Appendix Table 2. Comparative Efficacy or Effectiveness in Subgroups: Findings and Strength of Evidence

Outcome	Strength of Evidence*	Findings
Age		
Comparative efficacy	Moderate	Evidence from 11 trials indicates that efficacy does not differ substantially among second-generation antidepressants for treating MDD in patients aged ≥60 y.
Comparative harms	Low	Results from 6 studies indicate that adverse events may differ somewhat across second-generation antidepressants in elderly patients.
Sex		
Comparative efficacy	Insufficient	No evidence
Comparative effectiveness	Insufficient	No evidence
Comparative harms	Low	Two trials suggest differences between men and women in sexual side effects.
Race or ethnicity		
Comparative efficacy	Insufficient	No evidence
Comparative effectiveness	Insufficient	No evidence
Comparative harms	Insufficient	No evidence
Comorbid conditions		
Comparative efficacy	Low	Results from a subgroup analysis of 1 trial indicate significantly greater response with extended-release venlafaxine than fluoxetine in patients with MDD and comorbid generalized anxiety disorder.
Comparative effectiveness	Insufficient	No evidence
Comparative harms	Insufficient	No evidence

MDD = major depressive disorder.
* High strength of evidence indicates high confidence that the evidence reflects the true effect. Further research is very unlikely to change our confidence in the estimate of effect. Moderate strength of evidence indicates that the evidence reflects the true effect. Further research may change our confidence in the estimate of effect and may change the estimate. Low strength of evidence indicates that the evidence reflects the true effect. Further research is likely to change both the confidence in the estimate of effect and the estimate. Insufficient strength of evidence indicates that evidence is either unavailable or does not permit a conclusion.

Atypical Antipsychotic Augmentation in Major Depressive Disorder: A Meta-Analysis of Placebo-Controlled Randomized Trials

J. Craig Nelson, M.D.

George I. Papakostas, M.D.

Objective: The authors sought to determine by meta-analysis the efficacy and tolerability of adjunctive atypical antipsychotic agents in major depressive disorder.

Method: Searches were conducted of MEDLINE/PubMed (1966 to January 2009), the Cochrane database, abstracts of major psychiatric meetings since 2000, and online trial registries. Manufacturers of atypical antipsychotic agents without online registries were contacted. Trials selected were acute-phase, parallel-group, double-blind controlled trials with random assignment to adjunctive atypical antipsychotic or placebo. Patients had nonpsychotic unipolar major depressive disorder that was resistant to prior antidepressant treatment. Response, remission, and discontinuation rates were either reported or obtained. Data were extracted by one author and checked by the second. Data included study design, number of patients, patient characteristics, methods of establishing treatment resistance, drug doses, duration of the adjunctive trial, depression scale used, response and remission rates, and discontinuation rates for any reason or for adverse events.

Results: Sixteen trials with 3,480 patients were pooled using a fixed-effects meta-analysis. Adjunctive atypical antipsychotics were significantly more effective than placebo (response: odds ratio=1.69, 95% CI=1.46–1.95, z=7.00, N=16, p<0.00001; remission: odds ratio=2.00, 95% CI=1.69–2.37, z=8.03, N=16, p<0.00001). Mean odds ratios did not differ among the atypical agents and were not affected by trial duration or method of establishing treatment resistance. Discontinuation rates for adverse events were higher for atypical agents than for placebo (odds ratio=3.91, 95% CI=2.68–5.72, z=7.05, N=15, p<0.00001).

Conclusions: Atypical antipsychotics are effective augmentation agents in major depressive disorder but are associated with an increased risk of discontinuation due to adverse events.

(Am J Psychiatry 2009; 166:980–991)

D epression is among the most common medical disorders. In the United States approximately 1 in 6 individuals will suffer from major depressive disorder during their lifetime (1). Even though numerous treatments are available, only about one-third of patients receiving initial antidepressant treatment achieve remission (2). As a consequence, several treatment strategies have evolved for difficult-to-treat depression. One approach has been to augment antidepressants with an agent not approved for use as monotherapy in major depressive disorder.

Augmentation strategies have a long history. Use of stimulants and T$_3$ to augment tricyclic antidepressants was described four decades ago (3). Subsequently, use of several other agents for augmentation was described, but the evidence base comprised a limited number of controlled trials with small samples. Until recently lithium augmentation was the best studied augmentation strategy. Ten placebo-controlled trials were performed, but nine of them included no more than 35 patients (4). In 10 controlled lithium studies, the total number of patients was only 269 (4), and in the majority of these studies lith- ium was used to augment tricyclic antidepressants, which are not currently in widespread use.

The use of antipsychotic agents in depression has a long history (5), but recognition of the extrapyramidal side effects and the risk of tardive dyskinesia discouraged the use of the conventional antipsychotics. However, the advent of a newer generation of antipsychotic agents, which for the most part appeared to differ from conventional agents in their side effect and neuropharmacologic profile, rekindled interest in the use of this class of drugs in mood and anxiety disorders, including as adjunctive therapy. The first report of the use of an atypical antipsychotic for augmentation in major depressive disorder appeared in 1999. Ostroff and Nelson (6) described eight patients whose depression had failed to respond to selective serotonin reuptake inhibitors (SSRIs). Rapid effects were noted when low doses of risperidone were added. This observation was soon followed by the first placebo-controlled study. Shelton et al. (7) noted that the combination of olanzapine and fluoxetine was more effective than either drug alone in a sample of 30 patients with fluoxetine-resistant major

FIGURE 1. Results of Search for Articles on Trials of Atypical Antipsychotic Augmentation in Major Depressive Disorder

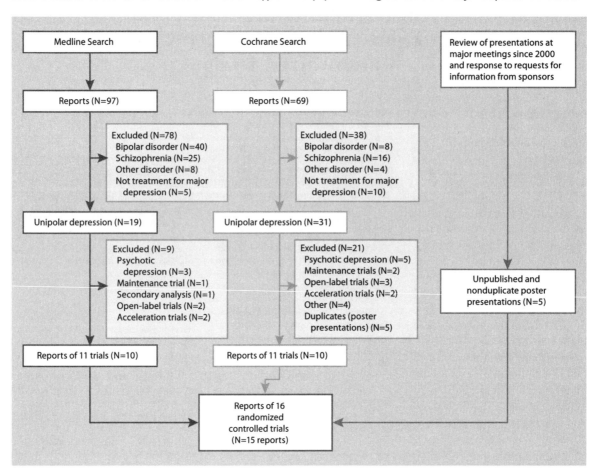

depression. Since those initial reports, the number and size of studies of augmentation with atypical antipsychotics has grown rapidly, and in 2008 aripiprazole became the first atypical agent and the first pharmacologic treatment of any type to be approved by the U.S. Food and Drug Administration (FDA) for use as an augmentation agent in major depressive disorder.

With the growth of the adjunctive use of atypical antipsychotics, interest in their efficacy and tolerability has increased. In 2007 Papakostas et al. (8) conducted a systematic review and meta-analysis of 10 placebo-controlled augmentation trials of atypical antipsychotics for major depressive disorder (N=1,500). The meta-analysis confirmed the efficacy of this strategy. Since that meta-analysis was published, however, six new trials with 2,007 subjects have been published or presented at major scientific meetings; these include three large trials of aripiprazole (9–11), as well as two large trials of extended-release quetiapine (12, 13), that increase the number of subjects treated with quetiapine from 109 to 1,028. Because the growth of evidence for the use of atypicals has been so rapid, an updated review and meta-analysis of the efficacy and tolerability of these agents is in order.

Given differences in the neuropharmacology of atypical antipsychotics (14–16), it is not clear that these agents would have similar efficacy in depression or that they would be effective in the same patients. Moreover, the dosages used in the adjunctive treatment of depression are often lower than those used in the treatment of psychotic disorders, and the prominent pharmacologic effects may differ between these dosage levels. All of the atypical antipsychotics display 5-HT$_2$ receptor antagonism, although their relative potency varies. Aripiprazole and ziprasidone also display 5-HT$_{1A}$ partial agonism (15). All of the atypical agents possess dopamine D$_2$ receptor affinity; aripiprazole acts as a partial agonist at this receptor (17), and the others have antagonist properties. The metabolite of quetiapine, *N*-desalkylquetiapine, has recently been shown to have moderate affinity for the norepinephrine reuptake transporter (18), but it is not clear that the metabolite achieves appreciable plasma concentrations in human subjects. Ziprasidone is associated with notable potency at the transporters for dopamine, norepinephrine, and serotonin (19). The olanzapine-fluoxetine combination is reported to produce a greater increase in extracellular levels of dopamine and norepinephrine in rat prefrontal cortex than ei-

TABLE 1. Placebo-Controlled Atypical Antipsychotic Augmentation Trials in Major Depressive Disorder

Authors (Reference)	Year	Atypical Antipsychotic	Anti-depressant	N[a]	Duration[b] (Weeks)	Prior Failed Trials	Rating Scale[c]
Shelton et al. (7)	2001	Olanzapine	Fluoxetine	20	8	Two historical trials and one prospective trial	MADRS
Shelton et al. (25)	2005	Olanzapine	Fluoxetine	288	8	One or more historical trials and one prospective trial	MADRS
Corya et al. (26)	2006	Olanzapine	Fluoxetine	286	12	One or more historical trials and one prospective trial	MADRS
Thase et al. (27)[d]	2006	Olanzapine	Fluoxetine	206	8	One or more historical trials and one prospective trial	MADRS
Thase et al. (27)[d]	2006	Olanzapine	Fluoxetine	200	8	One or more historical trials and one prospective trial	MADRS
Mahmoud et al. (28)	2007	Risperidone	Various	268	6	4-week prospective trial	HAM-D
Reeves et al. (29)	2008	Risperidone	Various	23	8	Historical trial of at least 3 weeks	MADRS
Keitner et al. (30)	2009	Risperidone	Various	95	4	One prospective trial of at least 5 weeks or a clearly documented trial	MADRS
Khullar et al. (31)	2006	Quetiapine	SSRI/SNRI	15	8	At least one historical trial of at least 6 weeks	MADRS
Mattingly et al. (32)	2006	Quetiapine	SSRI/SNRI	37	8	One prior trial of at least 4 weeks and at least 6 weeks in the current trial	MADRS
McIntyre et al. (33)	2006	Quetiapine	SSRI/SNRI	58	8	One or more trials of at least 6 weeks	HAM-D
Earley et al. (12)	2007	Quetiapine	SSRI/SNRI	487	6	One historical trial of at least 6 weeks	MADRS
El-Khalili et al. (13)	2008	Quetiapine	SSRI/SNRI	432	8	One historical trial of at least 6 weeks	MADRS
Berman et al. (9)	2007	Aripiprazole	SSRI/SNRI	353	6	1–3 historical trials and one prospective trial	MADRS
Marcus et al. (10)	2008	Aripiprazole	SSRI/SNRI	369	6	1–3 historical trials and one prospective trial	MADRS
Berman et al. (11)	2008	Aripiprazole	SSRI/SNRI	343	6	1–3 historical trials and one prospective trial	MADRS

[a] Number of randomized patients with at least one posttreatment rating.
[b] Duration of the acute-phase double-blind controlled trial.
[c] HAM-D=Hamilton Depression Rating Scale; MADRS=Montgomery-Åsberg Depression Rating Scale.
[d] This report included two separate trials of identical design.

ther agent alone or other combinations of antipsychotics and SSRIs (20). Each of these effects might contribute to clinical efficacy in depression. Alternatively, these effects as well as varying levels of α_1 adrenergic, antihistaminic, and antimuscarinic activity of these agents may produce differences in side effects.

In our meta-analysis, we hypothesized that adjunctive treatment with atypical antipsychotics would result in higher rates of response and remission than placebo but that this effect would be offset to some extent by an increase in discontinuation due to adverse events. We further hypothesized that sensitivity analyses would reveal that adjunctive trials of longer duration would be associated with larger drug-placebo differences and that studies using a prospective trial to confirm treatment resistance would have lower response rates but greater drug-placebo differences.

Method

We searched MEDLINE/PubMed (1966 to January 2009) for randomized placebo-controlled trials of atypical antipsychotic agents approved by the FDA for any indication. Search terms were "major depression" and "aripiprazole or olanzapine or paliperidone or quetiapine or risperidone or ziprasidone." The Cochrane Clinical Trials register was searched using identical terms. Poster presentations at major psychiatric meetings since 2000 were searched, and the manufacturers of atypical antipsychotic medications were asked for all published and unpublished reports of adjunctive trials in nonpsychotic major depressive disorder. Reports from different sources were then compared to identify nonduplicative trials.

Trial Selection

Trials were included if they were acute-phase, parallel-group, double-blind, placebo-controlled trials with random assignment to adjunctive treatment with an atypical antipsychotic or placebo. Patients had to have nonpsychotic major depressive disorder that was considered treatment resistant either by history or determined by a prospective trial. Response, remission, and discontinuation rates either were reported in published articles or poster presentations or were obtained from the sponsor or investigator.

Data Extraction

Data were extracted by one of the authors and checked for accuracy by the other. Data extracted included study design, number of patients, patient characteristics, methods used to establish treatment resistance, drug dosages, duration of the prospective adjunctive trial, response and remission rates, and rates of discontinuation for any reason and for adverse events. Response was defined as an improvement of ≥50% from baseline to endpoint on the Hamilton Depression Rating Scale (21) or the Montgomery-Åsberg Depression Rating Scale (22) in the intent-to-treat sample using the last-observation-carried-forward method. Remission was defined according to each individual trial in the intent-to-treat/last-observation-carried-forward sample.

Statistical Analysis

Across studies, the numbers of patients who responded, remitted, and dropped out and the number randomly assigned to each treatment group were statistically combined, using a fixed-effects meta-analytic model. Effects were expressed as odds ratios with their 95% confidence intervals (CIs), test of significance (Wald's z), number (N) of contrasts, and p values. Effects were calculated for each drug-placebo contrast, for each group of trials using the same drug, and as meta-analytic summaries for all drugs combined. A funnel plot in which the standard error of the log odds ratio against the log of the odds ratio was used to evaluate potential publication or retrieval bias.

Chi-square tests and the I^2 statistic derived from the chi-square values were used to test for heterogeneity among the studies. I^2

FIGURE 2. Meta-Analysis of Response Rates of Atypical Antipsychotic Agents in Treatment-Resistant Major Depressive Disorder[a]

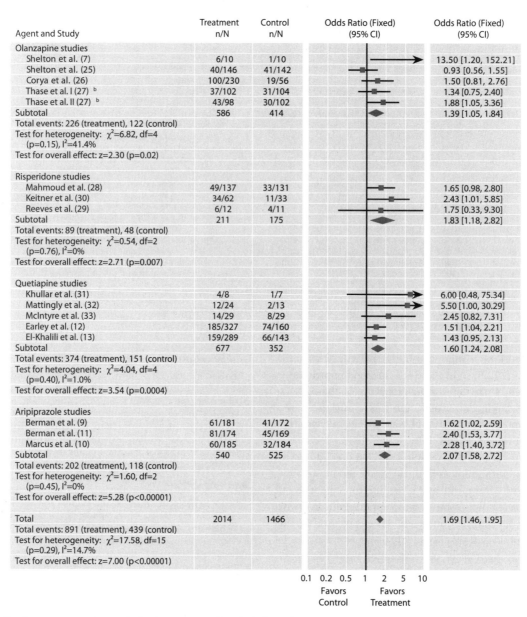

[a] Odds ratios for response on drug and placebo are grouped by atypical agent.
[b] This report included two separate trials of identical design.

approximates the proportion of total variation in the effect size estimates that is due to heterogeneity rather than sampling error (23). An alpha error <0.20 and an I² of at least 50% were taken as indicators of heterogeneity. In the Results section, the chi-square test and I² statistics for heterogeneity follow the 95% CI, z score, N, and p value for the odds ratio unless these values are provided in a figure.

In sensitivity analyses, we compared subgroups on potential differences between the different agents, duration of the adjunctive trial, and definition of treatment resistance (historical or prospective). Differences between two or more subgroups were investigated by subtracting the sum of the heterogeneity chi-square statistics of the subgroups from the overall chi-square statistic and comparing the result with a chi-square distribution with the value for degrees of freedom 1 less than the number of subgroups (24). Review Manager, version 4.2 (Cochrane Collaboration, Oxford, England), was used for statistical calculations.

Results

Figure 1 illustrates the search flow. The MEDLINE and Cochrane searches each found 10 nonduplicative reports of 11 randomized, double-blind controlled trials of acute-phase treatment with atypical antipsychotic augmentation in patients with nonpsychotic major depressive disor-

FIGURE 3. Meta-Analysis of Remission Rates of Atypical Antipsychotic Agents in Treatment-Resistant Major Depressive Disorder[a]

Agent and Study	Treatment n/N	Control n/N	Odds Ratio (Fixed) (95% CI)
Olanzapine studies			
Shelton et al. (7)	6/10	2/10	6.00 [0.81, 44.35]
Shelton et al. (25)	25/146	18/142	1.42 [0.74, 2.74]
Corya et al. (26) [b]	69/230	10/56	1.97 [0.94, 4.13]
Thase et al. I (27) [b]	24/102	18/104	1.47 [0.74, 2.91]
Thase et al. II (27) [b]	30/98	16/102	2.37 [1.20, 4.70]
Subtotal	586	414	1.83 [1.30, 2.56]
Total events: 154 (treatment), 64 (control)			
Test for heterogeneity: χ^2=2.90, df=4 (p=0.57), I^2=0%			
Test for overall effect: z=3.49 (p=0.0005)			
Risperidone studies			
Mahmoud et al. (28)	26/137	12/131	2.32 [1.12, 4.83]
Keitner et al. (30)	32/62	8/33	3.33 [1.30, 8.53]
Reeves et al. (29)	4/12	2/11	2.25 [0.32, 15.76]
Subtotal	211	175	2.63 [1.51, 4.57]
Total events: 62 (treatment), 22 (control)			
Test for heterogeneity: χ^2=0.38, df=2 (p=0.83), I^2=0%			
Test for overall effect: z=3.43 (p=0.0006)			
Quetiapine studies			
Khullar et al. (31)	3/8	0/7	9.55 [0.40, 225.19]
Mattingly et al. (32)	11/24	2/13	4.65 [0.84, 25.66]
McIntyre et al. (33)	9/29	5/29	2.16 [0.62, 7.49]
Earley et al. (12)	110/327	38/160	1.63 [1.06, 2.50]
El-Khalili et al. (13)	112/289	35/143	1.95 [1.25, 3.06]
Subtotal	677	352	1.89 [1.41, 2.54]
Total events: 245 (treatment), 80 (control)			
Test for heterogeneity: χ^2=2.61, df=4 (p=0.63), I^2=1.0%			
Test for overall effect: z=4.25 (p<0.0001)			
Aripiprazole studies			
Berman et al. (9)	47/181	27/172	1.88 [1.11, 3.19]
Berman et al. (11)	64/174	32/169	2.49 [1.52, 4.08]
Marcus et al. (10)	47/185	28/184	1.90 [1.13, 3.19]
Subtotal	540	525	2.09 [1.55, 2.81]
Total events: 158 (treatment), 87 (control)			
Test for heterogeneity: χ^2=0.77, df=2 (p=0.68), I^2=0%			
Test for overall effect: z=4.88 (p<0.00001)			
Total	2014	1466	2.00 [1.69, 2.37]
Total events: 619 (treatment), 253 (control)			
Test for heterogeneity: χ^2=8.16, df=15 (p=0.92), I^2=10%			
Test for overall effect: z=8.03 (p<0.00001)			

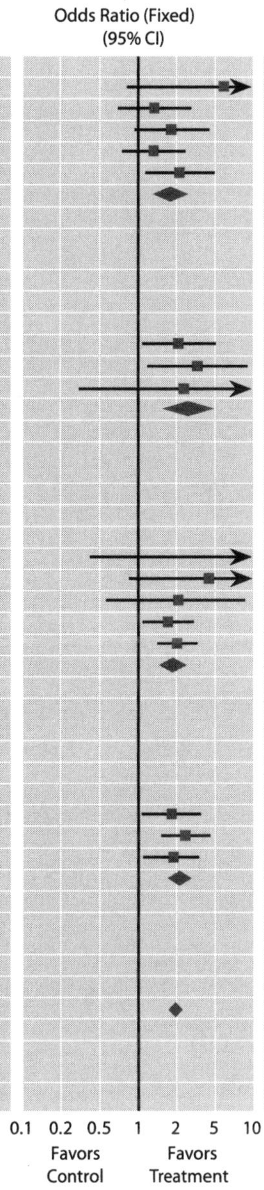

0.1 0.2 0.5 1 2 5 10 — Favors Control / Favors Treatment

[a] Odds ratios for remission on drug and placebo are grouped by atypical agent.
[b] This report included two separate trials of identical design.

der patients who had not responded to prior antidepressant treatment (either by history or in a prospective trial). The search of meeting abstracts and information provided by the manufacturers of atypical antipsychotics provided another five unpublished reports that were presented as posters. We excluded five trials of patients with psychotic depression, one relapse prevention trial, one secondary analysis, three open-label trials, two acceleration trials, and four other studies that did not investigate efficacy (focusing instead, for example, on effects on the hypothalamic-pituitary-adrenal axis).

The 15 reports of 16 trials included five trials with olanzapine (7, 25–27), three with risperidone (28–30), five with quetiapine (12, 13, 31–33), and three with aripiprazole (9–11). No acute-phase, double-blind trials of adjunctive ziprasidone or paliperidone in major depressive disorder were found. The 16 trials included a total of 3,480 patients, of whom 2,014 were randomly assigned to adjunctive treatment with an atypical antipsychotic and 1,466 to placebo. Other descriptive features of the trials are listed in Table 1. In one report for olanzapine (27), discontinuation rates were presented as combined data from two individ-

FIGURE 4. Meta-Analysis of Rates of Discontinuation for Any Reason for Atypical Antipsychotic Agents in Treatment-Resistant Major Depressive Disorder[a]

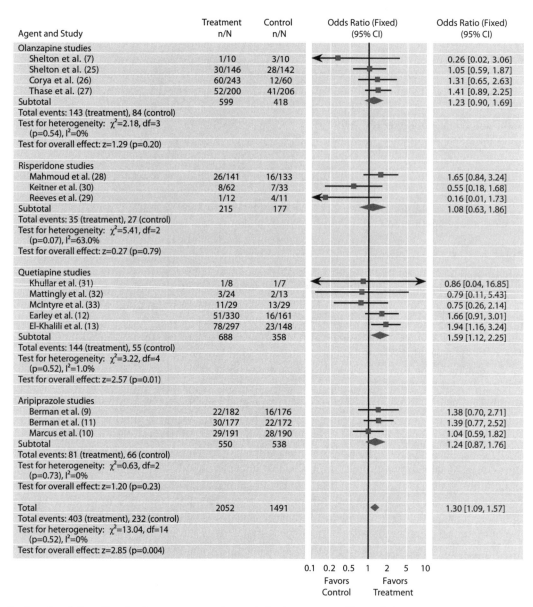

Agent and Study	Treatment n/N	Control n/N	Odds Ratio (Fixed) (95% CI)	Odds Ratio (Fixed) (95% CI)
Olanzapine studies				
Shelton et al. (7)	1/10	3/10		0.26 [0.02, 3.06]
Shelton et al. (25)	30/146	28/142		1.05 [0.59, 1.87]
Corya et al. (26)	60/243	12/60		1.31 [0.65, 2.63]
Thase et al. (27)	52/200	41/206		1.41 [0.89, 2.25]
Subtotal	599	418		1.23 [0.90, 1.69]
Total events: 143 (treatment), 84 (control)				
Test for heterogeneity: χ^2=2.18, df=3 (p=0.54), I^2=0%				
Test for overall effect: z=1.29 (p=0.20)				
Risperidone studies				
Mahmoud et al. (28)	26/141	16/133		1.65 [0.84, 3.24]
Keitner et al. (30)	8/62	7/33		0.55 [0.18, 1.68]
Reeves et al. (29)	1/12	4/11		0.16 [0.01, 1.73]
Subtotal	215	177		1.08 [0.63, 1.86]
Total events: 35 (treatment), 27 (control)				
Test for heterogeneity: χ^2=5.41, df=2 (p=0.07), I^2=63.0%				
Test for overall effect: z=0.27 (p=0.79)				
Quetiapine studies				
Khullar et al. (31)	1/8	1/7		0.86 [0.04, 16.85]
Mattingly et al. (32)	3/24	2/13		0.79 [0.11, 5.43]
McIntyre et al. (33)	11/29	13/29		0.75 [0.26, 2.14]
Earley et al. (12)	51/330	16/161		1.66 [0.91, 3.01]
El-Khalili et al. (13)	78/297	23/148		1.94 [1.16, 3.24]
Subtotal	688	358		1.59 [1.12, 2.25]
Total events: 144 (treatment), 55 (control)				
Test for heterogeneity: χ^2=3.22, df=4 (p=0.52), I^2=1.0%				
Test for overall effect: z=2.57 (p=0.01)				
Aripiprazole studies				
Berman et al. (9)	22/182	16/176		1.38 [0.70, 2.71]
Berman et al. (11)	30/177	22/172		1.39 [0.77, 2.52]
Marcus et al. (10)	29/191	28/190		1.04 [0.59, 1.82]
Subtotal	550	538		1.24 [0.87, 1.76]
Total events: 81 (treatment), 66 (control)				
Test for heterogeneity: χ^2=0.63, df=2 (p=0.73), I^2=0%				
Test for overall effect: z=1.20 (p=0.23)				
Total	2052	1491		1.30 [1.09, 1.57]
Total events: 403 (treatment), 232 (control)				
Test for heterogeneity: χ^2=13.04, df=14 (p=0.52), I^2=0%				
Test for overall effect: z=2.85 (p=0.004)				

0.1 0.2 0.5   1   2   5   10
Favors Control   Favors Treatment

[a] Odds ratios for rates of discontinuation for any reason on drug and placebo are grouped by atypical agent.

ual trials, so the two trials were presented as a single trial in the meta-analysis of discontinuation rates.

Response and Remission

The meta-analyses for response and remission are summarized in Figures 2 and 3. The odds ratio for response with drug versus placebo was 1.69 (95% CI=1.46–1.95, z= 7.00, N=16, p<0.00001). The risk difference by meta-analysis was 0.12 (95% CI=0.08–0.15, z=7.14, N=16, p<0.00001). The risk difference translates into a number needed to treat of nine. The test for heterogeneity indicated a lack of heterogeneity (χ^2=17.58, df=15, p=0.29, I^2=14.7%). The

overall pooled response rate for treatment with an atypical agent was 44.2%, compared with 29.9% for placebo.

Odds ratios for the trials grouped by atypical agent varied from 1.39 (95% CI=1.05–1.84) to 2.07 (95% CI=1.58–2.72), with considerable overlap among the confidence intervals. Testing the difference between the atypical subgroups indicated no significant differences (χ^2=4.58, df=3, p=0.21).

The odds ratio for remission was 2.00 (95% CI=1.69–2.37, z=8.03, N=16, p<0.00001). The risk difference for remission was 0.12 (95% CI=0.09–0.15), indicating a number needed to treat of nine. The test for heterogeneity was not

FIGURE 5. Meta-Analysis of Rates of Discontinuation Due to Adverse Events for Atypical Antipsychotic Agents in Treatment-Resistant Major Depressive Disorder[a]

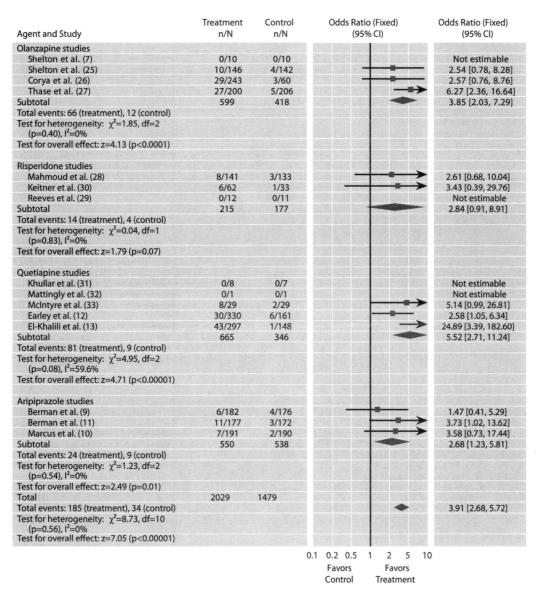

[a] Odds ratios for discontinuation rates due to adverse events on drug and placebo are grouped by atypical agent.

significant (χ^2=8.16, df=15, p=0.92, I^2=0%). The pooled remission rates were 30.7% for atypical antipsychotics, compared with 17.2% for placebo.

The odds ratios for remission varied from 1.83 to 2.63 among the drug subgroups, with overlapping confidence intervals. Testing the difference between the atypical subgroups indicated no significant differences (χ^2=1.50, df=3, p=0.68).

Discontinuation Rates

The odds ratio comparing drug and placebo groups for rates of discontinuation for any reason was 1.30 (95% CI= 1.09–1.57, z=2.85, p=0.004) (Figure 4). The test for hetero-

geneity was not significant (χ^2=13.04, df=14, p=0.52, I^2= 0%). The odds ratios for rates of discontinuation for any reason did not differ significantly among the drug subgroups (χ^2=1.60, df=3, p=0.66). The pooled actual rates of discontinuation for any reason were 19.6% in the atypical treatment group and 15.5% in the placebo group.

The odds ratio for the rate of discontinuation for adverse events with drug and placebo was 3.91 (95% CI= 2.68–5.72, z=7.05, N=15, p<0.00001) (Figure 5). The test for heterogeneity was not significant (χ^2=8.73, df=10, p=0.56, I^2=0%). The risk difference was 0.06 (95% CI=0.05–0.08), resulting in a number needed to harm of 17. The pooled adverse event discontinuation rates were 9.1% in the atyp-

FIGURE 6. Odds Ratios of Response Rates on Drug and Placebo in Atypical Antipsychotic Augmentation Trials, Grouped by Duration of the Acute-Phase Trial

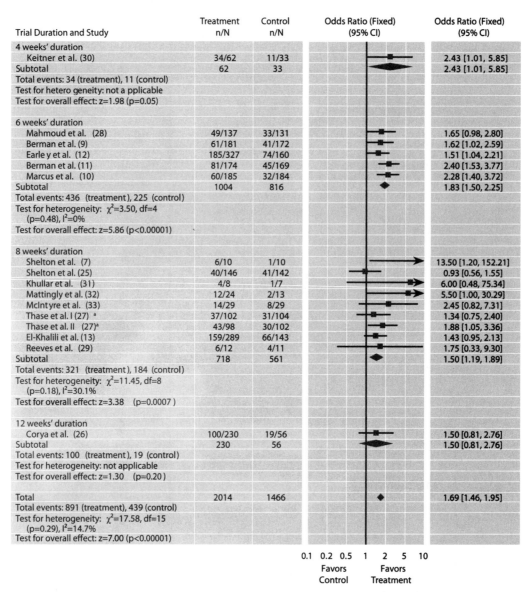

Trial Duration and Study	Treatment n/N	Control n/N	Odds Ratio (Fixed) (95% CI)
4 weeks' duration			
Keitner et al. (30)	34/62	11/33	2.43 [1.01, 5.85]
Subtotal	62	33	2.43 [1.01, 5.85]
Total events: 34 (treatment), 11 (control)			
Test for hetero geneity: not a pplicable			
Test for overall effect: z=1.98 (p=0.05)			
6 weeks' duration			
Mahmoud et al. (28)	49/137	33/131	1.65 [0.98, 2.80]
Berman et al. (9)	61/181	41/172	1.62 [1.02, 2.59]
Earle y et al. (12)	185/327	74/160	1.51 [1.04, 2.21]
Berman et al. (11)	81/174	45/169	2.40 [1.53, 3.77]
Marcus et al. (10)	60/185	32/184	2.28 [1.40, 3.72]
Subtotal	1004	816	1.83 [1.50, 2.25]
Total events: 436 (treatment), 225 (control)			
Test for heterogeneity: χ^2=3.50, df=4 (p=0.48), I^2=0%			
Test for overall effect: z=5.86 (p<0.00001)			
8 weeks' duration			
Shelton et al. (7)	6/10	1/10	13.50 [1.20, 152.21]
Shelton et al. (25)	40/146	41/142	0.93 [0.56, 1.55]
Khullar et al. (31)	4/8	1/7	6.00 [0.48, 75.34]
Mattingly et al. (32)	12/24	2/13	5.50 [1.00, 30.29]
McIntyre et al. (33)	14/29	8/29	2.45 [0.82, 7.31]
Thase et al. I (27) [a]	37/102	31/104	1.34 [0.75, 2.40]
Thase et al. II (27)[a]	43/98	30/102	1.88 [1.05, 3.36]
El-Khalili et al. (13)	159/289	66/143	1.43 [0.95, 2.13]
Reeves et al. (29)	6/12	4/11	1.75 [0.33, 9.30]
Subtotal	718	561	1.50 [1.19, 1.89]
Total events: 321 (treatment), 184 (control)			
Test for heterogeneity: χ^2=11.45, df=8 (p=0.18), I^2=30.1%			
Test for overall effect: z=3.38 (p=0.0007)			
12 weeks' duration			
Corya et al. (26)	100/230	19/56	1.50 [0.81, 2.76]
Subtotal	230	56	1.50 [0.81, 2.76]
Total events: 100 (treatment), 19 (control)			
Test for heterogeneity: not applicable			
Test for overall effect: z=1.30 (p=0.20)			
Total	2014	1466	1.69 [1.46, 1.95]
Total events: 891 (treatment), 439 (control)			
Test for heterogeneity: χ^2=17.58, df=15 (p=0.29), I^2=14.7%			
Test for overall effect: z=7.00 (p<0.00001)			

0.1 0.2 0.5 1 2 5 10

Favors Control — Favors Treatment

[a] This report included two separate trials of identical design.

ical antipsychotic group and 2.3% in the placebo group. The odds ratios for the subgroups varied from 2.68 to 5.52. Testing the difference between the atypical subgroups indicated no significant differences (χ^2=0.66, df=3, p=0.88).

Trial duration varied from 4 to 12 weeks. Duration of the trial did not significantly affect the odds ratio for response to drug and placebo (Figure 6). The odds ratios for trials of 4, 6, 8, and 12 weeks were 2.43 (95% CI=1.01–5.85), 1.83 (95% CI=1.50–2.25), 1.50 (95% CI=1.19–1.89), and 1.50 (0.81–2.76), respectively, and did not differ significantly (χ^2=2.63, df=3, p=0.45). This analysis, however, was limited because only one trial had a duration of 4 weeks and only one of 12 weeks.

We also examined whether the odds ratios for response differed in trials using history of drug failure rather than a prospective trial to establish treatment resistance (Figure 7). Ten of the trials required that patients have failed to respond in one prospective trial, and six required that patients have a history of nonresponse or failed to respond in the current trial. The odds ratio of the 10 trials requiring a failed prospective trial was 1.73 (95% CI=1.45–2.06), which did not differ from the trials using only historical data, in which the odds ratio was 1.61 (95% CI=1.24–2.08). The magnitude of the drug-placebo difference, estimated by the risk difference from the meta-analysis, was identical using the two methods, at 0.12. However, the pooled re-

FIGURE 7. Odds Ratios of Response Rates on Drug and Placebo in Atypical Antipsychotic Augmentation Trials, Grouped by Method of Establishing Treatment Resistance

Treatment Resistance Subcategory and Study	Treatment n/N	Control n/N	Odds Ratio (Fixed) (95% CI)	Odds Ratio (Fixed) (95% CI)
Historical failure only				
Khullar et al. (31)	4/8	1/7		6.00 [0.48, 75.34]
Mattingly et al. (32)	12/24	2/13		5.50 [1.00, 30.29]
McIntyre et al. (33)	14/29	8/29		2.45 [0.82, 7.31]
Earley et al. (12)	185/327	74/160		1.51 [1.04, 2.21]
El-Khalili et al. (13)	159/289	66/143		1.43 [0.95, 2.13]
Reeves et al. (29)	6/12	4/11		1.75 [0.33, 9.30]
Subtotal	689	363		1.61 [1.24, 2.08]
Total events: 380 (treatment), 155 (control)				
Test for heterogeneity: χ^2=4.05, df=5 (p=0.54), I^2=0%				
Test for overall effect: z=3.60 (p=0.0003)				
One prospective trial				
Mahmoud et al. (28)	49/137	33/131		1.65 [0.98, 2.80]
Shelton et al. (7)	6/10	1/10		13.50 [1.20, 152.21]
Shelton et al. (25)	40/146	41/142		0.93 [0.56, 1.55]
Corya et al. (26)	100/230	19/56		1.50 [0.81, 2.76]
Thase et al. I (27)[a]	37/102	31/104		1.34 [0.75, 2.40]
Thase et al. II (27)[a]	43/98	30/102		1.88 [1.05, 3.36]
Berman et al. (9)	61/181	41/172		1.62 [1.02, 2.59]
Berman et al. (11)	81/174	45/169		2.40 [1.53, 3.77]
Keitner et al. (30)	34/62	11/33		2.43 [1.01, 5.85]
Marcus et al. (10)	60/185	32/184		2.28 [1.40, 3.72]
Subtotal	1325	1103		1.73 [1.45, 2.06]
Total events: 511 (treatment), 284 (control)				
Test for heterogeneity: χ^2=13.30, df=9 (p=0.15), I^2=32.3%				
Test for overall effect: z=6.02 (p<0.00001)				
Total	2014	1466		1.69 [1.46, 1.95]
Total events: 891 (treatment), 439 (control)				
Test for heterogeneity: χ^2=17.58, df=15 (p=0.29), I^2=14.7%				
Test for overall effect: z=6.02 (p<0.00001)				

0.1 0.2 0.5 1 2 5 10
Favors Control — Favors Treatment

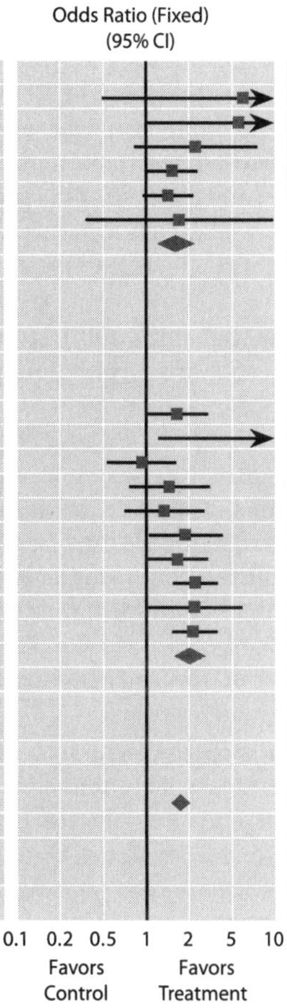

[a] This report included two separate trials of identical design.

sponse rates in trials requiring a failed prospective trial (38.6% [511/1,325] and 25.8% [284/1,103] for drug and placebo, respectively) were considerably lower than response rates in trials using historical data (55.2% [380/689] and 42.7% [155/363], respectively), suggesting that patients who did not respond in prospective treatment were more treatment resistant. All but two of the trials continued with the original antidepressant during the adjunctive trials. Two of the olanzapine trials switched to olanzapine plus fluoxetine after using a different antidepressant during the prospective trial. When these two trials were excluded from the analysis, the odds ratio for trials requiring nonresponse in a prospective trial was slightly higher at 1.93 (95% CI=1.58–2.36) but still not significantly different from that in the trials requiring historical nonresponse.

A funnel plot of the odds ratios for response plotted against standard error (log odds ratio) was asymmetric, with three of four small studies (N<25 per arm) showing high odds ratios (Figure 8). When these four trials were excluded, however, the odds ratio for response was relatively unaffected (1.64 [95% CI=1.42–191] compared with 1.69 [95% CI=1.46–196]).

Discussion

In this systematic review and meta-analysis, 15 reports of 16 adjunctive trials were pooled. Augmentation with atypical antipsychotic agents was significantly more effective than placebo for response and remission. The odds ratio for remission was 2.00, with a number needed to treat of nine. No significant differences in efficacy were noted among the different atypical agents (olanzapine, risperidone, quetiapine, and aripiprazole). The relative efficacy of the atypical agents compared with placebo in augmentation did not appear to be influenced by the duration of the adjunctive trial or by whether treatment resistance was determined using a prospective trial or historical nonresponse.

At present, this body of evidence is considerably larger than that for any other augmentation strategy in the treatment of major depressive disorder. For example, the 10 controlled trials of lithium cited earlier (4) included only 269 patients, whereas these 16 trials of atypical antipsychotics included 3,480 patients. In addition, the early trials of lithium and T_3 augmentation often required minimal evidence of treatment resistance, for example, 4 weeks of failure to respond to the initial antidepressant. The only placebo-controlled lithium augmentation trial to retrospectively and prospectively establish treatment resistance (34) failed to find lithium effective. All of the trials of atypicals required evidence of treatment resistance, and for several of the trials, patients had failed to respond to more than one antidepressant.

Although the funnel plot of the odds ratios was asymmetric for the smaller studies and thus suggestive of publication or retrieval bias, exclusion of the smaller studies from the meta-analysis had essentially no effect on the odds ratio. After a thorough literature search as well as contact with the manufacturers of all the atypical agents approved for use in the United States, we are reasonably confident that we have included all of the larger studies that have been completed. An asymmetric funnel plot is only *suggestive* of bias. It might be argued that smaller studies with a limited number of sites and careful patient selection may produce more valid results.

We used a fixed-effects model for the meta-analysis because the patient samples were reasonably homogeneous, the study designs were similar, and all studies used either the Hamilton Depression Rating Scale or the Montgomery-Åsberg Depression Rating Scale to rate response. Tests for heterogeneity were not statistically significant. Had we employed a random-effects model, the results for response (odds ratio=1.69, 95% CI=1.43–2.00, z=6.21, p<0.00001) and remission (odds ratio=1.99, 95 CI=1.68–2.36, z=7.95, p<0.00001) would have been nearly identical to those obtained using a fixed-effects model.

While the efficacy of the atypical agents for adjunctive therapy in major depressive disorder appears fairly well established, there are other considerations. The rate of discontinuation due to adverse events was significantly higher for the atypical group (9.1%) than the placebo group (2.3%). The risk difference by meta-analysis was 0.06, with a number needed to harm of 17. While the discontinuation rates did not differ significantly among the agents, rates of specific side effects may be quite different. In addition, during continuing treatment there may be other secondary effects that in the aggregate affect tolerability and patient acceptance. The atypical agents also are associated with a variety of relatively serious adverse effects, such as metabolic syndrome, extrapyramidal symptoms, and rare but serious symptoms such as tardive dyskinesia and neuroleptic malignant syndrome. As a consequence the risk-benefit ratio appears to be different from that of several alternative treatments for major depressive disorder. Because of these risks, the Texas Algorithm Group (M.H. Trivedi et al., unpublished 2007 data) placed the atypical antipsychotics below some other aug-

FIGURE 8. Funnel Plot of the Odds Ratios for Response Versus the Standard Error (Log Odds Ratio) in Trials of Atypical Antipsychotic Augmentation in Major Depressive Disorder

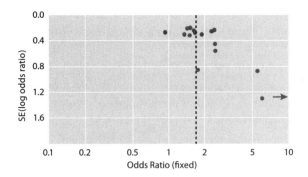

mentation agents (e.g., lithium and thyroid) even though the efficacy data are stronger for the atypicals. Finally, little is known about efficacy and safety of the atypicals during continuation and maintenance treatment in major depression.

There are limitations to this analysis. There may be other studies with different results that were not published or presented and thus were not included in our analysis. Definitions of treatment resistance are still evolving, and there is no standard for studies such as these. Yet the methods used to define treatment resistance in these trials of augmentation with atypical agents were more rigorous than those of previous augmentation trials. While the total number of patients included in these trials (N=3,480) is fairly large, the number of trials on which this trial-level data analysis is based is limited. This limitation is even more important when comparing subgroups. While risperidone was studied in three trials, the samples of two of the trials, 23 and 95, were relatively small, and the total number studied was 386. The other three agents were studied in at least 1,000 patients. While adjunctive olanzapine appears to be effective, the trials all examined adjunctive treatment with fluoxetine. The efficacy of olanzapine combined with other antidepressants has not been well studied.

In addition to factors limiting this analysis, there are several limitations to the existing clinical literature regarding the use of atypicals in depression. For each of these agents, limited data are available for establishing an effective dosage range during adjunctive treatment of depression. Even if efficacy in groups of patients is similar among these agents, it is not clear that patients of the same profile are responding. This would seem unlikely given the differences in neuropharmacology among these agents. Individual patients may respond better to one agent than to another; yet methods to tailor treatment to the patient have not been established. Given the cost and safety issues for the atypical agents, it will be important to compare their efficacy and safety with those of other, less expensive augmentation and combination strategies in depression.

Finally, all of the trials we reviewed were of short duration. Long-term efficacy and safety data are sorely needed. In addition, even if continuing adjunctive treatment is shown to reduce relapse rates, because of the increased side effect burden and cost of continuing two agents, there will be additional questions. For example, if a patient remits with adjunctive treatment, can the initial antidepressant be discontinued? If so, when and in which patients? Alternatively, can individuals be identified who will remain in remission if the atypical agent is withdrawn? These questions deserve study.

Received March 3, 2009; revision received April 23, 2009; accepted June 4, 2009 (doi: 10.1176/appi.ajp.2009.09030312). From the Department of Psychiatry, University of California San Francisco; Massachusetts General Hospital, Boston; and Harvard Medical School, Boston. Address correspondence and reprint requests to Dr. Nelson, Department of Psychiatry, University of California San Francisco, 401 Parnassus Ave., Box 0984-F, San Francisco, CA 94143; craign@lppi.ucsf.edu (e-mail).

Dr. Nelson has received grant support from or served as a speaker on advisory boards, or as a consultant for Abbott Laboratories, Acadia Pharmaceuticals, AstraZeneca, Biovail, Bristol-Myers Squibb, Corcept, Cyberonics, Eli Lilly, Forest Pharmaceuticals, GlaxoSmithKline, Health Resources and Services Administration, Janssen Pharmaceutica, Medtronics, Merck, NIMH, Novartis Pharmaceuticals, Organon, Orexigen, Otsuka, Pfizer U.S. Pharmaceuticals Group, Sepracor, Shire, and Sierra Neuropharmaceuticals. Dr. Papakostas has received grant support from or served as a speaker, on advisory boards, or as a consultant for Bristol-Myers Squibb, Eli Lilly, Evotec AG, GlaxoSmithKline, Inflabloc Pharmaceuticals, Jazz Pharmaceuticals, Lundbeck, NIMH, Otsuka, PAMLAB LLC, Pfizer U.S. Pharmaceuticals Group, Pierre Fabre Laboratories, Precision Human Biolaboratories, Shire Pharmaceuticals, Titan Pharmaceuticals, and Wyeth.

No external funding was received for the study design, trial search, data analysis, interpretation of the data, writing of the paper, or the decision to submit for publication.

References

1. Kessler RC, Berglund P, Demler O, Jin R, Koretz D, Merikangas KR, Rush AJ, Walters EE, Wang PS: The epidemiology of major depressive disorder: results from the National Comorbidity Survey replication (NCS-R). JAMA 2003; 289:3095–3105

2. Rush AJ, Trivedi MH, Wisniewski SR, Nierenberg AA, Stewart JW, Warden D, Niederehe G, Thase ME, Lavori PW, Lebowitz BD, McGrath PJ, Rosenbaum JF, Sackeim HA, Kupfer DJ, Luther J, Fava M: Acute and longer-term outcomes in depressed outpatients requiring one or several treatment steps: a STAR*D report. Am J Psychiatry 2006; 163:1905–1917

3. Nelson JC: Augmentation strategies for treatment of unipolar major depression, in Mood Disorders: Systematic Medication Management, vol 25, Modern Problems of Pharmacopsychiatry. Edited by Rush AJ. Basel, Karger, 1997, pp 34–55

4. Crossley NA, Bauer M: Acceleration and augmentation of antidepressants with lithium for depressive disorders: two meta-analyses of randomized, placebo-controlled trials. J Clin Psychiatry 2007; 68:935–940

5. Nelson JC: The use of antipsychotic drugs in the treatment of depression, in Treating Resistant Depression. Edited by Zohar J, Belmaker RH. New York, PMA Publishing, 1987, pp 131–146

6. Ostroff RB, Nelson JC: Risperidone augmentation of selective serotonin reuptake inhibitors in major depression. J Clin Psychiatry 1999; 60:256–259

7. Shelton RC, Tollefson GD, Tohen M, Stahl S, Gannon KS, Jacobs TG, Buras WR, Bymaster FP, Zhang W, Spencer KA, Feldman PD,

Meltzer HY: A novel augmentation strategy for treating resistant major depression. Am J Psychiatry 2001; 158:131–134

8. Papakostas GI, Shelton RC, Smith J, Fava M: Augmentation of antidepressants with atypical antipsychotic medications for treatment-resistant major depressive disorder: a meta-analysis. J Clin Psychiatry 2007; 68:826–831

9. Berman RM, Marcus RN, Swanink R, McQuade RD, Carson WH, Corey-Lisle PK, Khan A: The efficacy and safety of aripiprazole as adjunctive therapy in major depressive disorder: a multicenter, randomized, double-blind, placebo-controlled study. J Clin Psychiatry 2007; 68:843–853

10. Marcus R, McQuade R, Carson W, Hennicken D, Fava M, Simon J, Trivedi M, Thase M, Berman R: The efficacy and safety of aripiprazole as adjunctive therapy in major depressive disorder: a second multicenter, randomized, double-blind placebo-controlled study. J Clin Psychopharmacol 2008; 28:156–165

11. Berman RB, Fava M, Thase ME, Trivedi MH, Swanink R, McQuade RD, Carson WH, Adson D, Taylor L, Hazel J, Marcus RN: The third consecutive, positive, double-blind, placebo controlled trial of aripiprazole augmentation in the treatment of major depression, in American College of Neuropsychopharmacology 2008 Annual Meeting Abstracts (Scottsdale, Ariz, Dec 7–11, 2008). Nashville, Tenn, ACNP, 2008

12. Earley W, McIntyre A, Bauer M, Pretorius HW, Shelton R, Lindgren P, Brecher M: Efficacy and tolerability of extended release quetiapine fumarate (quetiapine extended release) as add-on to antidepressants in patients with major depressive disorder (MDD): results from a double-blind, randomized, phase III study, in American College of Neuropsychopharmacology 2007 Annual Meeting Abstracts (Boca Raton, Fla, Dec 9–13, 2007). Nashville, TN, ACNP, 2007

13. El-Khalili N, Joyce M, Atkinson S, Buynak R, Datto C, Lindgren P, Eriksson H, Brecher M: Adjunctive extended-release quetiapine fumarate (quetiapine-extended release) in patients with major depressive disorder and inadequate antidepressant response, in American Psychiatric Association 2008 Annual Meeting: New Research Abstracts (Washington, DC, May 3–8, 2008). Washington, DC, APA, 2008

14. Reynolds GP: Receptor mechanisms in the treatment of schizophrenia. J Psychopharmacology 2004; 18:340–345

15. Stahl SM, Shayegan DK: The psychopharmacology of ziprasidone: receptor-binding properties and real-world psychiatric practice. J Clin Psychiatry 2003; 64(suppl 19):6–12

16. Farah A: Atypicality of atypical antipsychotics. Prim Care Companion. J Clin Psychiatry 2005; 7:268–274

17. Tadori Y, Forbes RA, McQuade RD, Kikuchi T: Characterization of aripiprazole partial agonist activity at human dopamine D(3) receptors. Eur J Pharmacol 2008; 597:27–33

18. Jensen NH, Rodriguiz RM, Caron MG, Wetsel WC, Rothman RB, Roth BL: N-desalkylquetiapine, a potent norepinephrine reuptake inhibitor and partial 5-HT$_{1A}$ agonist, as a putative mediator of quetiapine's antidepressant activity. Neuropsychopharmacology 2008; 33:2303–2312

19. Tatsumi M, Jansen K, Blakely RD, Richelson E: Pharmacologic profile of neuroleptics at human monoamine transporters. Eur J Pharmacol 1999; 368:277–283

20. Zhang W, Perry KW, Wong DT, Potts BD, Bao J, Tollefson GD, Bymaster FP: Synergistic effects of olanzapine and other antipsychotic agents in combination with fluoxetine on norepinephrine and dopamine release in rat prefrontal cortex. Neuropsychopharmacology 2000; 23:250–262

21. Hamilton M: A rating scale for depression. J Neurol Neurosurg Psychiatry 1960; 23:56–61

22. Montgomery SA, Åsberg M: A new depression scale designed to be sensitive to change. Br J Psychiatry 1979; 134:382–389

23. Higgins JP, Thompson SG: Quantifying heterogeneity in a meta-analysis. Stat Med 2002; 21:1539–1558

24. Deeks J, Altman D, Bradburn M: Statistical methods for examining heterogeneity and combining results from several studies in meta-analysis, in Systematic Reviews in Health Care: Meta-Analysis in Context, 2nd ed. Edited by Egger M, Davey-Smith G, Altman D. London, BMJ Publishing Group, 2001, pp 285–312

25. Shelton RC, Williamson DJ, Corya SA, Sanger TM, Van Campen LE, Case M, Briggs SD, Tollefson GD: Olanzapine/fluoxetine combination for treatment-resistant depression: a controlled study of SSRI and nortriptyline resistance. J Clin Psychiatry 2005; 66:1289–1297

26. Corya SA, Williamson DJ, Sanger TM, Briggs SD, Case M, Tollefson GD: A randomized, double-blind comparison of olanzapine/fluoxetine combination, olanzapine, fluoxetine, and venlafaxine in treatment-resistant depression. Depress Anxiety 2006; 23:364–372

27. Thase M, Corya SA, Osuntokun O, Case M, Henley DB, Sanger TM, Watson SB, Dube S: A randomized, double-blind comparison of olanzapine/fluoxetine combination, olanzapine, and fluoxetine in treatment-resistant major depressive disorder. J Clin Psychiatry 2007; 68:224–236

28. Mahmoud RA, Pandina G, Turkoz I, Kosik-Gonzalez C, Canuso CM, Kujawa MJ, Gharabawi-Garibaldi GM: Risperdione for treatment-refractory major depressive disorder. Ann Intern Med 2007; 147:593–602

29. Reeves H, Batra S, May RS, Zhang R, Dahl DC, Li X: Efficacy of risperidone augmentation to antidepressant in the management of suicidality in major depressive disorder: a randomized, double-blind, placebo controlled pilot study. J Clin Psychiatry 2008; 69:1228–1336

30. Keitner GI, Garlow SJ, Ryan CE, Ninan PT, Solomon DA, Nemeroff CB, Keller MB: A randomized, placebo-controlled trial of risperidone augmentation for patients with difficult-to-treat unipolar, non-psychotic major depression. J Psychiatr Res 2009; 43:205–214

31. Khullar A, Chokka P, Fullerton D, McKenna S, Blackamn A: A double-blind, randomized, placebo-controlled study of quetiapine as augmentation therapy to SSRI/SNRI agents in the treatment of non-psychotic unipolar depression with residual symptoms, in American Psychiatric Association 2006 Annual Meeting: New Research Abstracts (Toronto, Canada, May 20–25, 2006). Washington, DC, APA, 2006

32. Mattingly G, Ilivicky H, Canale J, Anderson R: Quetiapine combination for treatment-resistant depression, in American Psychiatric Association 2006 Annual Meeting: New Research Abstracts (Toronto, Canada, May 20–25, 2006). Washington, DC, APA, 2006

33. McIntyre A, Gendron A, McIntyre A: Quetiapine adjunct to selective serotonin reuptake inhibitors or venlafaxine in patients with major depression, comorbid anxiety, and residual depressive symptoms: a randomized, placebo-controlled pilot study. Depress Anxiety 2007; 24:487–494

34. Nierenberg AA, Papakostas GI, Petersen T, Montoya HD, Worthington JJ, Tedlow J, Alpert JE, Fava M: Lithium augmentation of nortriptyline for subjects resistant to multiple antidepressants. J Clin Psychopharmacol 2003; 23:92–95

Combining Medications to Enhance Depression Outcomes (CO-MED): Acute and Long-Term Outcomes of a Single-Blind Randomized Study

A. John Rush, M.D.

Madhukar H. Trivedi, M.D.

Jonathan W. Stewart, M.D.

Andrew A. Nierenberg, M.D.

Maurizio Fava, M.D.

Benji T. Kurian, M.D.

Diane Warden, Ph.D.

David W. Morris, Ph.D.

James F. Luther, M.A.

Mustafa M. Husain, M.D.

Ian A. Cook, M.D.

Richard C. Shelton, M.D.

Ira M. Lesser, M.D.

Susan G. Kornstein, M.D.

Stephen R. Wisniewski, Ph.D.

Objective: Two antidepressant medication combinations were compared with selective serotonin reuptake inhibitor monotherapy to determine whether either combination produced a higher remission rate in first-step acute-phase (12 weeks) and long-term (7 months) treatment.

Method: The single-blind, prospective, randomized trial enrolled 665 outpatients at six primary and nine psychiatric care sites. Participants had at least moderately severe nonpsychotic chronic and/or recurrent major depressive disorder. Escitalopram (up to 20 mg/day) plus placebo, sustained-release bupropion (up to 400 mg/day) plus escitalopram (up to 20 mg/day), or extended-release venlafaxine (up to 300 mg/day) plus mirtazapine (up to 45 mg/day) was delivered (1:1:1 ratio) by using measurement-based care. The primary outcome was remission, defined

as ratings of less than 8 and less than 6 on the last two consecutive applications of the 16-item Quick Inventory of Depressive Symptomatology—Self-Report. Secondary outcomes included side effect burden, adverse events, quality of life, functioning, and attrition.

Results: Remission and response rates and most secondary outcomes were not different among treatment groups at 12 weeks. The remission rates were 38.8% for escitalopram-placebo, 38.9% for bupropion-escitalopram, and 37.7% for venlafaxine-mirtazapine, and the response rates were 51.6%–52.4%. The mean number of worsening adverse events was higher for venlafaxine-mirtazapine (5.7) than for escitalopram-placebo (4.7). At 7 months, remission rates (41.8%–46.6%), response rates (57.4%–59.4%), and most secondary outcomes were not significantly different.

Conclusions: Neither medication combination outperformed monotherapy. The combination of extended-release venlafaxine plus mirtazapine may have a greater risk of adverse events.

(Am J Psychiatry 2011; 168:689–701)

Major depressive disorder is a serious, disabling, life-shortening illness with a high lifetime risk: 7%–12% for men and 20%–25% for women (1). It is often recurrent, episodes frequently last more than 2 years (i.e., are chronic) (2), and interepisode recovery is often incomplete (3). Chronic episodes and recurrent courses are associated with worse prognoses and are more likely to need longer-term treatment (4–7).

Remission is the aim of treatment (8) because patients whose depression has remitted have better functioning and a better prognosis than those without remission (5). Antidepressant medications, when used as monotherapies in placebo-controlled registration trials, typically result in 30%–35% remission rates (8). Lower remission rates (25%–30%) are reported for patients with more chronic depressions (5, 6).

Could remission rates be increased with a combination of two antidepressant medications used together as ini-

tial treatment? Other branches of medicine often employ combination treatments at the outset of chronic illness, especially for the more severely ill (9, 10). In depression treatment, when a single antidepressant medication is not effective (7, 11), a second is often added to the first, with some evidence for efficacy (12). It also appears that some antidepressant medications work for some patients but not for others. A combination of two medications might therefore increase the spectrum of patients who could benefit from the combination (13). Furthermore, an unexpected synergy between medications might produce a rapid onset of benefit, so that fewer patients would drop out of treatment, which, in turn, might enhance remission rates. From a pharmacological perspective, a combination might affect a wider range of neurotransmitter or neuromodulator systems, which would enhance efficacy for some patients (14–16). Finally, clinical experience and a few small randomized, short-term trials (13, 17, 18) suggest that some combinations can be more effective than monotherapy. On the other hand, treatment guidelines do not recommend such an approach as a first treatment step, and the risk of serious adverse events or intrusive side effects has not been fully evaluated. Thus, combining antidepressants as a first-step treatment for depression needs proper evaluation.

The Combining Medications to Enhance Depression Outcomes (CO-MED) trial was designed as a proof-of-concept study to determine whether either of two different antidepressant medication combinations would produce a higher remission rate at 12 weeks and, secondarily, after 7 months than monotherapy with a selective serotonin reuptake inhibitor (SSRI) as a first-step treatment in outpatients with chronic or recurrent major depression. We also compared the treatment effects on patient retention, side effect burden, and quality of life.

Method

Study Overview

CO-MED was a 7-month single-blind, randomized, placebo-controlled trial that compared the efficacy of each of two medication combinations with escitalopram plus placebo in a 1:1:1 ratio as first-step treatment, including acute-phase (12 weeks) and long-term continuation (total 7 months) treatment. We planned a study group of 660 outpatients with nonpsychotic major depression from six primary and nine psychiatric care sites to allow detection of roughly a 15% difference in remission rates between each combination and escitalopram-placebo (with an expected remission rate of 35%). This difference was viewed as sufficiently large to affect practice since it approximates the benefit of a single antidepressant medication over placebo in successful antidepressant registration trials (8).

Site Selection

Clinical sites were selected on the basis of our prior experience and their performance in the Sequenced Treatment Alternatives to Relieve Depression trial to ensure 1) adequate patient flow, 2) committed administrative support, 3) adequate minority representation, and 4) adequate representation of both primary and psychiatric care sites.

Recruitment

Potential participants were screened at each clinical site with each site's standard procedure (variable across sites). Most sites used two to nine questions from the Patient Health Questionnaire (19, 20). Patients identified by screening saw their study clinicians and clinical research coordinator to determine study eligibility following written informed consent.

Participants

Broad inclusion and minimal exclusion criteria ensured a reasonably representative participant group. The outpatient enrollees were 18–75 years old and met the DSM-IV-TR (21) criteria for either recurrent or chronic (current episode lasting at least 2 years) major depression according to a clinical interview and confirmed with a DSM-IV-based symptom checklist completed by the clinical research coordinator. Eligible participants had to have an index episode lasting at least 2 months and had to score at least 16 on the 17-Item Hamilton Depression Rating Scale (HAM-D) (22). Those with any psychotic illness or bipolar disorder and those in need of hospitalization were ineligible. (For a complete list of exclusion criteria, see http://clinicaltrials.gov/ct2/show/NCT00590863.)

The study protocol and all consent and study procedures were approved by the institutional review boards at the national coordinating center (University of Texas Southwestern Medical Center at Dallas), the University of Pittsburgh data coordinating center, and each participating regional center and relevant clinical site.

Baseline Data

Sociodemographic and illness features were recorded at baseline. The anxiety subscale of the HAM-D was used to establish the presence of anxious features at baseline (23). This anxiety/somatization factor, derived from a factor analysis of the HAM-D conducted by Cleary and Guy (24), includes six items from the original 17-item version: item 10 (anxiety, psychic), item 11 (anxiety, somatic), item 12 (somatic symptoms, gastrointestinal), item 13 (somatic symptoms, general), item 15 (hypochondriasis), and item 17 (insight). A HAM-D anxiety/somatization factor score of 7 or higher indicated anxiety. The HAM-D administered at baseline by research outcome assessors (not located at any clinical site) was used to define anxious features. The self-report Psychiatric Diagnostic Screening Questionnaire (25) was used to establish the presence of current axis I disorders. The Self-Administered Comorbidity Questionnaire (26) established the presence, severity, and functional impact of a range of common concurrent general medical conditions.

Antidepressant Treatment

A 12-week study period was chosen for the primary analysis to provide sufficient time for maximal dosing (if needed) and to allow most cases of depression that could remit to do so (27). Treatment visits were planned at baseline and weeks 1, 2, 4, 6, 8, 10, 12, 16, 20, 24, and 28. No washout was required, but clinicians could choose a washout period if they thought it to be clinically advisable. Dose adjustments were based on measurement-based care following an operations manual to provide personally tailored but vigorous dosing (28). Dose adjustments were based on the score on the 16-item Quick Inventory of Depressive Symptomatology—Clinician-Rated (QIDS-C) (29), which was extracted from the 30-item Inventory of Depressive Symptomatology—Clinician-Rated (IDS-C) (30), and the score on the Frequency, Intensity, and Burden of Side Effects Rating Scale (31) obtained at each visit.

Treatment was randomly assigned, stratified by clinical site according to a web-based randomization system (32). Random block sizes of three and six were used to minimize the probability of identifying the next treatment assignment. Dosing schedules were based on prior reports (33–35). Doses were increased only in the context of acceptable side effects. Participants could exit the study if unacceptable or intolerable side effects occurred and could not be resolved with dose reduction or medication treatment of the side effects.

Escitalopram plus placebo (monotherapy). Escitalopram treatment was begun at 10 mg/day (one pill) and could be increased to 20 mg/day (two pills) at 4 weeks if the score on the QIDS-C was higher than 5 (if side effects allowed). Pill placebo was started at week 2, with the option to increase it to two pills at week 4 if the QIDS-C score was higher than 5 (if side effects allowed).

Bupropion plus escitalopram. The dose of sustained-release bupropion was 150 mg/day initially and was increased to 300 mg/day at the week 1 visit. Escitalopram was begun at 10 mg/day at the week 2 visit. At week 4, the bupropion dose was raised to 400 mg/day (200 mg b.i.d.) and/or the escitalopram dose was raised to 20 mg/day if the score on the QIDS-C was higher than 5 (if side effects allowed). At week 6 and beyond, doses could be increased up to a maximum of 400 mg/day (200 mg b.i.d.) for bupropion and 20 mg/day for escitalopram if the QIDS-C score was above 5 (if side effects allowed).

Venlafaxine plus mirtazapine. Treatment with extended-release venlafaxine was begun at 37.5 mg/day for 3 days and then raised to 75 mg/day. At week 1, the dose was raised to 150 mg/day. At week 2, if the score on the QIDS-C was above 5, mirtazapine was added at a dose of 15 mg/day. At week 4, if the QIDS-C score was above 5, the venlafaxine dose was raised to 225 mg/day and/or the mirtazapine dose was increased to 30 mg/day. At week 6, if the QIDS-C score was higher than 5, the mirtazapine dose could be raised to 45 mg/day, the maximum dose. At week 8, if the score was above 5, the venlafaxine dose could be raised to 300 mg/day, the maximum allowed.

Medication Blinding

The first medication given in each treatment group was open label (both participant and study personnel were unblinded), while each second medication was given in a single-blind fashion (participant only) to ensure that the participants all took two types of pills. Specifically, in the escitalopram-placebo cell, placebo administration was blinded. For the bupropion-escitalopram combination, escitalopram was blinded. For venlafaxine-mirtazapine, mirtazapine was blinded. The participants remained blinded to the second medication throughout the 7-month study. The research coordinators and physicians were not blinded, to maximize safety and facilitate informed flexible dosing decisions.

Concurrent Treatments

Only protocol antidepressant medications were allowed. Treatments with possible antidepressant effects were proscribed, as were anxiolytics, sedative-hypnotics, and depression-targeted, empirically validated psychotherapies for depression. Other therapies (e.g., supportive, couples, occupational) were allowed, as were medications for any general medical condition. Given the inhibition of the 2D6 isoenzyme by sustained-release bupropion, we alerted clinicians about nonprotocol medications (e.g., type 1C antiarrhythmics, beta-blockers) for which serum or dose adjustments might be needed. Medications to treat antidepressant medication side effects were allowed; administration was based on clinician judgment.

Research Outcomes

Outcome measures were assessed at baseline and all treatment visits. The primary outcome, symptom remission, was based on the score on the 16-item Quick Inventory of Depressive Symptomatology—Self-Report (QIDS-SR) at 12 weeks (29). The designation of remission was based on the last two consecutive measurements during the 12-week acute-phase trial to ensure that a single "good week" was not falsely signaling remission. At least one of these ratings had to be less than 6, while the other had to be less than 8. If participants exited before 12 weeks, their last two consecutive scores were used to determine remission. Those without two post-baseline measures were considered not to have remission.

Physicians were advised that participants could exit the study if they had received a maximally tolerated dose(s) for 4 or more weeks by week 8 without obtaining at least a 30% reduction from the baseline score on the QIDS-C. They could enter continuation treatment (weeks 12–28) if they had received an acceptable benefit (defined as a QIDS-C score of 9 or less by week 12) or if they reached a score of 10–13 and the clinician and participant judged the benefit to be substantial enough to recommend treatment continuation. Thus, virtually all participants entering the continuation phase had at least a 40% reduction in the QIDS-C score. If a participant exited the study at any time, a study exit form was completed. Clinical research coordinators attempted to contact all participants who did not come for a final exit visit.

Secondary outcomes included attrition, anxiety as reflected in the score on the anxiety subscale of the IDS-C (30), functioning as measured by the Work and Social Adjustment Scale (36), quality of life as measured by the Quality of Life Inventory (37), side effect burden as measured by the Frequency, Intensity, and Burden of Side Effects Rating Scale (31), and specific side effects as measured by the Systematic Assessment for Treatment Emergent Events—Systematic Inquiry (38). Manic symptoms were assessed by using the Altman Self-Rating Mania Scale (39), and cognitive and executive dysfunction was assessed by means of the Cognitive and Physical Functioning Questionnaire (40).

Statistical Analyses

Descriptive statistics, including measures of central tendency and dispersion, were computed for continuous data. Frequency distributions were estimated for categorical data.

Outcome analyses were conducted with the full group, on the basis of the intention-to-treat principle. Each combination therapy was compared to the monotherapy. To control for the overall type I error rate, a type I error rate of 0.025 was planned for the comparison of each combination treatment with monotherapy. The analytic approach for the two comparisons was identical. A chi-square test was used to compare the remission rates across the treatment groups. Fisher's exact test was used when the expected cell frequencies were less than 5. For binary outcomes (e.g., remission), bivariate logistic regression models were fit to estimate the effect of treatment on outcome. Multivariable logistic regression models were then fit to control for the effect of regional center and baseline characteristics that were not balanced across treatment groups. A similar approach was used for discrete outcomes with more than two levels, except a polytomous logistic regression model was used. For continuous outcomes, a t test was used to compare the means when distributions were normal, and the nonparametric Kruskal-Wallis test was used when distributions were nonnormal. Linear regression models were used to compare the means after controlling for regional center and baseline characteristics not balanced across treatment groups. A general linear model with a negative binomial distribution and log link was estimated for outcomes with severely nonnormal distributions (the last number of worsening adverse events indicated by the Systematic Assessment for Treatment Emergent Effects and the score on the IDS-C anxiety subscale).

Results

Baseline Characteristics

Figure 1 contains a chart specifying how the study group was formed. From March 2008 through February 2009, the study enrolled 665 participants. They were moderately to severely ill, as indicated by a mean HAM-D score of 23.8 (SD=4.8) and a score on the QIDS-SR of 15.5 (SD=4.3). About half of the participants were unemployed, and two-thirds were female (Table 1). Over three-quarters had recurrent major depression (Table 2). More than one-half of the participants were in a chronic current major depressive episode. About one-third had both recurrent and chronic depression. Almost one in 10 had made a prior suicide attempt, and for over 40% the illness had begun before age 18. Most (75%) had anxious features. Concurrent comorbid axis I and axis III disorders were common (Table 3).

Outcomes at 12 Weeks

During the first 12 weeks, the participants were in treatment for an average of 10 weeks (Table 4). Of the 665 par-

FIGURE 1. Recruitment and Treatment of Depressed Patients in a Comparison of Antidepressant Monotherapy With Two Antidepressant Combinations

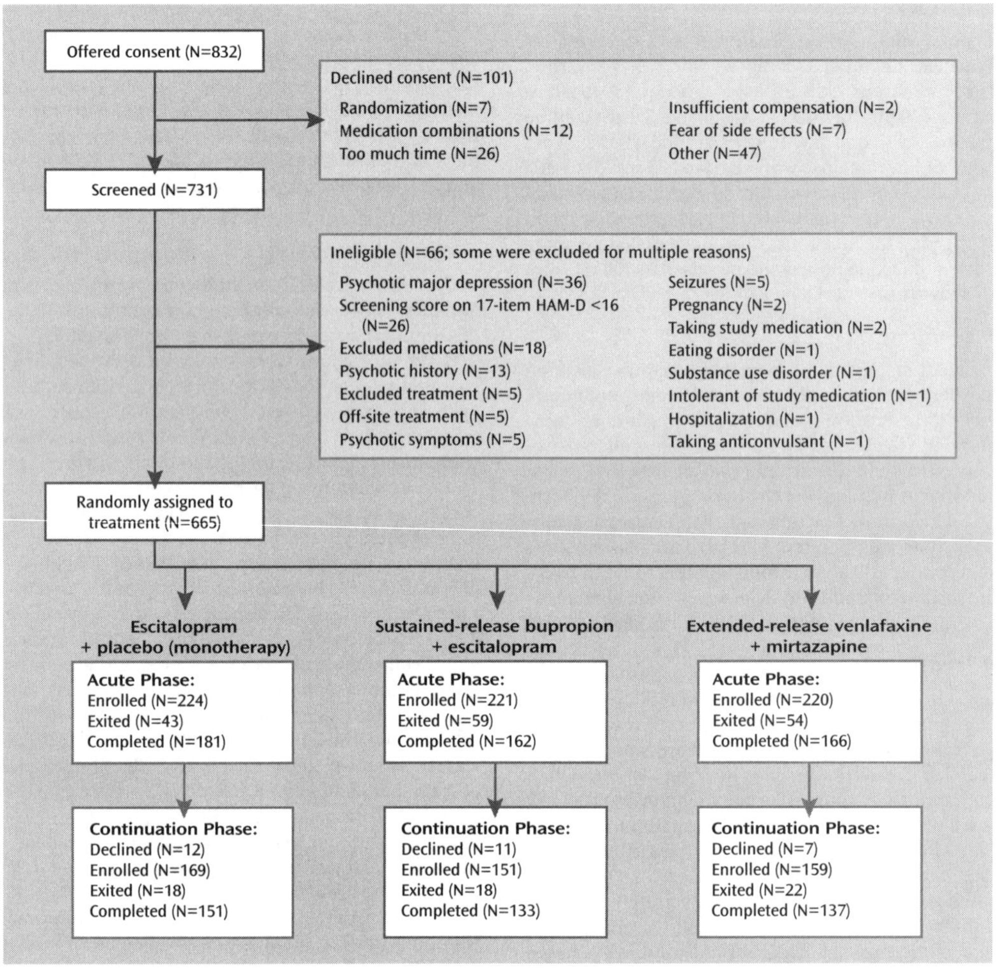

TABLE 1. Baseline Sociodemographic Characteristics of Depressed Patients in a Comparison of Antidepressant Monotherapy With Two Antidepressant Combinations

Characteristic[a]	Patient Group								Comparison With Monotherapy[b]	
	Total (N=665)		Monotherapy: Escitalopram Plus Placebo (N=224)		Sustained-Release Bupropion Plus Escitalopram (N=221)		Extended-Release Venlafaxine Plus Mirtazapine (N=220)		Bupropion Plus Escitalopram	Venlafaxine Plus Mirtazapine
	N	%	N	%	N	%	N	%	p	p
Sex									0.43	<0.05[c]
Male	213	32.0	81	36.2	72	32.6	60	27.3		
Female	452	68.0	143	63.8	149	67.4	160	72.7		
Race									0.90	0.84
White	431	67.0	147	67.7	142	67.0	142	66.4		
Black	174	27.1	56	25.8	58	27.4	60	28.0		
Other	38	5.9	14	6.5	12	5.7	12	5.6		
Hispanic	101	15.2	37	16.5	36	16.3	28	12.7	0.95	0.26
Employed	331	49.8	99	44.2	119	53.8	113	51.4	<0.05[c]	0.14
	Mean	SD	Mean	SD	Mean	SD	Mean	SD	p	p
Age (years)	42.7	13.0	43.6	13.1	42.4	13.5	42.1	12.4	0.34	0.22
Education (years)	13.8	3.0	13.8	3.2	13.8	2.6	13.7	3.1	0.85	0.82
Monthly household income (dollars)	2,678	5,353	2,449	3,696	2,828	5,037	2,759	6,832	0.81	0.28

[a] For some variables, data were not available for all subjects.
[b] Chi-square analysis for categorical data and t tests for continuous data.
[c] Significantly different from monotherapy.

TABLE 2. Baseline Clinical Characteristics of Depressed Patients in a Comparison of Antidepressant Monotherapy With Two Antidepressant Combinations

	All (N=665)		Monotherapy: Escitalopram Plus Placebo (N=224)		Sustained-Release Bupropion Plus Escitalopram (N=221)		Extended-Release Venlafaxine Plus Mirtazapine (N=220)		Comparison With Monotherapy[b]	
									Bupropion Plus Escitalopram	Venlafaxine Plus Mirtazapine
Characteristic[a]										
	N	%	N	%	N	%	N	%	p	p
First episode before age 18	296	44.6	96	43.0	95	43.0	105	47.9	0.99	0.31
Recurrent depression	517	78.0	171	76.7	174	78.7	172	78.5	0.61	0.64
Ever attempted suicide	59	9.2	14	6.5	23	10.7	22	10.3	0.13	0.16
Abused before age 18										
Emotionally	261	39.3	94	42.2	88	39.8	79	35.9	0.62	0.18
Physically	131	19.7	45	20.2	42	19.0	44	20.0	0.76	0.97
Sexually	145	21.9	43	19.3	50	22.6	52	23.7	0.39	0.26
Chronic depression (index episode duration ≥2 years)	368	55.5	121	54.3	121	54.8	126	57.5	0.92	0.49
Chronic or recurrent depression									0.81	0.53
Chronic only	146	22.0	52	23.3	47	21.3	47	21.5		
Recurrent only	295	44.5	102	45.7	100	45.2	93	42.5		
Both	222	33.5	69	30.9	74	33.5	79	36.1		
Anxious features (HAM-D)	497	74.7	156	69.6	177	80.1	164	74.5	0.02[c]	0.25
Atypical features (IDS-C)	103	15.5	33	14.7	38	17.2	32	14.5	0.48	0.96
Melancholic features (IDS-C)	124	20.5	42	20.5	36	18.0	46	23.0	0.53	0.54
	Mean	SD	Mean	SD	Mean	SD	Mean	SD	p	p
Age at first episode (years)	24.0	14.1	24.4	14.4	23.9	13.7	23.7	14.2	0.85	0.53
Years since first episode	18.7	13.6	19.3	14.4	18.5	13.4	18.4	13.1	0.69	0.76
Index episode duration (months)	61.7	104.8	66.4	114.4	58.1	100.8	60.6	98.5	0.91	0.77
Scores on clinical ratings										
HAM-D	23.8	4.8	23.4	4.9	23.8	4.6	24.3	5.0	0.34	<0.05[c]
IDS-C	38.0	9.1	37.0	8.8	37.8	9.2	39.3	9.3	0.39	0.02[c]
QIDS-C	15.8	3.4	15.6	3.4	15.7	3.5	16.1	3.5	0.72	0.13
QIDS-SR	15.5	4.3	15.2	4.0	15.3	4.6	15.9	4.2	0.77	0.10
Altman Self-Rating Mania Scale (39)	1.5	2.3	1.6	2.4	1.6	2.2	1.3	2.2	0.79	0.21
Cognitive and Physical Functioning Questionnaire (40)	27.6	5.9	27.4	5.7	27.7	6.1	27.8	5.8	0.62	0.39
Quality of Life Inventory (37)	−1.2	1.9	−1.2	1.9	−1.1	1.9	−1.3	1.9	0.85	0.41
Work and Social Adjustment Scale (36)	26.9	8.8	26.2	8.8	26.7	9.2	27.9	8.4	0.50	0.04[c]

[a] For some variables, data were not available for all subjects. HAM-D, 17-item Hamilton Depression Rating Scale (22). IDS-C, 30-item Inventory of Depressive Symptomatology—Clinician-Rated (30). QIDS-C, 16-item Quick Inventory of Depressive Symptomatology—Clinician-Rated (29). QIDS-SR, 16-item Quick Inventory of Depressive Symptomatology—Self-Report (29).
[b] Chi-square analysis for categorical data and t tests for continuous data.
[c] Significantly different from monotherapy.

ticipants, 86.0% (N=572) completed at least 4 weeks of treatment. Overall, 78.3% (N=521) completed week 8 and 72.2% (N=480) completed at least 12 weeks of treatment. For the escitalopram-placebo group, the escitalopram dose was close to the maximum target dose of 20 mg/day. For bupropion-escitalopram, the comparable mean exit escitalopram dose during acute treatment was significantly lower, at 12.5 mg/day (SD=8.3) (χ^2=31.15, df=1, p<0.0001). Also of note, while the venlafaxine dose was close to 200 mg/day by 12 weeks, the mean mirtazapine dose was only 20.0 mg/day (SD=15.7) (Table 4).

As shown in Table 5 and Figure 2, the treatment groups did not differ in either remission or response rates, nor did they differ in the percentage of change in QIDS-SR score

(baseline to exit or 12 weeks) or in effects on quality of life. The venlafaxine-mirtazapine combination was associated with more side effect burden than escitalopram-placebo. Patients taking venlafaxine-mirtazapine had more adverse symptoms (ear aches, blurred vision, irritability, etc.) present at baseline that became worse during treatment, as measured by the Systematic Assessment for Treatment Emergent Events (mean number of effects=5.7, SD=5.8), than the monotherapy group (Table 5).

Outcomes at 7 Months

Overall, while 72.2% of the 665 participants (N=480) completed at least 12 weeks of treatment, 65.6% completed 16 weeks or more, 61.4% completed 20 weeks, 55.6%

TABLE 3. Baseline Axis I and III Disorders of Depressed Patients in a Comparison of Antidepressant Monotherapy With Two Antidepressant Combinations

Illness Variable[a]	All (N=665)		Monotherapy: Escitalopram Plus Placebo (N=224)		Sustained-Release Bupropion Plus Escitalopram (N=221)		Extended-Release Venlafaxine Plus Mirtazapine (N=220)		Bupropion Plus Escitalopram	Venlafaxine Plus Mirtazapine
	N	%	N	%	N	%	N	%	p	p
Comorbid axis I disorders[c]										
Agoraphobia	69	10.4	20	8.9	28	12.7	21	9.5	0.21	0.83
Alcohol abuse	67	10.1	23	10.3	24	10.9	20	9.1	0.83	0.68
Bulimia	78	11.7	27	12.1	22	10.0	29	13.2	0.48	0.73
Drug abuse	35	5.3	15	6.7	12	5.4	8	3.6	0.58	0.15
Generalized anxiety	131	19.7	39	17.4	43	19.5	49	22.3	0.58	0.20
Hypochondriasis	29	4.4	9	4.0	12	5.4	8	3.6	0.49	0.84
Obsessive-compulsive	79	11.9	27	12.1	25	11.3	27	12.3	0.81	0.95
Panic	65	9.8	16	7.1	25	11.3	24	10.9	0.13	0.17
Posttraumatic stress	81	12.2	29	12.9	32	14.5	20	9.1	0.64	0.20
Social phobia	178	26.8	60	26.8	59	26.7	59	26.8	0.99	1.00
Somatoform	21	3.2	7	3.1	7	3.2	7	3.2	0.98	0.98
Number of comorbid axis I disorders									0.27	0.66
0	296	44.6	107	47.8	85	38.6	104	47.3		
1	159	23.9	51	22.8	67	30.5	41	18.6		
2	92	13.9	27	12.1	29	13.2	36	16.4		
3	50	7.5	16	7.1	19	8.6	15	6.8		
≥4	67	10.1	23	10.3	20	9.1	24	10.9		
Number of comorbid axis III disorders[d]									0.25	0.86
0	161	24.2	55	24.7	59	26.7	47	21.4		
1	198	29.8	66	29.6	67	30.3	65	29.5		
2	154	23.2	54	24.2	43	19.5	57	25.9		
3	77	11.6	20	9.0	32	14.5	25	11.4		
≥4	74	11.1	28	12.6	20	9.0	26	11.8		
	Mean	SD	Mean	SD	Mean	SD	Mean	SD	p	p
Axis III comorbidity score[d]	3.4	3.5	3.5	3.7	3.0	3.1	3.6	3.8	0.41	0.56

[a] For some variables, data were not available for all subjects.
[b] Chi-square analysis for categorical data and t tests for continuous data.
[c] From the Psychiatric Diagnostic Screening Questionnaire (25).
[d] From the Self-Administered Comorbidity Questionnaire (26).

completed 24 weeks, and 58.0% completed 28 weeks. Attrition rates over the 7-month period did not differ among treatment groups. Average drug doses were basically unchanged from 12 weeks to 7 months of treatment, regardless of treatment group (Table 4).

At 7 months (or study exit, if earlier), the three groups were not different in terms of remission rate (range: 41.8%–46.6%), response rate (range: 57.4%–59.4%), or attrition rate. Nor did the groups differ in the percentage of change in QIDS-SR (baseline to exit or 7 months), quality of life, or work and social adjustment.

Table 6 compares the side effect frequency, intensity, and burden in the escitalopram monotherapy group and each of the combination groups. Overall, there were modestly more side effects with escitalopram-bupropion than with escitalopram-placebo in both the 12-week and 7-month comparisons. On the other hand, the venlafaxine-mirtazapine group had greater side effect frequency and intensity at 12 weeks and greater side effect frequency,

intensity, and burden at 7 months as compared to escitalopram-placebo.

Discussion

The study has four key findings: 1) remission and response rates were not different at 12 weeks, 2) remission and response rates were not different at 7 months, 3) the effects of the three treatments on quality of life and on work and social adjustment were not different, and 4) extended-release venlafaxine plus mirtazapine was associated with a greater side effect burden at 12 weeks and 7 months than escitalopram plus placebo and a higher number of worsening adverse events than escitalopram plus placebo at 7 months. We found no clinical advantage over escitalopram-placebo from either combination of antidepressant medications in terms of either remission or response rates at either 12 weeks or 7 months. The remission rates approximated those expected on the basis of monotherapy

TABLE 4. Treatment Characteristics at 12 Weeks and 7 Months of Depressed Patients in a Comparison of Antidepressant Monotherapy With Two Antidepressant Combinations

Characteristic[a]	All (N=665)		Monotherapy: Escitalopram Plus Placebo (N=224)		Sustained-Release Bupropion Plus Escitalopram (N=221)		Extended-Release Venlafaxine Plus Mirtazapine (N=220)		Comparison With Monotherapy[c] Bupropion Plus Escitalopram	Venlafaxine Plus Mirtazapine
12 weeks	N	%	N	%	N	%	N	%	p	p
Weeks in treatment										
<4	93	14.0	30	13.5	33	14.9	30	13.7	0.66	0.94
<8	144	21.7	43	19.3	55	24.9	46	21.0	0.16	0.66
	Mean	SD	Mean	SD	Mean	SD	Mean	SD	p	p
Weeks in treatment	9.9	3.9	10.0	3.9	9.6	4.0	10.0	3.8	0.13	0.88
Number of postbaseline visits	5.3	2.2	5.4	2.1	5.1	2.2	5.3	2.2	0.21	0.88
Maximum open dose (mg/day)	—	—	17.6	4.5	324.0	80.4	207.6	69.2	—	—
Last open dose (mg/day)	—	—	16.8	5.3	287.7	121.2	192.3	82.2	—	—
Maximum blinded dose (mg/day)[d]	—	—	1.4	0.7	14.0	7.2	25.3	32.0	—	—
Last blinded dose (mg/day)[d]	—	—	1.3	0.7	12.5	8.3	20.0	15.7	—	—
7 months	N	%	N	%	N	%	N	%	p	p
Weeks in treatment <12	185	27.8	56	25.1	72	32.6	57	26.0	0.09	0.83
	Mean	SD	Mean	SD	Mean	SD	Mean	SD	p	p
Weeks in treatment	19.9	10.5	20.5	10.3	19.1	10.8	20.1	10.4	0.38	0.77
Number of postbaseline visits	7.7	3.7	7.9	3.6	7.4	3.8	7.7	3.7	0.26	0.81
Maximum open dose (mg/day)	—	—	17.9	4.4	328.5	81.7	217.3	73.3	—	—
Last open dose (mg/day)	—	—	15.6	6.9	271.0	136.8	177.6	94.0	—	—
Maximum blinded dose (mg/day)[d]	—	—	1.5	0.7	14.2	7.3	26.7	32.2	—	—
Last blinded dose (mg/day)[d]	—	—	0.7	0.9	11.5	8.6	18.0	16.4	—	—

[a] For some variables, data were not available for all subjects.
[b] Medications listed first are referred to as "open," while those listed second are referred to as "blinded."
[c] Chi-square analysis for categorical data and t tests for continuous data.
[d] For the subgroup receiving escitalopram plus placebo, the unit of measurement is pills.

studies of chronic depression (5, 6). Both combination treatments had more side effects (in terms of frequency, intensity, or burden) than escitalopram-placebo in both the acute and continuation phases. Attrition rates, however, were not different across the three treatment groups in either phase of treatment. The venlafaxine-mirtazapine group was at particularly greater risk for side effects. In fact, it had significantly greater worsening of side effects than escitalopram-placebo despite the fact that the mirtazapine dose was not high (about 20 mg/day).

Prior reports have suggested that the response to either medication combination would exceed the effects of monotherapy. An open study of 49 patients (41) given escitalopram (up to 40 mg/day) plus sustained-release bupropion (400–450 mg/day) found a 63% remission rate at week 8. Blier et al. (18) compared mirtazapine, paroxetine, and the combination in a 6-week double-blind, randomized, controlled trial conducted at two research clinics with clinically referred patients and symptomatic volunteers (N=61). Remission rates at 6 weeks were 19% for mirtazapine, 26% for paroxetine, and 43% for the combination. Most of these patients had melancholic symptom features and either had nonrecurrent depression or had an index episode lasting less than 1 year. Drug doses

included up to 45 mg/day of mirtazapine and paroxetine amounts that could exceed 30 mg/day (average final or exit doses not reported).

In a recent, larger 6-week double-blind acute randomized, controlled trial, Blier et al. (13) compared fluoxetine (20 mg/day) with mirtazapine (30 mg/day) in combination with fluoxetine (20 mg/day), extended-release venlafaxine (225 mg/day), or sustained-release bupropion (150 mg/day). Each combination had a remission rate (46%–58%) that exceeded that of fluoxetine alone (25%). In the study, 76% of the participants met melancholia criteria, 63% had recurrent major depression, and 61% had an index episode longer than 1 year. It is interesting that the response rates were not significantly different (54% for fluoxetine, 68% for mirtazapine-fluoxetine, 73% for mirtazapine-venlafaxine, 65% for mirtazapine-bupropion). Of note, this 6-week study may have been too brief to allow the full benefit of fluoxetine to be expressed (42).

There are several other possible explanations for why our findings differ from those of Blier et al. (13). The studies differ in terms of length of treatment, primary outcome, and scales used to assess outcomes. Our results are not accounted for by either differential attrition across the three treatments or baseline differences. On the other

TABLE 5. Outcomes at 12 Weeks and 7 Months of Depressed Patients in a Comparison of Antidepressant Monotherapy With Two Antidepressant Combinations

Characteristic[a]	All (N=665)		Monotherapy: Escitalopram Plus Placebo (N=224)		Sustained-Release Bupropion Plus Escitalopram (N=221)		Extended-Release Venlafaxine Plus Mirtazapine (N=220)		Comparison With Monotherapy[b]	
									Bupropion Plus Escitalopram	Venlafaxine Plus Mirtazapine
12 weeks	N	%	N	%	N	%	N	%	p	p
Early termination	182	27.4	55	24.6	70	31.7	57	25.9	0.10	0.75
Remission[c]	256	38.5	87	38.8	86	38.9	83	37.7	0.99	0.81
Last QIDS-SR score ≤5	242	36.6	81	36.2	82	37.4	79	36.2	0.78	0.99
Reduction in QIDS-SR score ≥50%	334	51.9	113	51.8	111	51.6	110	52.4	0.97	0.91
Maximum side effect burden[d]									0.07	<0.0001[e]
No impairment	128	20.2	46	21.6	44	21.0	38	18.1		
Minimal/mild	276	43.6	110	51.6	90	42.9	76	36.2		
Moderate/marked	167	26.4	48	22.5	55	26.2	64	30.5		
Severe/intolerable	62	9.8	9	4.2	21	10.0	32	15.2		
Last side effect burden[d]									0.66	0.64
No impairment	344	54.7	117	55.5	118	56.5	109	52.2		
Minimal/mild	215	34.2	74	35.1	69	33.0	72	34.4		
Moderate/marked	53	8.4	16	7.6	14	6.7	23	11.0		
Severe/intolerable	17	2.7	4	1.9	8	3.8	5	2.4		
At least one serious adverse event	27	4.1	8	3.6	7	3.2	12	5.5	0.82	0.34
At least one psychiatric serious adverse event	7	1.1	1	0.4	1	0.5	5	2.3	1.00	0.12
	Mean	SD	Mean	SD	Mean	SD	Mean	SD	p	p
Last QIDS-SR score	8.1	5.4	7.9	5.2	8.1	5.3	8.4	5.7	0.74	0.34
Percent change in QIDS-SR score	−45.6	35.1	−46.5	35.2	−44.6	34.6	−45.8	35.8	0.59	0.85
Score on IDS-C anxiety subscale	2.6	2.1	2.4	2.0	2.6	2.1	2.8	2.3	0.28	0.10
Last Quality of Life Inventory (37) score	0.2	2.3	0.1	2.4	0.3	2.1	0.1	2.4	0.57	0.92
Last Work and Social Adjustment Scale (36) score	14.9	12.3	14.9	11.9	13.9	11.9	15.9	13.0	0.43	0.53
Last number of symptom worsenings[f]	5.1	5.1	4.7	4.9	5.0	4.4	5.7	5.8	0.12	0.04[e]
7 months	N	%	N	%	N	%	N	%	p	p
Early termination	244	36.7	78	34.8	84	38.0	82	37.3	0.49	0.60
Remission[c]	298	44.8	103	46.0	103	46.6	92	41.8	0.90	0.38
Last QIDS-SR score ≤5	292	44.4	101	45.3	101	46.3	90	41.5	0.83	0.42
Reduction in QIDS-SR score ≥50%	374	58.4	129	59.4	125	58.4	120	57.4	0.83	0.68
Maximum side effect burden[d]									0.14	<0.0001[e]
No impairment	115	18.2	43	20.2	41	19.5	31	14.8		
Minimal/mild	269	42.5	107	50.2	88	41.9	74	35.2		
Moderate/marked	184	29.1	52	24.4	60	28.6	72	34.3		
Severe/intolerable	65	10.3	11	5.2	21	10.0	33	15.7		
Last side effect burden[d]									0.77	0.02[e]
No impairment	374	59.3	135	63.7	128	61.0	111	53.1		
Minimal/mild	184	29.2	60	28.3	60	28.6	64	30.6		
Moderate/marked	59	9.4	13	6.1	15	7.1	31	14.8		
Severe/intolerable	14	2.2	4	1.9	7	3.3	3	1.4		
At least one serious adverse event	46	6.9	16	7.1	13	5.9	17	7.7	0.60	0.82

(continued)

hand, our participants differed from those studied by Blier et al. Neither participant group was treatment resistant. However, participants in our study were required to have chronic and/or recurrent depression. In fact, there were far more chronically ill participants in our study than in the one by Blier et al. In addition, 62%–85% of their participants had melancholic features (compared to only 20% in this study). Some reports (17, 43) suggest better effica-

cy, i.e., drug-placebo differences, for inpatients (who are more likely to have melancholic features) with combination medications or dual-action medications. In addition, a meta-analysis by Perry (44) revealed that broader-action agents (e.g., tricyclic antidepressants) have far greater efficacy than SSRIs in melancholic depression.

To evaluate the potential impact of chronicity on outcome, we reanalyzed the data. Chronicity was associated

TABLE 5. Outcomes at 12 Weeks and 7 Months of Depressed Patients in a Comparison of Antidepressant Monotherapy With Two Antidepressant Combinations (*continued*)

Characteristic[a]	All (N=665)		Monotherapy: Escitalopram Plus Placebo (N=224)		Sustained-Release Bupropion Plus Escitalopram (N=221)		Extended-Release Venlafaxine Plus Mirtazapine (N=220)		Comparison With Monotherapy[b] Bupropion Plus Escitalopram	Venlafaxine Plus Mirtazapine
7 months (*continued*)	Mean	SD	Mean	SD	Mean	SD	Mean	SD	p	p
Last QIDS-SR score	7.6	5.6	7.3	5.4	7.3	5.4	8.1	5.9	0.98	0.26
Percent change in QIDS-SR score	−49.5	36.0	−50.9	34.5	−49.8	37.0	−47.8	36.7	0.98	0.49
Score on IDS-C anxiety subscale	2.5	2.1	2.4	2.1	2.6	2.1	2.5	2.2	0.19	0.34
Last Quality of Life Inventory (37) score	0.5	2.4	0.4	2.6	0.6	2.1	0.4	2.4	0.27	0.87
Last Work and Social Adjustment Scale (36) score	13.8	12.5	13.5	12.0	13.0	12.2	15.0	13.2	0.62	0.31
Last number of worsening adverse events[f]	4.9	5.3	4.7	5.4	4.8	5.2	5.4	5.3	0.47	<0.05[e]

[a] For some variables, data were not available for all subjects. IDS-C, 30-item Inventory of Depressive Symptomatology—Clinician-Rated (30). QIDS-SR, 16-item Quick Inventory of Depressive Symptomatology—Self-Report (29).
[b] Chi-square analysis for categorical data and t tests for continuous data.
[c] Defined as at least one of the last two consecutive QIDS-SR scores ≤5 and the other ≤7.
[d] From the Frequency, Intensity, and Burden of Side Effects Rating Scale (31).
[e] Significantly different from monotherapy.
[f] From the Systematic Assessment for Treatment Emergent Effects—Systematic Inquiry (38).

FIGURE 2. Rates of Remission and Response for Depressed Patients in a Comparison of Antidepressant Monotherapy With Two Antidepressant Combinations[a]

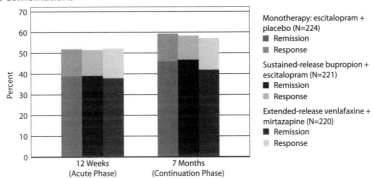

[a] Remission was defined as scores of less than 8 and less than 6 on the 16-item Quick Inventory of Depressive Symptomatology—Self-Report (QIDS-SR) (29) at the last two consecutive assessments. Response was defined as a reduction of at least 50% in QIDS-SR score.

with lower remission rates across all three treatment cells. Specifically, in the bupropion-escitalopram group, 37.2% of the patients with episodes of chronic depression had remissions, whereas the remission rate was 41.0% for non-chronic depression. Analogous rates were 35.5% versus 43.1% for escitalopram-placebo and 34.9% versus 41.9% for venlafaxine-mirtazapine. We conducted a similar analysis to compare patients with and without melancholic features from the current study. Melancholic features were associated with more axis I comorbidity, greater symptom severity, and more suicidal plans and thoughts. However, remission rates ranged from 30.0% to 39.1% for those with melancholic features and from 37.5% to 39.5% for those without. There were no differences across medication groups. Thus, neither the difference in the proportion with chronic illness nor the difference in melancholia seems to

account for why our results differ from those of Blier et al. (13). While we enrolled the kinds of patients (i.e., those with chronic or recurrent depression) for whom most clinicians would be likely to consider antidepressant medication combinations (45), we cannot rule out potential impact on outcomes from one or more unknown baseline features.

This group with chronic and/or recurrent depression had high rates of self-reported emotional, sexual, or physical abuse before age 18, and a high proportion had anxious features. While these features could have reduced the overall benefit of any one treatment, they would be unlikely to obscure differences between treatment cells, given their proportional distribution across the cells.

Perhaps the differences between the present study and the results reported by Blier et al. (13) are due to the specific antidepressant medications and doses that we used and to

TABLE 6. Odds Ratios and Beta Coefficients From Regression Models of Outcomes at 12 Weeks and 7 Months of Depressed Patients in a Comparison of Antidepressant Monotherapy With Two Antidepressant Combinations

	Comparison with Monotherapy: Escitalopram Plus Placebo (N=224)							
	Sustained-Release Bupropion Plus Escitalopram (N=221)				Extended-Release Venlafaxine Plus Mirtazapine (N=220)			
	Unadjusted		Adjusted[b]		Unadjusted		Adjusted[c]	
Outcome[a]	Odds Ratio	p	Odds Ratio	p	Odds Ratio	p	Odds Ratio	p
12 weeks								
Early termination	1.42	0.10	1.46	0.09	1.08	0.75	1.00	1.00
Side effects[d]								
Maximum frequency	1.51	0.02[e]	1.42	0.06	2.12	<0.0001[e]	2.05	<0.0001[e]
Maximum intensity	1.82	<0.001[e]	1.73	0.003[e]	1.97	0.0002[e]	1.86	0.0008[e]
Maximum burden	1.37	0.09	1.28	0.18	1.96	0.0002[e]	1.87	0.0008[e]
Last frequency	1.25	0.23	1.12	0.57	1.70	<0.004[e]	1.62	<0.02[e]
Last intensity	1.31	0.15	1.19	0.36	1.68	<0.005[e]	1.58	<0.02[e]
Last burden	0.99	0.96	0.90	0.61	1.19	0.36	1.11	0.61
At least one serious adverse event[f]	0.88	0.82	—	—	1.56	0.35	—	—
At least one psychiatric serious adverse event[f]	1.01	1.00	—	—	5.19	0.14	—	—
Last QIDS-SR score ≤5	1.06	0.78	1.08	0.72	1.00	0.99	1.14	0.54
Reduction in QIDS-SR score ≥50%	0.99	0.97	0.96	0.85	1.02	0.91	1.03	0.87
Last Work and Social Adjustment Scale (36) score[g]	0.93	0.67	0.98	0.93	1.15	0.43	0.95	0.80
	β	p	β	p	β	p	β	p
Maximum number of worsening adverse events[h]	0.07	0.26	0.08	0.19	0.11	0.06	0.11	0.06
Last number of worsening adverse events[h]	0.07	0.46	0.06	0.54	0.20	<0.04[e]	0.14	0.14
Last QIDS-SR score	0.17	0.74	0.13	0.80	0.50	0.34	0.02	0.97
Percent change in QIDS-SR score	1.82	0.59	2.44	0.47	0.66	0.85	0.22	0.95
Score on IDS-C anxiety subscale	0.10	0.25	0.06	0.44	0.16	0.06	0.09	0.24
Last Quality of Life Inventory (37) score	0.13	0.57	0.12	0.60	−0.03	0.92	0.14	0.54
7 months	Odds Ratio	p	Odds Ratio	p	Odds Ratio	p	Odds Ratio	p
Early termination	1.15	0.49	1.15	0.49	1.11	0.60	1.07	0.75
Side effects[d]								
Maximum frequency	1.53	<0.02[e]	1.44	<0.05[e]	2.31	<0.0001[e]	2.20	<0.0001[e]
Maximum intensity	1.79	<0.002[e]	1.67	<0.006[e]	2.26	<0.0001[e]	2.12	<0.0001[e]
Maximum burden	1.34	0.11	1.26	0.22	2.15	<0.0001[e]	2.02	0.0002[e]
Last frequency	1.40	0.08	1.32	0.16	1.80	<0.002[e]	1.76	<0.004[e]
Last intensity	1.53	<0.03[e]	1.48	<0.05[e]	1.94	0.0004[e]	1.99	0.0005[e]
Last burden	1.15	0.48	1.09	0.69	1.63	<0.02[e]	1.61	0.02[e]
At least one serious adverse event	0.81	0.60	—	—	1.09	0.82	—	—
At least one psychiatric serious adverse event	0.60	0.50	—	—	1.44	0.54	—	—
Last QIDS-SR score ≤5	1.04	0.83	1.02	0.93	0.86	0.42	0.98	0.95
Reduction in QIDS-SR score ≥50%	0.96	0.83	0.92	0.69	0.92	0.68	0.99	0.97
Last Work and Social Adjustment Scale (36) score[g]	0.96	0.81	1.05	0.79	1.25	0.20	1.06	0.74
	β	p	β	p	β	p	β	p
Maximum number of worsening adverse events[h]	0.05	0.37	0.06	0.26	0.10	0.10	0.10	0.09
Last number of worsening adverse events[h]	0.03	0.76	0.04	0.73	0.14	0.19	0.13	0.22
Last QIDS-SR score	−0.04	0.94	−0.05	0.93	0.76	0.16	0.22	0.66
Percent change in QIDS-SR score	1.14	0.74	2.09	0.54	3.17	0.36	2.12	0.53
Score on IDS-C anxiety subscale	0.10	0.27	0.06	0.49	0.07	0.41	0.02	0.77
Last Quality of Life Inventory (37) score	0.26	0.27	0.24	0.28	−0.04	0.87	0.11	0.64

[a] IDS-C, 30-item Inventory of Depressive Symptomatology—Clinician-Rated (30). QIDS-C, 16-item Quick Inventory of Depressive Symptomatology—Clinician-Rated (29). QIDS-SR, 16-item Quick Inventory of Depressive Symptomatology—Self-Report (29).
[b] Adjusted for regional center, employment, and anxious features.
[c] Adjusted for regional center, sex, baseline score on IDS-C, and baseline score on Work and Social Adjustment Scale.
[d] From the Frequency, Intensity, and Burden of Side Effects Rating Scale (31).
[e] Significant odds (categorical measures) or beta (continuous measures) for the combination.
[f] Adjusted models are unestimable.
[g] An extremely nonnormal distribution required binning.
[h] From the Systematic Assessment for Treatment Emergent Events—Systematic Inquiry (38).

the doses that were administered. There is evidence for the efficacy of venlafaxine plus mirtazapine (13, 35) and bupropion plus escitalopram (16, 34). Carpenter et al. (46) found that mirtazapine, when used as an adjunct to previously ineffective SSRIs alone, was more effective than placebo in treating depression. In fact, Blier et al. (13) used the venlafaxine-mirtazapine combination and Stewart et al. (41) used bupropion plus escitalopram in their trials, although the doses were higher in both of them. The rationale for a higher venlafaxine dose is that the effect on the norepinephrine system (17, 47) is only realized at doses of at least 225 mg/day. Mirtazapine has antagonistic effects that are modest at 15 mg/day and more clearly evident at 30 mg/day. Thus, as suggested by Blier (personal communication), the doses in CO-MED may have been insufficient in a large enough proportion of participants to preclude the benefit otherwise available from the combination. In an attempt to evaluate that notion, we identified the 86 participants who reached 225 mg/day of venlafaxine and 30 mg/day of mirtazapine at any time during treatment. Their remission rate was 33.7% at 12 weeks and 41.9% at 7 months. These results do not suggest that underdosing was the cause of the poor performance of this combination.

It remains an unanswered question whether these larger doses (if they are required to achieve an advantage for antidepressant combinations) are achievable in practice with more representative patients who have chronic and/or recurrent major depressive disorder and more concurrent axis I and III disorders.

This study had several limitations. While larger than many studies, the study group may not be representative of the universe of outpatients with chronic and/or recurrent major depression. As noted, the doses used may not have been sufficient to realize the full potential value of combination antidepressant medications. The results for the continuation treatment phase are limited by the fact that the subjects were not rerandomized or stratified by level of improvement following the acute phase. Finally, the clinicians were not blind to treatment, and a structured interview was not used to establish axis I diagnoses.

In summary, in outpatients with chronic and/or recurrent major depressive disorder, there appears to be no advantage to either medication combination over escitalopram alone as a first-step treatment for nonresistant depression. Some combinations may incur a risk of higher side effect burden. This conclusion is conditioned on the doses employed.

Received Nov. 16, 2010; revision received Feb. 10, 2011; accepted Feb. 14, 2011 (doi: 10.1176/appi.ajp.2011.10111645). From the Duke–National University of Singapore Graduate Medical School, Singapore; the Department of Psychiatry, University of Texas Southwestern Medical Center at Dallas; the Epidemiology Data Center, Graduate School of Public Health, University of Pittsburgh; the Depression Clinical and Research Program, Massachusetts General Hospital, Boston; New York State Psychiatric Institute and the Department of Psychiatry, College of Physicians and Surgeons, Columbia University, New York; the Depression Research and Clinic Program, Semel Institute for Neuroscience and Human Behavior, UCLA; the Department of Psychiatry, Vanderbilt University, Nashville, Tenn.; the Department of Psychiatry, Harbor-UCLA Medical Center and the Los Angeles Biomedical Research Institute, Torrance, Calif.; and the Department of Psychiatry, Virginia Commonwealth University, Richmond. Address correspondence and reprint requests to Dr. Trivedi, Department of Psychiatry, University of Texas Southwestern Medical Center at Dallas, 5323 Harry Hines Blvd., Dallas, TX 75390-9119; madhukar.trivedi@utsouthwestern.edu (e-mail).

Dr. Rush has received consulting fees from Advanced Neuromodulation Systems, Best Practice Project Management, Brain Resource, Otsuka, and the University of Michigan; he has received consultant/speaker fees from Forest; he has received consultant fees from and owns stock in Pfizer; he has received author royalties from Guilford Publications, Healthcare Technology Systems, and the University of Texas Southwestern Medical Center; and he has received research support from the National Institute of Mental Health. Dr. Trivedi has received research support from the Agency for Healthcare Research and Quality, Corcept, Cyberonics, Merck, NARSAD, the National Institute of Mental Health, the National Institute on Drug Abuse, Novartis, Pharmacia & Upjohn, Predix (EPIX), Solvay, and Targacept; he has received consulting and speaker fees from Abbott, Abdi Ibrahim, Akzo (Organon), AstraZeneca, Bristol-Myers Squibb, Cephalon, Eli Lilly, Evotec, Fabre Kramer, Forest, GlaxoSmithKline, Janssen, Johnson & Johnson, Meade Johnson, Medtronic, Neuronetics, Otsuka, Parke-Davis, Pfizer, Sepracor, Shire Development, VantagePoint, and Wyeth. Dr. Fava has received research support from Abbott, Alkermes, Aspect Medical Systems, AstraZeneca, BioResearch, BrainCells, Bristol-Myers Squibb, CeNeRx BioPharma, Cephalon, Clinical Trials Solutions, Clintara, Covidien, Eli Lilly, EnVivo, Euthymics Bioscience, Forest, Ganeden Biotech, GlaxoSmithKline, Icon Clinical Research, i3 Innovus/Ingenix, Johnson & Johnson, Lichtwer, Lorex, NARSAD, the National Center for Complementary and Alternative Medicine, the National Institute on Drug Abuse, NIMH, Novartis, Organon, Pamlab, Pfizer, Pharmavite, Photothera, RCT Logic, Roche, Sanofi-Aventis, Shire, Solvay, Synthelabo, and Wyeth; he has served as adviser or consultant to Abbott, Affectis, Alkermes, Amarin, Aspect Medical Systems, AstraZeneca, Auspex, Bayer, Best Practice Project Management, BioMarin, Biovail, BrainCells, Bristol-Myers Squibb, CeNeRx BioPharma, Cephalon, Clinical Trials Solutions, CNS Response, Compellis, Cypress, DiagnoSearch Life Sciences, Dinippon Sumitomo, DOV, Edgemont, Eisai, Eli Lilly, ePharmaSolutions, EPIX, Euthymics Bioscience, Fabre-Kramer, Forest, GenOmind, GlaxoSmithKline, Grunenthal, i3 Innovus/Ingenix, Janssen, Jazz, Johnson & Johnson, Knoll, Labopharm, Lorex, Lundbeck, MedAvante, Merck, MSI Methylation Sciences, Naurex, Neuronetics, NextWave, Novartis, Nutrition 21, Orexigen, Organon, Otsuka, Pamlab, Pfizer, PharmaStar, Pharmavite, PharmoRx, Precision Human Biolaboratory, Prexa, PsychoGenics, Psylin Neurosciences, Puretech Ventures, RCT Logic, Rexahn, Ridge Diagnostics, Roche, Sanofi-Aventis, Schering-Plough, Sepracor, Servier, Solvay, Somaxon, Somerset, Sunovion, Synthelabo, Takeda, Tal Medical, Tetragenex, Transcept, TransForm, and Vanda; he has received speaking or publishing fees from Adamed, Advanced Meeting Partners, the American Psychiatric Association, the American Society of Clinical Psychopharmacology, AstraZeneca, Belvoir Media Group, Boehringer Ingelheim, Bristol-Myers Squibb, Cephalon, CME Institute/Physicians Postgraduate Press, Eli Lilly, Forest, GlaxoSmithKline, Imedex, MGH Psychiatry Academy/Primedia, MGH Psychiatry Academy/Reed Elsevier, Novartis, Organon, Pfizer, PharmaStar, United BioSource, and Wyeth; he owns stock in Compellis; he has a patent for SPCD, a patent application for a combination of azapirones and bupropion in major depressive disorder, and a patent for research and licensing of SPCD with RCT Logic and Lippincott, Williams & Wilkins; and he receives copyright royalties for the MGH CPFQ, SFI, ATRQ, DESS, and SAFER. Dr. Kurian has received research support from Evotec, Pfizer, and Targacept. Dr. Warden has owned stock in Bristol-Myers Squibb and Pfizer in the past 5 years. Dr. Husain has received research support from Cyberonics, Magstim, Neuronetics, NIH/NIMH, the Stanley Foundation, and St. Jude Medical; he has also served on advisory boards for AstraZeneca, BMS, Forest, and Novartis. Dr. Cook has served as an adviser and consultant for Ascend Media, Bristol-Myers Squibb, Cyberonics, Janssen, NeuroSigma, and the U.S. Departments of Defense and of Justice; he has served on the speakers bureaus for Bristol-Myers Squibb, Neuronetics, and Wyeth/Pfizer; he has received research support from Aspect Medical Systems/Covidien, Cyberonics, Eli Lilly, Neuronetics,

NIH, Novartis, Pfizer, and Sepracor; his patents on biomedical devices are assigned to the Regents of the University of California. Dr. Shelton has received grant/research support from Abbott, AstraZeneca, Eli Lilly, GlaxoSmithKline, Janssen, Pamlab, Pfizer, Sanofi, and Wyeth; he has been a paid consultant to Evotec, Janssen, and Sierra Neuropharmaceuticals; and he has served on speakers bureaus for Abbott, Bristol-Myers Squibb, Eli Lilly, GlaxoSmithKline, Janssen, and Wyeth. Dr. Lesser has received research support from Aspect Medical Systems and NIMH. Dr. Kornstein has received grants/research support from Boehringer-Ingelheim, Bristol-Myers Squibb, Eli Lilly, Forest, the National Institute of Mental Health, Novartis, Pfizer, Rexahn, Takeda, and Wyeth; she has served on advisory boards for Bristol-Myers Squibb, Dey, Eli Lilly, Forest, Pfizer, PGx Health, Takeda, and Wyeth; and she has received book royalties from Guilford Press. Dr. Wisniewski reports financial relationships with Cyberonics (2005–2009), ImaRx Therapeutics (2006), Bristol-Myers Squibb (2007–2008), Organon (2007), Case-Western University (2007), Singapore Clinical Research Institute (2009), Dey (2010), and Venebio (2010). The other authors report no financial relationships with commercial interests.

Funded by NIMH under contract N01 MH-90003 to the University of Texas Southwestern Medical Center at Dallas (principal investigators, A.J. Rush and M.H. Trivedi). Forest Pharmaceuticals, GlaxoSmithKline, Organon, and Wyeth Pharmaceuticals provided medications for this trial at no cost.

The content of this publication does not necessarily reflect the views or policies of the U.S. Department of Health and Human Services, nor does mention of trade names, commercial products, or organizations imply endorsement by the U.S. government. NIMH had no role in the drafting or review of the manuscript or in the collection or analysis of the data.

The authors thank the clinical staff at each clinical site for their assistance with this project; all of the study participants; Eric Nestler, M.D., Ph.D., and Carol A. Tamminga, M.D., for administrative support; and Jon Kilner, M.S., M.A., for editorial support.

References

1. Kessler RC, Berglund P, Demler O, Jin R, Koretz D, Merikangas KR, Rush AJ, Walters EE, Wang PS: The epidemiology of major depressive disorder: results from the National Comorbidity Survey Replication (NCS-R). JAMA 2003; 289:3095–3105

2. Depression Guideline Panel: Clinical Practice Guideline, number 5: Depression in Primary Care, Volume 1: Detection and Diagnosis: AHCPR Publication 93-0550. Rockville, Md, Agency for Health Care Policy and Research, 1993

3. Keller MB, Klein DN, Hirschfeld RMA, Kocsis JH, McCullough JP, Miller I, First MB, Holzer CP III, Keitner GI, Marin DB, Shea T: Results of the DSM-IV mood disorders field trial. Am J Psychiatry 1995; 152:843–849

4. Rush AJ, Kraemer HC, Sackeim HA, Fava M, Trivedi MH, Frank E, Ninan PT, Thase ME, Gelenberg AJ, Kupfer DJ, Regier DA, Rosenbaum JF, Ray O, Schatzberg AF: Report by the ACNP Task Force on Response and Remission in Major Depressive Disorder. Neuropsychopharmacology 2006; 31:1841–1853

5. Keller MB, Gelenberg AJ, Hirschfeld RM, Rush AJ, Thase ME, Kocsis JH, Markowitz JC, Fawcett JA, Koran LM, Klein DN, Russell JM, Kornstein SG, McCullough JP, Davis SM, Harrison WM: The treatment of chronic depression, part 2: a double-blind, randomized trial of sertraline and imipramine. J Clin Psychiatry 1998; 59:598–607

6. Keller MB, McCullough JP, Klein DN, Arnow B, Dunner DL, Gelenberg AJ, Markowitz JC, Nemeroff CB, Russell JM, Thase ME, Trivedi MH, Zajecka J: A comparison of nefazodone, the cognitive behavioral-analysis system of psychotherapy, and their combination for the treatment of chronic depression. N Engl J Med 2000; 342:1462–1470

7. Mischoulon D, Nierenberg AA, Kizilbash L, Rosenbaum JF, Fava M: Strategies for managing depression refractory to selective serotonin reuptake inhibitor treatment: a survey of clinicians. Can J Psychiatry 2000; 45:476–481

8. Depression Guideline Panel: Clinical Practice Guideline, number 5: Depression in Primary Care: Volume 2. Treatment of Major Depression: AHCPR Publication 93-0551. Rockville, Md, Agency for Health Care Policy and Research, 1993

9. Patel A, ADVANCE Collaborative Group, MacMahon S, Chalmers J, Neal B, Woodward M, Billot L, Harrap S, Poulter N, Marre M, Cooper M, Glasziou P, Grobbee DE, Hamet P, Heller S, Liu LS, Mancia G, Mogensen CE, Pan CY, Rodgers A, Williams B: Effects of a fixed combination of perindopril and indapamide on macrovascular and microvascular outcomes in patients with type 2 diabetes mellitus (the ADVANCE trial): a randomised controlled trial. Lancet 2007; 370:829–840

10. Mourad JJ, Waeber B, Zannad F, Laville M, Duru G, Andréjak M, Investigators of the STRATHE trial: Comparison of different therapeutic strategies in hypertension: a low-dose combination of perindopril/indapamide versus a sequential monotherapy or a stepped-care approach. J Hypertens 2004; 22:2379–2386; correction, 2007; 25:258

11. Rush AJ, Trivedi MH, Wisniewski SR, Nierenberg AA, Stewart JW, Warden D, Niederehe G, Thase ME, Lavori PW, Lebowitz BD, McGrath PJ, Rosenbaum JF, Sackeim HA, Kupfer DJ, Luther J, Fava M: Acute and longer-term outcomes in depressed outpatients requiring one or several treatment steps: a STAR*D report. Am J Psychiatry 2006; 163:1905–1917

12. Rush AJ, Trivedi MH, Wisniewski SR, Stewart JW, Nierenberg AA, Thase ME, Ritz L, Biggs MM, Warden D, Luther JF, Shores-Wilson K, Niederehe G, Fava M: Bupropion-SR, sertraline, or venlafaxine-XR after failure of SSRIs for depression. N Engl J Med 2006; 354:1231–1242

13. Blier P, Ward HE, Tremblay P, Laberge L, Hébert C, Bergeron R: Combination of antidepressant medications from treatment initiation for major depressive disorder: a double-blind randomized study. Am J Psychiatry 2010; 167:281–288

14. Kalia M: Neurobiological basis of depression: an update. Metabolism 2005; 54(5 suppl 2):24–27

15. Fava M, Rush AJ: Current status of augmentation and combination treatments for major depressive disorder: a literature review and a proposal for a novel approach to improve practice. Psychother Psychosom 2006; 75:139–153

16. Trivedi MH, Fava M, Wisniewski SR, Thase ME, Quitkin F, Warden D, Ritz L, Nierenberg AA, Lebowitz BD, Biggs MM, Luther JF, Shores-Wilson K, Rush AJ: Medication augmentation after the failure of SSRIs for depression. N Engl J Med 2006; 354:1243–1252

17. Nelson JC, Mazure CM, Jatlow PI, Bowers MB Jr, Price LH: Combining norepinephrine and serotonin reuptake inhibition mechanisms for treatment of depression: a double-blind, randomized study. Biol Psychiatry 2004; 55:296–300

18. Blier P, Gobbi G, Turcotte JE, de Montigny C, Boucher N, Hebert C, Debonnel G: Mirtazapine and paroxetine in major depression: a comparison of monotherapy versus their combination from treatment initiation. Eur Neuropsychopharmacol 2009; 19:457–465

19. Kroenke K, Spitzer RL, Williams JB: The Patient Health Questionnaire-2: validity of a two-item depression screener. Med Care 2003; 41:1284–1292

20. Kroenke K, Spitzer RL, Williams JBW: The PHQ-9: validity of a brief depression severity measure. J Gen Intern Med 2001; 16:606–613

21. American Psychiatric Association: Diagnostic and Statistical Manual of Mental Disorders, 4th Edition, Text Revision (DSM-IV-TR). Washington, DC, APA, 2000

22. Hamilton M: A rating scale for depression. J Neurol Neurosurg Psychiatry 1960; 23:56–61

23. Fava M, Rush AJ, Alpert JE, Balasubramani GK, Wisniewski SR, Carmin CN, Biggs MM, Zisook S, Leuchter A, Howland R, Warden D, Trivedi MH: Difference in treatment outcome in outpa-

tients with anxious versus nonanxious depression: a STAR*D report. Am J Psychiatry 2008; 165:342–351

24. Cleary P, Guy W: Factor analysis of the Hamilton Depression Scale. Drugs Exp Clin Res 1977; 1:115–120

25. Rush AJ, Zimmerman M, Wisniewski SR, Fava M, Hollon SD, Warden D, Biggs MM, Shores-Wilson K, Shelton RC, Luther JF, Thomas B, Trivedi MH: Comorbid psychiatric disorders in depressed outpatients: demographic and clinical features. J Affect Disord 2005; 87:43–55

26. Sangha O, Stucki G, Liang MH, Fossel AH, Katz JN: The Self-Administered Comorbidity Questionnaire: a new method to assess comorbidity for clinical and health services research. Arthritis Rheum 2003; 49:156–163

27. Trivedi MH, Rush AJ, Wisniewski SR, Nierenberg AA, Warden D, Ritz L, Norquist G, Howland RH, Lebowitz B, McGrath PJ, Shores-Wilson K, Biggs MM, Balasubramani GK, Fava M, STAR*D Study Team: Evaluation of outcomes with citalopram for depression using measurement-based care in STAR*D: implications for clinical practice. Am J Psychiatry 2006; 163:28–40

28. Trivedi MH, Rush AJ, Gaynes BN, Stewart JW, Wisniewski SR, Warden D, Ritz L, Luther JF, Stegman D, DeVeaugh-Geiss J, Howland R: Maximizing the adequacy of medication treatment in controlled trials and clinical practice: STAR*D measurement-based care. Neuropsychopharmacology 2007; 32:2479–2489

29. Rush AJ, Bernstein IH, Trivedi MH, Carmody TJ, Wisniewski S, Mundt JC, Shores-Wilson K, Biggs MM, Woo A, Nierenberg AA, Fava M: An evaluation of the Quick Inventory of Depressive Symptomatology and the Hamilton Rating Scale for Depression: A Sequenced Treatment Alternatives to Relieve Depression trial report. Biol Psychiatry 2006; 59:493–501

30. Rush AJ, Gullion CM, Basco MR, Jarrett RB, Trivedi MH: The Inventory of Depressive Symptomatology (IDS): psychometric properties. Psychol Med 1996; 26:477–486

31. Wisniewski SR, Rush AJ, Balasubramani GK, Trivedi MH, Nierenberg AA: Self-rated global measure of the frequency, intensity, and burden of side effects. J Psychiatr Pract 2006; 12:71–79

32. Wisniewski SR, Eng H, Meloro L, Gatt R, Ritz L, Stegman D, Trivedi M, Biggs MM, Friedman E, Shores-Wilson K, Warden D, Bartolowits D, Martin JP, Rush AJ: Web-based communications and management of a multi-center clinical trial: the Sequenced Treatment Alternatives to Relieve Depression (STAR*D) project. Clin Trials 2004; 1:387–398

33. Fava M: Augmentation and combination strategies in treatment-resistant depression. J Clin Psychiatry 2001; 62(suppl 18):4–11

34. Leuchter AF, Lesser IM, Trivedi MH, Rush AJ, Morris DW, Warden D, Fava M, Wisniewski SR, Luther JF, Perales M, Gaynes BN, Stewart JW: An open pilot study of the combination of escitalopram and bupropion-SR for outpatients with major depressive disorder. J Psychiatr Pract 2008; 14:271–280

35. McGrath PJ, Stewart JW, Fava M, Trivedi MH, Wisniewski SR, Nierenberg AA, Thase ME, Davis L, Biggs MM, Shores-Wilson K, Luther JF, Niederehe G, Warden D, Rush AJ, STAR*D Study Team: Tranylcypromine versus venlafaxine plus mirtazapine following three failed antidepressant medication trials for depression: a STAR*D report. Am J Psychiatry 2006; 163:1531–1541

36. Mundt JC, Marks IM, Shear MK, Greist JH: The Work and Social Adjustment Scale: a simple measure of impairment in functioning. Br J Psychiatry 2002; 180:461–464

37. Frisch MB, Clark MP, Rouse SV, Rudd MD, Paweleck JK, Greenstone A, Kopplin DA: Predictive and treatment validity of life satisfaction and the Quality of Life Inventory. Assessment 2005; 12:66–78

38. Levine J, Schooler NR: General versus specific inquiry with SAFTEE (letter). J Clin Psychopharmacol 1992; 12:448

39. Altman EG, Hedeker D, Peterson JL, Davis JM: The Altman Self-Rating Mania Scale. Biol Psychiatry 1997; 42:948–955

40. Fava M, Iosifescu DV, Pedrelli P, Baer L: Reliability and validity of the Massachusetts General Hospital Cognitive and Physical Functioning Questionnaire. Psychother Psychosom 2009; 78:91–97

41. Stewart JW, McGrath PJ, Deliyannides RA, Quitkin FM: Does dual antidepressant therapy as initial treatment hasten and increase remission from depression? J Psychiatr Pract 2009; 15:337–345

42. Quitkin FM, Petkova E, McGrath PJ, Taylor B, Beasley C, Stewart J, Amsterdam J, Fava M, Rosenbaum J, Reimherr F, Fawcett J, Chen Y, Klein D: When should a trial of fluoxetine for major depression be declared failed? Am J Psychiatry 2003; 160:734–740

43. Poirier MF, Boyer P: Venlafaxine and paroxetine in treatment-resistant depression: double-blind, randomised comparison. Br J Psychiatry 1999; 175:12–16

44. Perry PJ: Pharmacotherapy for major depression with melancholic features: relative efficacy of tricyclic versus selective serotonin reuptake inhibitor antidepressants. J Affect Disord 1996; 39:1–6

45. Khan A, Dager SR, Cohen S, Avery DH, Scherzo B, Dunner DL: Chronicity of depressive episode in relation to antidepressant-placebo response. Neuropsychopharmacology 1991; 4:125–130

46. Carpenter LL, Yasmin S, Price LH: A double-blind, placebo-controlled study of antidepressant augmentation with mirtazapine. Biol Psychiatry 2002; 51:183–188

47. Maes M, Libbrecht I, van Hunsel F, Campens D, Meltzer HY: Pindolol and mianserin augment the antidepressant activity of fluoxetine in hospitalized major depressed patients, including those with treatment resistance. J Clin Psychopharmacol 1999; 19:177–182

Clinical Guidance: Effectiveness and Safety of Combining Antidepressants

Rush et al. compared two combination therapies, 300 mg/day of extended-release venlafaxine plus 45 mg/day of mirtazapine and 20 mg/day of escitalopram plus 400 mg/day of sustained-release bupropion, to escitalopram alone in a 12-week trial in chronically depressed patients. Remission rates (38%) and response rates (52%) did not differ among the three treatment arms. Patients who received venlafaxine plus mirtazapine experienced more side effects. In an editorial, Coryell (p. 664) points out that the difference between these results and the more encouraging results of an earlier study by Blier et al. (Am J Psychiatry 2010; 167:281–288) are not clear.

Linking Molecules to Mood: New Insight Into the Biology of Depression

Vaishnav Krishnan, M.D., Ph.D.

Eric J. Nestler, M.D., Ph.D.

Major depressive disorder is a heritable psychiatric syndrome that appears to be associated with subtle cellular and molecular alterations in a complex neural network. The affected brain regions display dynamic neuroplastic adaptations to endocrine and immunologic stimuli arising from within and outside the CNS. Depression's clinical and etiological heterogeneity adds a third level of complexity, implicating different pathophysiological mechanisms in different patients with the same DSM diagnosis. Current pharmacological antidepressant treatments improve depressive symptoms through complex mechanisms that are themselves incompletely understood. This review summarizes the current knowledge of the neurobiology of depression by combining insights from human clinical studies and molecular explanations from animal models. The authors provide recommendations for future research, with a focus on translating today's discoveries into improved diagnostic tests and treatments.

(Am J Psychiatry 2010; 167:1305–1320)

Understanding the molecular mechanisms underlying major depressive disorder is essential because one in six individuals in the United States will develop depressive symptoms requiring treatment (1), depression significantly complicates chronic illness (2), and depression is the leading cause of disability worldwide (3). However, exploring the molecular underpinnings of depression brings substantial challenges. In contrast to the clear-cut phenotypes encountered in substance dependence or obesity, the strictest guidelines for diagnosing depression include elements that are difficult to capture in animal models, e.g., "insomnia or hypersomnia nearly every day" (4). Unlike Parkinson's or Alzheimer's disease, depression lacks any clear consensus neuropathology, rare familial genetic causes, or highly penetrant vulnerability genes, providing no obvious starting points for molecular investigations. In spite of its heritability, the search for genetic causes has not been successful to date. Consequently, progress in understanding the molecular biology of depression has been slow, particularly in comparison to other multifactorial syndromes, such as type 2 diabetes mellitus and cancer. Thus, the burden of depression will continue to increase (3), especially during the extra years of life gained from improved outcomes in cardiovascular disease, cancer, and other domains.

Nevertheless, it is an exciting time to be a depression researcher. Advances in molecular tools and ongoing improvements in behavioral techniques have allowed for genuinely novel insights into depression's neurobiological correlates. Methods to capture and artificially stimulate or inhibit the electrophysiological activity of individual types of neurons in the brain in vivo have added new dimensions to available approaches, permitting us for the first time to describe and manipulate the previously enigmatic neurophysiological correlates of concepts such as "reward" and "anxiety." Coupled with experimental advances in treatment, these developments suggest we can anticipate that developing tomorrow's therapies will no longer rely solely on modifications of existing agents that were discovered by serendipity six decades ago. Our aim in this review is to provide a framework to interpret continuing advances in the basic science of depression.

Insights From Human Studies

While animal experiments offer a unique opportunity to test cellular and molecular hypotheses, human clinical investigation continues to provide insights about depression that are inaccessible in animals. Postmortem studies designed to capture the neuropathology of depression have largely focused on certain cortical and hippocampal regions, which show a number of subtle differences, such as smaller neuronal size, fewer glial cells, shorter dendrites, and lower levels of trophic factors (5–7). These results agree with evidence of volume loss in these regions as shown by structural magnetic resonance imaging (MRI)

(8, 9). Molecular techniques such as DNA microarray profiling have been applied to specific regions, including the amygdala and locus ceruleus, to document gene expression alterations associated with depression (10, 11). Within the coming years, we can hope for a more comprehensive list of depression's neuropathological changes, particularly with the advent of centralized brain collections, which are able to furnish larger samples while simultaneously excluding traditional sources of confound, such as suicide, comorbid substance abuse, and a bipolar diagnosis. When elegantly combined with animal models or neuroimaging data, these postmortem depression studies provide the opportunity to demonstrate true causal relationships (12–15).

Functional MRI and positron emission tomography (PET) have shown how depressive behavior can be correlated with hypermetabolism of the subgenual cingulate cortex and amygdala (16) as well as hypometabolism of the dorsal prefrontal cortex and striatal regions (8). In an attempt to integrate these anatomic data, there have been several formulations of a "depression circuit" (Figure 1). After years of largely empirical reports, we now approach the possibility of testing and refining these circuit models in humans, thanks to recent experimental interventional advances such as deep brain stimulation and repetitive transcranial magnetic stimulation (rTMS). For cases of treatment-resistant depression, deep brain stimulation has been successfully applied to the subgenual cingulate cortex (18, 19) and the ventral striatum/nucleus accumbens (20–22) without known permanent adverse effects in the subjects studied to date. Refinements in stimulation variables for rTMS applied to the dorsolateral prefrontal cortex have significantly improved the magnitude and endurance of observed antidepressant effects (23). While these techniques are safer than earlier rudimentary approaches to "psychosurgery," the precise mechanisms by which deep brain stimulation and rTMS act are still incompletely understood. It is not known, for example, whether the local effects of deep brain stimulation work through excitation or inhibition or effects on fibers of passage (24). Recently developed optogenetic tools make it possible to activate or inhibit particular neuronal cell types and/or their terminals within defined brain regions (25), allowing for a deeper exploration of the neurophysiological mechanisms underlying the therapeutic effects of deep brain stimulation. Thus, as deep brain stimulation and rTMS are scaled down and characterized in laboratory animals, one can expect clinical improvements in patient selection, technique, and localization.

With heritability estimates of approximately 40% (26), two main techniques have been utilized to explore the genetics of depression. Candidate genes, identified through an investigator's best guess about etiological mechanisms, have been examined through linkage and genetic association studies (27). Single nucleotide polymorphisms (SNPs) in specific genes, such as GNB3 (for guanine nucleotide-binding protein 3) or MTHFR (for methylene tetrahydrofolate reductase), have survived stringent statistical requirements of meta-analyses. While their odds ratios are too weak for diagnostics or risk stratification, these and other genes may offer new clues into disease pathophysiology (28). Genome-wide association studies are inherently unbiased, as they currently can simultaneously examine up to one million SNPs. While such trials have identified SNPs in previously unappreciated molecules, such as Piccolo (a presynaptic nerve terminal protein) or GRM7 (metabotropic glutamate receptor 7), these findings are themselves of relatively poor statistical significance and are not replicated across studies (27). Several explanations have been put forth, including vague DSM diagnostic criteria, considerable disease heterogeneity, and the relatively potent contribution of ongoing life stressors and epigenetic plasticity. We remain hopeful that within the coming decade, that newer technologies will have greater success and replicability, including "whole-exome" studies (which exclude noncoding regions, representing 99% of the genome) as well as whole-genome sequencing. Of course, a key unanswered question is whether these genetic data should be correlated with DSM diagnostic categories, more broadly across several DSM diagnoses, or with more carefully defined behavioral, endocrine, neurochemical, or neuroimaging phenotypes. Identifying such genes will be hugely beneficial for the generation of bona fide animal models of depression.

An important insight gained from everyday clinical practice is the observation that monoamine reuptake inhibitors and other modulators of monoaminergic function improve symptoms in about 50% of depressed patients and produce a remission in 30%–40% of patients (29). These data illustrate the tremendous genetic heterogeneity of treatment response, and efforts are under way to identify pharmacogenetic predictors of a favorable treatment response to monoaminergic agents (30, 31). Since monoamine enhancers improve depressive symptoms, it was suggested historically that depression is caused by deficits in monoaminergic transmission. This "monoamine hypothesis" continues to be a prominent preoccupation of the field. However, after more than a decade of PET studies (positioned aptly to quantitatively measure receptor and transporter numbers and occupancy) (32), monoamine depletion studies (which transiently and experimentally reduce brain monoamine levels) (33), and genetic association analyses examining polymorphisms in monoaminergic genes (28, 34, 35), there is little evidence to implicate true deficits in serotonergic, noradrenergic, or dopaminergic neurotransmission in the pathophysiology of depression. This is not surprising, as there is no a priori reason that the mechanism of action of a treatment is the opposite of disease pathophysiology (36). Thus, currently available agents likely restore mood by modulating distinct processes that are

FIGURE 1. Two Heuristic Formulations of Neural "Depression Circuits"[a]

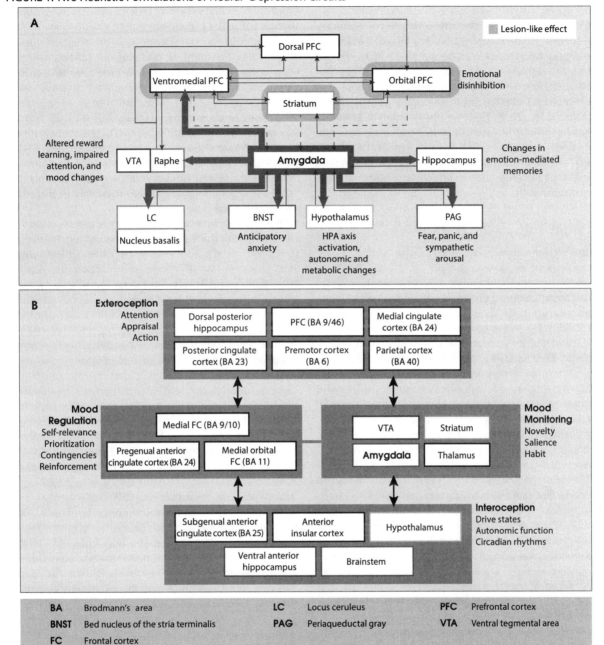

[a] Part A represents an amygdala-centric circuit (8) largely inspired by structural brain imaging and postmortem studies. According to this model, the emotional symptoms of depression can be brought about by functional impairment ("lesion-like" effects) of the striatum or the prefrontal and orbital prefrontal cortex (and/or their associated white matter tracts), resulting in disinhibition of the amygdala and downstream structures. Alternatively, they can arise from functional hypersensitivity of the amygdala (thick arrows), which gives rise to dysregulation of prefrontal cortical structures. (Part A used by permission from Elsevier.) Part B represents a circuit model (17) generated with a greater emphasis on functional imaging results. The main nodes consist of four clusters of brain regions with strong anatomical connections to each other. This model compartmentalizes depressive endophenotypes into exteroceptive (cognitive), interoceptive (visceral-motor), mood-regulating, and mood-monitoring functions. Both formulations should be seen as offering a simplified heuristic framework for further research into depression's diagnosis, pathophysiology, and treatment. They do not convey the cellular and molecular heterogeneity of each node within the circuit (for example, the ventral tegmental area comprises several types of dopaminergic and GABA-ergic neurons defined by differences in connectivity and receptor expression). Part B used by permission of the American Society for Clinical Investigation.)

unrelated to the primary pathology of depression, just as diuretics improve the symptoms of congestive heart failure without affecting cardiac myocytes directly. Similarly, the success of intravenous ketamine in rapidly alleviating depressive symptoms in treatment-resistant depression (37) has prompted an exploration of the cellular and neuroanatomical substrates for ketamine's actions and the search for ketamine-like therapies that lack psychotomimetic side effects. However, formulating a "glutamatergic hypothesis of depression" is grossly simplistic and only fuels inaccurate public misconceptions of depression's "chemical imbalance," particularly since more than one-half of all neurons in the brain utilize glutamate as a neurotransmitter.

Animal Models of Depression

The design, application, and relative strengths and limitations of depression models have been discussed in several reviews (1, 38). Without definitive knowledge of pathophysiological processes, these models are often evaluated for their *face, construct,* and *pharmacological* validity (1), as are models of other clinically defined neuropsychiatric syndromes, such as autism and schizophrenia. *Face validity* is a model's symptomatic homology to human depression. Today's depression models achieve this goal to a considerable extent: rodent and primate models have successfully recapitulated states of social withdrawal, hypophagia and weight loss, anhedonia, circadian changes, and abnormalities of the HPA axis, although these phenotypes are generally transient and not all present simultaneously.

The more challenging *construct validity* is the ability of a model to replicate etiological factors implicated in depression, which are themselves not entirely understood. Most paradigms use some form of stress (of a physical or a psychosocial form), given the known association between independent stressful life events and depressive episodes (39). More recently, a greater emphasis has been placed on replicating both environmental risk factors (such as stressful life events) and genetic risk factors (although these remain largely unknown) in the same model.

Pharmacological or *predictive validity* is met when a model's depression-like behaviors are reversed by currently available antidepressant modalities, and several models in use today display this type of predictability with the therapeutic delay that characterizes antidepressant responses in humans. However, given that all available pharmacological agents are monoamine modulators and only a minority of patients experience remission after first-line therapies (29), the requirement for pharmacological reversibility is perhaps desirable but not mandatory. Since the mechanisms underlying the delayed antidepressant effects of medication and nonmedication treatments (exercise, electroconvulsive seizures, etc.) remain largely unknown, animal models have been employed to dissect these mechanisms (i.e., models of antidepressant action),

with the caveat that these therapies are applied to laboratory animals that generally lack depression-like behavior or any particular genetic vulnerability to depression.

A potential fourth criterion that has received considerably less attention is *pathological validity*, whereby depression-related physiological, molecular, and cellular abnormalities in animals are validated by demonstrating identical changes in postmortem brain samples from depressed humans. This is a genuinely difficult requirement but has been gaining increasing popularity with the more widespread access to postmortem samples (12–15). Ideally, this criterion might be better addressed through functional imaging studies with depressed patients, but this will require substantial improvements in molecular imaging capabilities.

From an evolutionary perspective, depression may be an analogue of the "involuntary defeat strategy," occurring when an animal perceives defeat in a hierarchical struggle for resources (40). Hyperarousal, psychomotor retardation, reduced motivation, and sleep alterations in the setting of losing are postulated to have an adaptive advantage in that they serve to protect losers from further attack and focus cognitive resources on planning ways out of complex social problems (41, 42). Most behavioral endpoints in depression models aim to quantitatively assay some type of experimentally induced defeat or despair (Figure 2), even though this aspect of mammalian behavior is likely physiological (i.e., adaptive) rather than pathological. Additionally, while despair behavior is often extrapolated as being depression-like, it is clearly a huge inference to make from rodent models, and most stressors also produce anxiety-like changes that are exaggerated manifestations of the fight-or-flight response (reduced exploration, freezing, hyperthermia, HPA axis activation, etc.). For example, repeated social subordination in mice (social defeat) leads to a long-lasting phenotype of reduced social interaction with other mice. This impairment in sociability can be interpreted as a reduced motivation to interact (an abnormality of reward) or as a heightened avoidance of novel social stimuli (a pathological anxiety response). Distinguishing between these alternative hypotheses is difficult and may even be irrelevant, particularly given the poorly defined neurobiological distinctions between anxiety and depression and their highly variable clinical presentation. In either case, the model employs a naturalistic social-stress-induced behavior that is quantifiable and amenable to experimental manipulation (12–14, 43–52).

The forced-swim and tail-suspension tests are the simplest and most widely used models of depression and antidepressant action. While these approaches have been rightly criticized for involving acute stress and acute antidepressant responses, they have permitted the rapid behavioral screening of novel chemical antidepressants and the phenotyping of genetically altered mutant mice. In certain instances, they have directed the field toward fundamentally novel molecular hypotheses. For example, an antidepressant-like phenotype in the forced-

FIGURE 2. Common Behavioral Endpoints in Rodent Depression Studies[a]

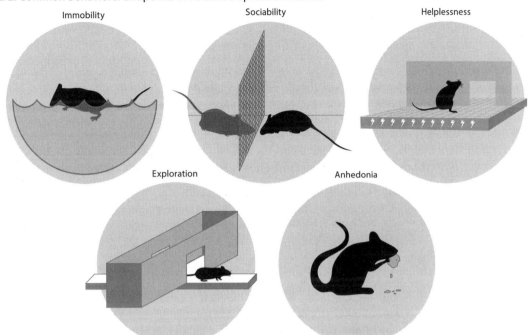

Immobility   Sociability   Helplessness

Exploration   Anhedonia

[a] These quantitative and automatable behavioral endpoints are widely used in experiments with rats or mice as measures of depression-related behavior. They can be employed following chronic stress paradigms such as social defeat, to phenotype genetic mutant mice, to validate antidepressant treatments, or to provide tools for localizing genomic mediators of complex behaviors in quantitative trait locus analyses. The most popular endpoint is immobility, which is interpreted as a measure of behavioral despair or freezing in response to an inescapable stressor, such as forced swimming or tail suspension. A closely related endpoint is helplessness, which can be inferred through the learned helplessness paradigm, where animals receive a series of inescapable electrical shocks in one compartment and on subsequent testing days display a deficit in their motivation to avoid these shocks when a clear escape route is provided. Anhedonia in mice can be measured in several ways, including simple measures of preference (measuring the relative preference for palatable rewards such as a dilute sucrose solution or a high-fat chow), quantitative indices of sexual behavior such as latency to mount a receptive female, and intracranial self-stimulation, where one directly measures motivation (lever pressing) to receive a highly rewarding electrical shock. Reductions in exploratory behavior are often interpreted as elevations in anxiety and can be quantified by measuring the amount of time spent in aversive portions of a field of exploration, such as the open arms of an elevated plus-shaped maze. One can also measure deficits in sociability, which may reflect impairments in natural reward or social anxiety. These assays have been employed in stress paradigms, mutant mouse models, and models of secondary depression, such as that seen, for example, with obesity, breast cancer, or chronic interferon treatment. A common practice is to generate behavioral profiles by employing a broad battery of these tests following stress, genetic, or pharmacological manipulations; these behavioral profiles can also include changes in weight and appetite, as well as deficits in self-grooming (deteriorations in fur coat).

swim test (decreased immobility and greater struggling or swimming) was observed in mice deficient in acid-sensing ion channel 1a (ASIC-1a), a pH-sensitive ion channel expressed in the brain (53). Subsequent studies have shown that ASIC-1a expressed in the amygdala participates in eliciting a fear response to a variety of aversive cues culminating in acidemia (53, 54), implicating inhibitors of ASIC-1a (a previously unappreciated target) as potential therapeutics against anxiety and depressive disorders. Analogous approaches have identified several other novel molecular targets, including p11 (a calcium-binding chaperone molecule that promotes serotonin signaling through the serotonin 1B receptor subtype [15]), TREK-1 (a distinct type of potassium channel that is enriched in depression-related limbic brain regions [55, 56]), ghrelin (a stomach-derived endocrine mediator of energy homeostasis [46]), and many others.

In the following sections, we focus on neurobiological themes that exhibit therapeutic promise. The two main

values of using rats and mice to study depression are 1) the ability to describe and characterize neuroplasticity with exquisite spatial and temporal precision and 2) the opportunity to utilize molecular innovations to demonstrate the causative effects of those neuroplastic changes on assays of depression- and antidepressant-like behavior.

Neurogenic and Neurotrophic Theories

The first description of continually dividing neuronal progenitors in the adult mammalian brain offered the promise of solutions for a host of neurodegenerative disorders that so far lack definitive cures (57). Exploring the physiologic role of endogenous neurogenesis, particularly that which occurs in the hippocampal dentate gyrus, has important relevance to the study of psychiatric disease (58). The journey from a hippocampal stem cell in the subgranular zone to a mature dentate gyrus granule cell neuron with appropriate synaptic connections occurs in stages defined by specific cellular markers, with the rates of proliferation and survival modulated by numerous stimuli. Unpredictable stressors, glucocorticoids, drugs of abuse, and high-energy electromagnetic radiation negatively influence this process, while antidepressants, voluntary exercise, and environmental enrichment accelerate adult hippocampal neurogenesis (59).

Laboratory rodents have been used extensively to explore the regulation of these new hippocampal neurons and their contribution to depression-related phenotypes. In models of antidepressant action, cranial irradiation (which severely impairs the mitotic potential of hippocampal stem cells) and aging (another robust negative regulator of adult hippocampal neurogenesis) impair some but not all of the effects of monoamine reuptake inhibitors (60–63), suggesting that these agents may function through neurogenesis-dependent and -independent processes (64). Clearly, only the actions of antidepressants that involve hippocampal circuitry could be mediated through enhanced neurogenesis. Indeed, one study was able to demonstrate the antidepressant effect of a direct intracerebral infusion of bone-marrow-derived mesenchymal stem cells, which both themselves transform into neurons and generate diffusible permissive factors that accelerate endogenous neurogenesis (65). These preliminary results support the idea that enhancing hippocampal neurogenesis (pharmacologically or by way of cellular transplantation) can serve to boost or augment the antidepressant response. At the same time, impairments in the rates of neurogenesis do not appear to be involved in the core features of depression. Following cranial irradiation, mice are unimpaired across several indices of depression-related behavior (60, 62). Consistent with its proposed role in hippocampal-dependent learning (57, 59), adult hippocampal neurogenesis may play a pathological role in the establishment of aversive memories of traumatic stressors and the sequelae of posttraumatic stress (66). As the field struggles to clarify the functional relevance of these new neurons, stress-induced reductions in hippocampal proliferation are best interpreted as a marker of hippocampal plasticity (which may be impaired in some types of depression).

Another widespread endpoint for assaying the effects of stress, antidepressants, and genetic manipulations is the measurement of levels of brain-derived neurotrophic factor (BDNF) in the hippocampus. This practice, stemming from the "neurotrophic hypothesis" of depression (67), is based on three main observations: an impairment of hippocampal BDNF signaling produces certain depression-related behaviors and impairs the actions of antidepressants (68–70), experimental increases in hippocampal BDNF levels produce antidepressant-like effects (71–73), and hippocampal BDNF levels are low in postmortem samples from depressed humans (6). BDNF is one of numerous growth factors that have been implicated in depression, including fibroblast growth factor, vascular endothelial growth factor, and nonacronymic VGF (1). Through modulation of their levels and downstream signaling, these growth factors appear to transduce stressors into lowered rates of adult hippocampal neurogenesis, atrophic changes, and impaired synaptic plasticity of hippocampal neurons, which might (in theory) explain the cognitive impairments and hippocampal atrophy seen in depression (67).

Translating these BDNF findings may not be straightforward. Aside from the challenges associated with synthesizing a specific agonist of BDNF, enhancing BDNF function in the nucleus accumbens and amygdala can have detrimental effects on measures of anhedonia, anxiety, and social interaction in rodents (1, 71). A naturally occurring SNP in BDNF (G196A, Val66Met) results in dramatic alterations in intracellular trafficking of BDNF and its activity-dependent release (1). Meta-analyses show that while the Met allele marginally increases the risk for depression in men but not women, it is also associated with a better antidepressant response (74, 75). A hippocampus-specific increase in BDNF activity may improve certain cognitive symptoms of depression and facilitate hippocampal neurogenesis (60). While we possess the technology to deliver specific genes into the human brain through viral vectors (76), the beneficial effects of BDNF would have to outweigh potential negative effects, i.e., lower seizure threshold, altered indices of learning and memory, and increased likelihood of malignant transformation (77, 78). Nevertheless, understanding the roles of these growth factors in depression's pathophysiology remains an extremely active area of research, with an emphasis now placed on extrahippocampal trophic signaling and exploring downstream signaling pathways (79), which may have greater pharmaceutical application.

Contribution of Epigenetic Modifications

Biological theories of depression's etiology have traditionally focused on the interplay between genetic risks and environmental/social hazards, with gene-environment interactions invoked to explain how relatively weak genetic vulnerabilities combined with the right environmental triggers may lead to significant psychiatric impairment (80). However, the significant discordance of depression between monozygotic twins (who often share the same environment as well as genes), the remarkably slow progress in identifying genetic risk factors, and depression's twofold female predominance suggest the presence of a third, nongenetic and nonenvironmental component to variability (81). Epigenetic modifications have been implicated as a significant contributor to this third source of variability and are broadly divided into those that modify DNA directly (e.g., DNA methylation), those that alter histones (e.g., histone acetylation or methylation), and those that involve noncoding

RNAs (such as microRNAs) that regulate gene expression (82). In changing DNA's tertiary structure, they adjust interactions between DNA and associated proteins such as transcription factors and RNA polymerases, thereby ultimately altering levels of mRNA expressed by given genes. Pathological epigenetic events have been implicated in numerous chronic diseases, most notably cancer, in which aberrant epigenetic changes promote genetic instability (83).

Through combining animal models with an explosion of novel molecular tools, several epigenetic events have been linked to depression-related behavior and antidepressant action. In rats, offspring born to mothers that display low levels of maternal licking and grooming behavior display exaggerated corticosteroid responses to stress and increased anxiety, which are mediated in part by increased methylation (and subsequent repression) of the glucocorticoid receptor gene promoter in the hippocampus. This type of epigenetic mark is stable to adulthood, reversed by chemical inhibitors of DNA methylation, and entirely dependent on the maternal behavior of the fostering, rather than biological, mother (i.e., independent of germ-line transmission) (84). Early life stress applied to mice produces hypomethylation of the arginine vasopressin (AVP) gene in the hypothalamic paraventricular nucleus, resulting in hypersecretion of AVP, pathologically enhanced serum corticosterone level, and increased depression-like behavior (85). Histone acetylation, a mark of active transcription, is increased at certain BDNF promoters when socially defeated mice receive a course of chronic imipramine, and this hyperacetylation event is mediated by the down-regulation of histone deacetylase 5 (HDAC5) (47). While overexpression of HDAC5 in the hippocampus counteracts the effects of antidepressants, mice that are globally deficient in HDAC5 display an enhanced vulnerability to chronic stress (49).

These examples illustrate the complexity in translating these epigenetic changes into clinical phenomena: while certain perturbations robustly alter epigenetic marks on one gene in one brain region, other brain regions may have opposing changes at distinct genes. Furthermore, most enzymes affected by epigenetic changes occur in several isoforms, each with its own tissue specificity and regulatory factors (e.g., HDAC5 is part of a family of 11 HDAC isoforms that are expressed across all major organ systems [86]), further complicating the development of selective small-molecule antagonists. In spite of this complexity, epigenetic modulators show some promise as treatments for depression. In animal models, systemically or locally administered HDAC inhibitors display antidepressant properties without obvious adverse effects on health (12, 82), suggesting that HDAC inhibitors may function by modulating a global acetylation/deacetylation balance across several brain regions. Of course, histone acetylation functions in concert with several other markers of gene repression and activation, including histone methylation, phosphorylation, sumoylation, and ubiquitination (86).

Thus, to comprehensively describe and appreciate the intricacies of depression-related epigenetic plasticity, we can expect a continued evolution in molecular and bioinformatic techniques. Rather than examining candidate genes such as those for BDNF and glucocorticoid receptors, the field has begun to transition toward genome-wide approaches to studying chromatin regulation (48), shifting the focus from "epigenetic marks" to "epigenomic signatures." As these technologies characterized in mouse and rat models begin to be applied to human postmortem tissue from depressed individuals (87), the ultimate goal would be to use transcriptional and epigenetic profiling as biomarkers to distinguish clinical categories of depressive illness, to determine responsivity to various antidepressant classes, and to differentiate treatment-sensitive from treatment-resistant illness. These profiles may offer new insights into subtype-specific pathophysiology and therapies and aid in the validation of our current animal models.

Role of Dopaminergic Reward Circuits

The dramatic reinforcing properties of direct intracranial self-stimulation in rodents led to the appreciation of a series of subcortical regions critical for reward and appetitive behavior (88). The two main structures implicated by intracranial self-stimulation are the lateral hypothalamus and medial forebrain bundle, the latter containing ascending dopaminergic projections from the ventral tegmental area to the nucleus accumbens (88). Under baseline conditions, dopaminergic neurons in the ventral tegmental area oscillate between tonic patterns of activity (low-frequency regular action potentials) and phasic activity patterns (bursts of action potentials) (89). Unexpected rewards produce a transient increase in phasic firing (encoding a "reward prediction error"), which is sufficient to reinforce antecedent behaviors (25). All major classes of abused drugs appear to "signal" a reward, at least in part, by artificially enhancing dopamine transmission in the nucleus accumbens (for example, cocaine blocks the dopamine transporter) (88).

Given depression's prominent features of anhedonia and appetite alterations, this circuit has become an obvious focus of attention for basic molecular and electrophysiological studies. In rodents, long-term antidepressant administration reduces the firing rates of dopamine neurons in the ventral tegmental area (90). In contrast, psychosocial stressors activate firing in the ventral tegmental area and increase nucleus accumbens dopamine levels (13, 50, 91), and this may represent a positive coping strategy to enhance motivation during stressful situations (88). One mechanism for this enhanced excitability of the ventral tegmental area may be the reduced activation of the protein kinase AKT, which leads to reductions in local inhibitory neurotransmission (14). Variations in the neuroplastic adaptations expressed by these neurons may also contribute to individual differences in the responsiveness

FIGURE 3. Effects of Deep Brain Stimulation on Brain Metabolic Activity in Treatment-Resistant Depression[a]

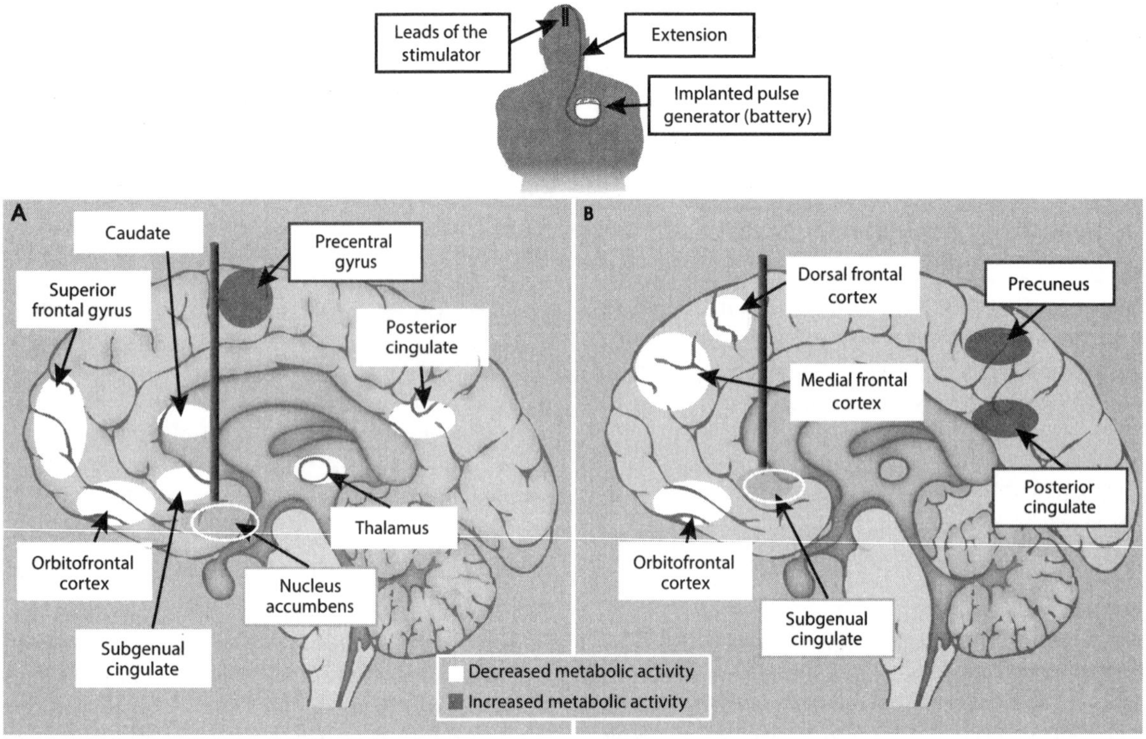

[a] Part A: applied to the nucleus accumbens and nearby regions, deep brain stimulation produces significant clinical improvement and changes in metabolic activity across an array of neural substrates (as measured by fluorodeoxyglucose PET studies before and 6 months after implantation of the stimulators) (19, 20). Among responders, reduced glucose metabolism (white ovals\circles) is observed in the orbitofrontal cortex, superior frontal gyrus, and posterior and subgenual cingulate cortical areas. Part B: the subgenual (also known as subcallosal) cingulate cortex is itself another target for deep brain stimulation in depression (18, 19), and poststimulation PET studies reveal similar patterns of decreases in frontal cortical metabolism. In addition, stimulation applied here normalizes the heightened blood flow to this region that is associated with depressive episodes (not shown). These data, together with results from rodent studies of deep brain stimulation (99), suggest that continuous stimulation in these areas may alleviate severe depressive symptoms by enhancing inhibition across a circuit of cortical and subcortical structures.

to stress. In the mouse social defeat paradigm, while stress-susceptible mice display enhanced activity in the ventral tegmental area and subsequent BDNF release, stress-resilient mice overcome this excitability change by up-regulating potassium channel subunits expressed by dopamine neurons in the ventral tegmental area that maintain normal tonic firing rates (13, 44). Stress-induced increases in nucleus accumbens BDNF may mediate pathological reward learning such that, following a series of aversive social encounters, the positive rewarding value of social interaction is now modified to have a negative valence (1). Enhanced mesolimbic dopaminergic signaling may explain the reported efficacy of antidopaminergic agents as adjunct antidepressants (92), and by enhancing basal dopaminergic and BDNF signaling, this model may also explain the significant comorbidity of substance dependence and depressive disorders (93, 94).

Nucleus accumbens neurons, anatomically situated to integrate reward-related dopaminergic signals as well as glutamatergic input from the prefrontal cortex, hippocampus, and amygdala (21), themselves display numerous stress- and antidepressant-induced changes (88). One

example is the modulation of cAMP response element binding protein (CREB): while prolonged social isolation stress reduces CREB activity and generates a predominantly anxious phenotype (95), active stressors or drugs of abuse *increase* CREB activity and promote anhedonia in the presence of a host of natural and drug rewards (88). Neuroimaging studies with depressed humans show that quantitative indices of anhedonia are associated with low nucleus accumbens volume (96) as well as hypoactivation during simple tasks of incentive reward (97, 98). In an attempt to reverse this nucleus accumbens hypoactivation, bilateral deep brain stimulation to this and nearby regions has been successfully applied to several cases of treatment-resistant depression (Figure 3). Consistent with the centralized location of the stimulation, responders displayed normalized PET indices of activity in the nucleus accumbens and the larger ventral striatum, in addition to lower activity in the subgenual cingulate cortex and other prefrontal cortical regions (20, 21). In rats, deep brain stimulation applied to the nucleus accumbens with simultaneous electrophysiological recordings from multiple distant sites has suggested that the therapeutically relevant effects are due to the synchronization of inhibition across a network of cortical and subcortical regions (99), possibly explaining anatomically distant effects of deep brain stimulation. In this way, the application and validation of deep brain stimulation in depression models offers opportunities to improve our circuit models (Figure 1) and shed light on the neurobiological correlates of treatment resistance.

Sex, Steroids, and Immunity

The network of neural substrates involved in depression's symptoms displays a remarkable degree of plasticity in response to a host of peripherally derived chemical stimuli, and advancing our understanding of the endocrinology and immunology of depression offers exciting therapeutic avenues. Considerable research in the field has focused on a central role of a pathologically dysregulated HPA axis (1), whereby stress-induced hypercortisolemia leads to the central down-regulation of glucocorticoid receptors, impairing cortisol's negative feedback and enhancing levels of corticotropin-releasing hormone (CRH) and adrenocorticotrophic hormone (ACTH) (36). This vicious cycle sustains elevated cortisol levels, possibly leading to hippocampal atrophy and reduced rates of neurogenesis, as well as predisposing depressed individuals to insulin resistance and abdominal obesity (100, 101). A large body of clinical and preclinical evidence supports this model. Depressed patients display dexamethasone nonsuppression that is reversed by antidepressant treatment (102), enhanced CSF levels of CRH (103), and alterations in diurnal cortisol rhythms (104). Mice that are treated chronically with glucocorticoids develop anhedonia in conjunction with other molecular correlates of depression (105). In line with these data, chronic glucocorticoid administration reduces hippocampal volume and impairs cognition in humans (106), while the glucocorticoid receptor antagonist mifepristone improves psychotic and depressive symptoms in patients with psychotic major depression (107). Antagonizing CRH signaling, particularly through the CRH1 receptor subtype, leads to strong anxiolytic effects in several rodent models (108). While the validation of CRH1 antagonists for depression and anxiety disorders remains an active area of clinical research, previously tested pharmacological prototypes have failed for a variety of reasons, including off-target hepatotoxicity (109, 110).

This "cortisol hypothesis" represents a vibrant part of the preclinical depression literature: with commercially available glucocorticoid immunoassays, experimental manipulations are often validated as being "prodepressant" or "antidepressant" depending on their effects on baseline or stress-induced glucocorticoid levels. However, several key points argue for a reappraisal of this practice: 1) true hypercortisolemia is rarely observed in outpatient depressed populations and may be associated only with depression severe enough to require hospitalization (111,

112); 2) depressed patients with atypical features and victims of posttraumatic stress tend to display hypocortisolemia (111, 113, 114); and 3) mice designed to display reduced central glucocorticoid receptor signaling (mimicking hypercortisolemic states) and those that centrally overexpress glucocorticoid receptors display identical behavioral and endocrinological phenotypes (115, 116). In spite of the strong immunosuppressant properties of glucocorticoids, levels of circulating proinflammatory cytokines (taken as a quantitative marker of systemic glucocorticoid-receptor-mediated signaling) are usually elevated in major depression (117); these cytokines include interleukin 1 (IL-1), IL-6, and tumor necrosis factor α. They are themselves sufficient to impair glucocorticoid receptor signaling, and thus, rather than directly affecting HPA function, stress likely leads to glucocorticoid *insufficiency* through cytokine intermediates (102). Under certain circumstances, this reduced glucocorticoid-receptor-mediated signaling may promote hypercortisolemia, severe insomnia, and hypophagia (melancholic features) but in other conditions may lead to hypocortisolemia, hyperphagia, and fatigue (atypical features). Cytokines themselves play powerful roles in depression-related neuroplasticity: chronic stress produces significant changes in immune function (118), and cytokines induce depression-like behavior when injected into rodents (119). IL-1β is one such cytokine: through the actions of the transcription factor nuclear factor κB, stress-induced increases in IL-1β lead to reductions in hippocampal neurogenesis and anhedonic phenotypes (120).

The greater female predisposition to depression, as well as its greater incidence in postpartum and perimenopausal periods, argue strongly for a thorough understanding of the role of gonadal hormones in affective regulation. The heightened female vulnerability to experience depressive episodes is limited to the postpubertal and premenopausal period, and accordingly, much of the field's emphasis has focused on the neurobiology of estrogen. Studies in rodent models have demonstrated that estrogen has antidepressant properties and also augments antidepressant actions of monoaminergic agents. Conversely, mice lacking aromatase (required for the generation of estrogenic steroids) or estrogen receptor β display aberrant stress-related behavior (121). Consistent with the broad central expression of estrogen receptor β, the antidepressant effects of estrogen signaling have been linked to several neurobiological substrates, including hippocampal neurogenesis, BDNF signaling, serotonergic neurotransmission, and HPA axis function (122).

While this body of evidence may explain how significant fluctuations in hormone levels can trigger depressive episodes, it does not account for the heightened female vulnerability to depression, which is likely as much about female vulnerability factors in responses to depressogenic stimuli as about male resiliency factors. For instance, in comparison to males, female rodents display passive cop-

FIGURE 4. Genetic Model for Studying Gender Differences in Depression-Related Behavior[a]

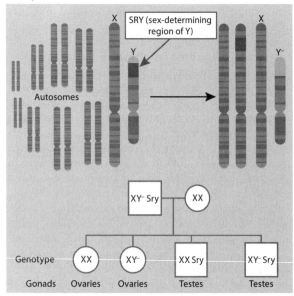

[a] The neurobiology underlying the greater female vulnerability to depression (or the relative resilience in males) remains largely unknown. The vast majority of research in the field has focused on how gonadal hormones (i.e., estrogens, progesterones, and testosterones) affect stress-related behavior. However, studies using the "four core genotypes" model shown here illustrate that important sexually dimorphic anatomic and behavioral traits are unrelated to gonadal output and are localized to the many genes contained on sex chromosomes. This mouse model was developed through a spontaneous mutation in the Y chromosome resulting in the loss of SRY (sex-determining region of the Y chromosome), effectively giving rise to gonadally female XY mice. The Sry gene was then subsequently inserted into an autosome, resulting in "XY⁻ Sry" mice that remain gonadally and chromosomally male. Mating these males with standard XX females results in the four core genotypes, comparisons between which have allowed for a dissociation of chromosomal and gonadal mediators of a variety of behavioral and physiological phenotypes (125). Studies using this model generally involve a gonadectomy prior to experimentation to control for confounds related to menstrual cycling in females.

ing strategies and a more pronounced HPA axis activation in response to a variety of stressors. These features can be "masculinized" by providing testosterone during puberty, demonstrating how gender differences in behavioral physiology can be hardwired during certain critical periods (123). Ovariectomy also promotes active stress-related coping, an effect that may be related to estrogen signaling within the nucleus accumbens (124). Aside from hormonal influences, it is important to recognize that gender differences also likely arise from numerous genes on sex chromosomes that are unrelated to gonadal function. Through standard genetic engineering techniques, one can create mice that are chromosomally male (i.e., XY) while having female gonads, and vice versa (Figure 4). Studies with this model have shown that while the development and maturation of male copulatory behaviors and sexually dimorphic brain structures depend on gonadal output, other genes on sex chromosomes independently

drive other behavioral traits that are relevant to depression, including habit formation, parental and aggressive behaviors, and social interaction (125, 126).

Mediators of Energy Homeostasis

The appetite and metabolic abnormalities associated with depression and depression-related entities range from severe hypophagia and anorexia to binge eating and obesity. A thorough understanding of such complex phenomena requires knowledge about physiological mechanisms of energy homeostasis, which refers to processes that maintain equilibrium between caloric intake and energy expenditure. In mammals, this is achieved largely through the action of circulating hormones that relay information about peripheral energy levels to the brain (127). Two such hormones that have received tremendous attention are leptin and ghrelin (Figure 5). Leptin is synthesized in white adipose tissue and is secreted in times of nutritional excess. Many obese individuals display a hyperleptinemia associated with central leptin resistance (131). In contrast, ghrelin is synthesized by gastric fundus cells and released during times of energy scarcity, and its secretion stimulates caloric intake and energy storage (127). The principal homeostatic site of action of leptin and ghrelin is the hypothalamic arcuate nucleus, where they exert anorexigenic and orexigenic effects, respectively, through a biologically elegant system of neuropeptides. It is interesting that receptors for leptin and ghrelin and receptors for other feeding-related peptides (such as melanin-concentrating hormone, neuropeptide Y, agouti-related peptide, α-melanocyte-stimulating hormone, and orexin [hypocretin]) are expressed in several depression-related limbic substrates. In rodents, chronic stress decreases serum leptin levels (132) and increases serum ghrelin (46). The systemic administration of either hormone produces antidepressant effects on the forced-swim test, enhances hippocampal neurogenesis, and improves learning and memory in behavioral and cellular (i.e., long-term potentiation) assays (46, 132–136). Whereas ghrelin and leptin have identical actions in the hippocampus, dopaminergic neurons of the ventral tegmental area are excited by ghrelin and inhibited by leptin (130, 137, 138), which illustrates how their hypothalamic effects on appetite are complemented in the ventral tegmental area through opposite modulation of reward sensitivity.

In addition to persistent deficits in social interaction and anhedonia, mice subjected to chronic social defeat stress display an initial weight loss followed by a prolonged hyperphagic phase, during which they rapidly regain their body weight and eventually gain more weight than do control or stress-resilient animals. This phenomenon is at least partially mediated by both reduced serum leptin levels and central leptin resistance, which ultimately weaken central melanocortinergic signaling, i.e., through the

FIGURE 5. Mediators of Energy Homeostasis Implicated in Metabolic and Affective Illness[a]

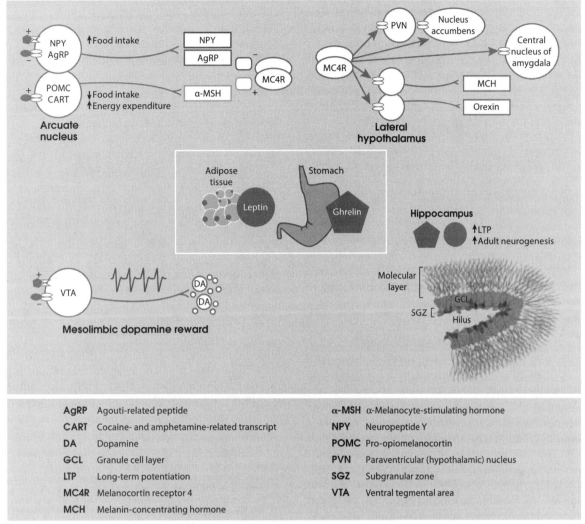

AgRP	Agouti-related peptide	**α-MSH**	α-Melanocyte-stimulating hormone
CART	Cocaine- and amphetamine-related transcript	**NPY**	Neuropeptide Y
DA	Dopamine	**POMC**	Pro-opiomelanocortin
GCL	Granule cell layer	**PVN**	Paraventricular (hypothalamic) nucleus
LTP	Long-term potentiation	**SGZ**	Subgranular zone
MC4R	Melanocortin receptor 4	**VTA**	Ventral tegmental area
MCH	Melanin-concentrating hormone		

[a] Leptin (synthesized by white adipose tissue) and ghrelin (synthesized in the stomach) provide two canonical examples of how endocrine hormones that signal information about peripheral energy state can also exert effects on depression-related behaviors. Leptin and ghrelin receptors are expressed in the hypothalamic arcuate nucleus, which contains two main types of neurons, defined by their neuropeptides. These two neuronal types differentially express neuropeptides that act on the same melanocortin receptor (MC4R) with opposing effects : AgRP, an endogenous antagonist, and α-MSH, an endogenous agonist (α-MSH is a product of the POMC gene). AgRP neurons also express NPY, while α-MSH neurons also express CART. NPY and AgRP are orexigenic, while α-MSH and CART are anorexigenic. Leptin reduces food intake and increases energy expenditure by inhibiting NPY/AgRP-releasing neurons and exciting α-MSH/CART neurons. Ghrelin acts by promoting the release of NPY and AgRP. MC4Rs are expressed widely in the brain, and their reach includes the paraventricular nucleus (influencing the release of numerous neuropeptides, including corticotropin-releasing hormone and thyrotropin-releasing hormone), the lateral hypothalamus (containing MCH- and orexin-secreting neurons, which regulate food intake and arousal), and extrahypothalamic sites such as the nucleus accumbens and amygdala (where they are thought to influence mood regulation) (51, 128). Synthetic antagonists of MC4R are antidepressant and anxiolytic (129), as are agonists of NPY (122). In the ventral tegmental area, direct infusions of leptin and ghrelin exert opposing effects on food intake through their contrasting effects on dopaminergic neuronal firing. Their actions in the ventral tegmental area are believed to control the motivational or hedonic aspects of food intake (130) and are likely altered in other reward-related disorders, such as depression and substance dependence. In contrast to their effects in the ventral tegmental area, leptin and ghrelin appear to have identical effects on hippocampal plasticity: they both positively modulate long-term potentiation (an electrophysiological assay for activity-dependent synapse strengthening) and enhance adult hippocampal neurogenesis through receptors expressed on hippocampal progenitor cells. (Diagram of hippocampal plasticity comes from Eisch et al. [59] and is used by permission of the Society for Neuroscience.)

melanocortin 4 receptor (Figure 5). This hypoleptinemia seems to be mediated by enhanced β₃-adrenergic signaling, which promotes sympathetically mediated lipolysis. Coadministration of β₃-adrenergic antagonists during social defeat prevents the weight gain and reduced leptin but worsens social deficits (51), suggesting that enhanced β₃-adrenergic signaling has an adaptive function at the expense of metabolic derangements.

Understanding the hedonic impact of homeostatic signals provides numerous targets for pharmaceutical development in depressive disorders, particularly in cases associated with significant metabolic abnormalities. An obvious example would be in cases of HIV- or cancer-related cachexia, where artificially enhancing ghrelin or attenuating melanocortin signaling would have therapeutic hyperphagic and antidepressant effects. Nonpeptide antagonists of the melanocortin 4 receptor have already been shown to exert antidepressant and anxiolytic effects in animal models (129). Conversely, patients with comorbid depression and obesity (139) might benefit from therapies designed to alleviate central leptin resistance (a challenging objective). Elucidating such therapies will require a deep understanding of the anatomy and physiology of leptin receptor signaling and of numerous other feeding-related peptides. This is an exciting area of active research.

Conclusions and Perspectives on the Future

Today's approaches to dissecting the neurobiology of depression employ an unprecedented array of experimental techniques in humans and animals, including genome-wide DNA sequencing, chromatin immunoprecipitation to study epigenetic factors, functional brain imaging, optogenetic electrophysiological tools, viral-mediated gene transfer, and an impressive assortment of genetic mutant mice. The list of molecular players involved in depression's phenotypes has now expanded to include genes from diverse aspects of cellular physiology, such as numerous neurotransmitter and neuropeptide systems, steroid hormones, neurotrophic and cytokine signaling cascades, ion channels, histone deacetylases, circadian genes (88, 108), transcription factors (e.g., CREB, nuclear factor κB, and ΔFosB [43]), p11, and many others. Most of the new targets are derived from experiments in rodents and while these studies are scientifically sound, the targets themselves may or may not be therapeutically relevant or feasible for human depression. Beyond the synthetic obstacles to designing safe and effective small-molecule modulators or viral vectors for use in depressed humans, a key challenge will be to prioritize these targets and develop collaborative efforts to rule them in or out at a reasonable pace.

A large and unacceptable divide continues to exist between animal studies and human clinical investigation. An important example involves our appreciation of cortical contributions to depression: while human neuroimaging studies repeatedly implicate cortical subregions, such as the subgenual cingulate and orbitofrontal cortex, the vast majority of rodent studies limit their analyses to the hippocampus or amygdala. While studying cortical circuits in rodents is more challenging, the human findings clearly demonstrate the high priority of this work. Many reports in the basic literature focus on drastic behavioral and neurobiological phenotypes in constitutive knockout mice, even though homozygous human "knockouts" pre-

sumably are a negligible contribution to clinical depression. As progress in delineating the genetics of depression continues, it will be crucial to complement knockout studies by examining molecular and epigenetic mechanisms underlying individual variability and understanding the cellular and physiological consequences of psychiatrically relevant human SNPs. Finally, pathological validation using postmortem brain tissue provides a crucial link between our inherently limited laboratory models and the molecular enigmas of human depression.

Human studies must also mature. Observational studies that measure serum BDNF or glucocorticoid levels can expand to include multiple measures such as serum leptin, ghrelin, and thyroid hormone levels and metabolic status, to name just a few, as well as segregating patients into depressive subtypes. Brain imaging experiments continue to largely focus on volume or activity measures of particular brain regions or on monoamine receptor/transporter occupancy. It is essential to vastly expand the range of proteins that can be assessed in the living brain so that proteins at the heart of pathophysiological models in rodents can at last be analyzed in depressed patients. As informed clinicians and scientists in the field, we have a responsibility to expand the horizon of our investigations and constantly reassess our analytic methods and theoretical paradigms. We should look well beyond monoamines, cortisol, BDNF, and the hippocampus to determine tomorrow's novel medical and surgical therapeutic avenues for depression.

Received March 25, 2010; revision received May 17, 2010; accepted June 25, 2010 (doi: 10.1176/appi.ajp.2009.10030434). From the Departments of Psychiatry, Neuroscience, and Internal Medicine, University of Texas Southwestern Medical Center; and the Fishberg Department of Neuroscience, Mount Sinai School of Medicine, New York. Address correspondence and reprint requests to Dr. Krishnan, vaishnav.krishnan@alumni.utsouthwestern.edu (e-mail).

Dr. Nestler reports receiving grants from NIMH and consulting income from Merck and PsychoGenics. Dr. Krishnan reports no financial relationships with commercial interests.

Preparation of this review was supported by grants P50 MH-61772 and R01 MH-51399 from NIMH.

Dr. Krishnan thanks the University of Texas Southwestern's Medical Scientist Training Program for support and mentorship.

References

1. Krishnan V, Nestler EJ: The molecular neurobiology of depression. Nature 2008; 455:894–902

2. Evans DL, Charney DS, Lewis L, Golden RN, Gorman JM, Krishnan KR, Nemeroff CB, Bremner JD, Carney RM, Coyne JC, Delong MR, Frasure-Smith N, Glassman AH, Gold PW, Grant I, Gwyther L, Ironson G, Johnson RL, Kanner AM, Katon WJ, Kaufmann PG, Keefe FJ, Ketter T, Laughren TP, Leserman J, Lyketsos CG, McDonald WM, McEwen BS, Miller AH, Musselman D, O'Connor C, Petitto JM, Pollock BG, Robinson RG, Roose SP, Rowland J, Sheline Y, Sheps DS, Simon G, Spiegel D, Stunkard A, Sunderland T, Tibbits P Jr, Valvo WJ: Mood disorders in the medically ill: scientific review and recommendations. Biol Psychiatry 2005; 58:175–189

3. Lopez AD, Murray CC: The global burden of disease, 1990–2020. Nat Med 1998; 4:1241–1243

4. American Psychiatric Association: Diagnostic and Statistical Manual of Mental Disorders, 4th ed. Washington, DC, APA, 1994

5. Hercher C, Turecki G, Mechawar N: Through the looking glass: examining neuroanatomical evidence for cellular alterations in major depression. J Psychiatr Res 2009; 43:947–961

6. Karege F, Vaudan G, Schwald M, Perroud N, La Harpe R: Neurotrophin levels in postmortem brains of suicide victims and the effects of antemortem diagnosis and psychotropic drugs. Brain Res Mol Brain Res 2005; 136:29–37

7. Soetanto A, Wilson RS, Talbot K, Un A, Schneider JA, Sobiesk M, Kelly J, Leurgans S, Bennett DA, Arnold SE: Association of anxiety and depression with microtubule-associated protein 2- and synaptopodin-immunolabeled dendrite and spine densities in hippocampal Ca3 of older humans. Arch Gen Psychiatry 2010; 67:448–457

8. Savitz J, Drevets WC: Bipolar and major depressive disorder: neuroimaging the developmental-degenerative divide. Neurosci Biobehav Rev 2009; 33:699–771

9. Videbech P, Ravnkilde B: Hippocampal volume and depression: a meta-analysis of MRI studies. Am J Psychiatry 2004; 161:1957–1966

10. Bernard R, Kerman IA, Thompson RC, Jones EG, Bunney WE, Barchas JD, Schatzberg AF, Myers RM, Akil H, Watson SJ: Altered expression of glutamate signaling, growth factor, and glia genes in the locus coeruleus of patients with major depression. Mol Psychiatry 2010; April 13 [Epub ahead of print]

11. Sibille E, Wang Y, Joeyen-Waldorf J, Gaiteri C, Surget A, Oh S, Belzung C, Tseng GC, Lewis DA: A molecular signature of depression in the amygdala. Am J Psychiatry 2009; 166:1011–1024

12. Covington HE 3rd, Maze I, LaPlant QC, Vialou VF, Ohnishi YN, Berton O, Fass DM, Renthal W, Rush AJ 3rd, Wu EY, Ghose S, Krishnan V, Russo SJ, Tamminga C, Haggarty SJ, Nestler EJ: Antidepressant actions of histone deacetylase inhibitors. J Neurosci 2009; 29:11451–11460

13. Krishnan V, Han MH, Graham DL, Berton O, Renthal W, Russo SJ, Laplant Q, Graham A, Lutter M, Lagace DC, Ghose S, Reister R, Tannous P, Green TA, Neve RL, Chakravarty S, Kumar A, Eisch AJ, Self DW, Lee FS, Tamminga CA, Cooper DC, Gershenfeld HK, Nestler EJ: Molecular adaptations underlying susceptibility and resistance to social defeat in brain reward regions. Cell 2007; 131:391–404

14. Krishnan V, Han MH, Mazei-Robison M, Iniguez SD, Ables JL, Vialou V, Berton O, Ghose S, Covington HE 3rd, Wiley MD, Henderson RP, Neve RL, Eisch AJ, Tamminga CA, Russo SJ, Bolanos CA, Nestler EJ: AKT signaling within the ventral tegmental area regulates cellular and behavioral responses to stressful stimuli. Biol Psychiatry 2008; 64:691–700

15. Svenningsson P, Chergui K, Rachleff I, Flajolet M, Zhang X, El Yacoubi M, Vaugeois JM, Nomikos GG, Greengard P: Alterations in 5-Ht1b receptor function by P11 in depression-like states. Science 2006; 311:77–80

16. Ressler KJ, Mayberg HS: Targeting abnormal neural circuits in mood and anxiety disorders: from the laboratory to the clinic. Nat Neurosci 2007; 10:1116–1124

17. Mayberg HS: Targeted electrode-based modulation of neural circuits for depression. J Clin Invest 2009; 119:717–725

18. Mayberg HS, Lozano AM, Voon V, McNeely HE, Seminowicz D, Hamani C, Schwalb JM, Kennedy SH: Deep brain stimulation for treatment-resistant depression. Neuron 2005; 45:651–660

19. Lozano AM, Mayberg HS, Giacobbe P, Hamani C, Craddock RC, Kennedy SH: Subcallosal cingulate gyrus deep brain stimulation for treatment-resistant depression. Biol Psychiatry 2008; 64:461–467

20. Bewernick BH, Hurlemann R, Matusch A, Kayser S, Grubert C, Hadrysiewicz B, Axmacher N, Lemke M, Cooper-Mahkorn D,

Cohen MX, Brockmann H, Lenartz D, Sturm V, Schlaepfer TE: Nucleus accumbens deep brain stimulation decreases ratings of depression and anxiety in treatment-resistant depression. Biol Psychiatry 2010; 67:110–116

21. Schlaepfer TE, Cohen MX, Frick C, Kosel M, Brodesser D, Axmacher N, Joe AY, Kreft M, Lenartz D, Sturm V: Deep brain stimulation to reward circuitry alleviates anhedonia in refractory major depression. Neuropsychopharmacology 2008; 33:368–377

22. Malone DA Jr, Dougherty DD, Rezai AR, Carpenter LL, Friehs GM, Eskandar EN, Rauch SL, Rasmussen SA, Machado AG, Kubu CS, Tyrka AR, Price LH, Stypulkowski PH, Giftakis JE, Rise MT, Malloy PF, Salloway SP, Greenberg BD: Deep brain stimulation of the ventral capsule/ventral striatum for treatment-resistant depression. Biol Psychiatry 2009; 65:267–275

23. Gross M, Nakamura L, Pascual-Leone A, Fregni F: Has repetitive transcranial magnetic stimulation (RTMS) treatment for depression improved? a systematic review and meta-analysis comparing the recent vs the earlier RTMS studies. Acta Psychiatr Scand 2007; 116:165–173

24. Montgomery EB Jr, Gale JT: Mechanisms of action of deep brain stimulation (DBS). Neurosci Biobehav Rev 2008; 32:388–407

25. Tsai HC, Zhang F, Adamantidis A, Stuber GD, Bonci A, de Lecea L, Deisseroth K: Phasic firing in dopaminergic neurons is sufficient for behavioral conditioning. Science 2009; 324:1080–1084

26. Kendler KS, Gatz M, Gardner CO, Pedersen NL: A Swedish national twin study of lifetime major depression. Am J Psychiatry 2006; 163:109–114

27. Shyn SI, Hamilton SP: The genetics of major depression: moving beyond the monoamine hypothesis. Psychiatr Clin North Am 2010; 33:125–140

28. López-León S, Janssens ACJW, González-Zuloeta Ladd AM, Del-Favero J, Claes SJ, Oostra BA, van Duijn CM: Meta-analyses of genetic studies on major depressive disorder. Mol Psychiatry 2007; 13:772–785

29. Trivedi MH, Rush AJ, Wisniewski SR, Nierenberg AA, Warden D, Ritz L, Norquist G, Howland RH, Lebowitz B, McGrath PJ, Shores-Wilson K, Biggs MM, Balasubramani GK, Fava M, STAR*D Study Team: Evaluation of outcomes with citalopram for depression using measurement-based care in STAR*D: implications for clinical practice. Am J Psychiatry 2006; 163:28–40

30. Garriock HA, Kraft JB, Shyn SI, Peters EJ, Yokoyama JS, Jenkins GD, Reinalda MS, Slager SL, McGrath PJ, Hamilton SP: A genomewide association study of citalopram response in major depressive disorder. Biol Psychiatry 2010; 67:133–138

31. Uher R, Huezo-Diaz P, Perroud N, Smith R, Rietschel M, Mors O, Hauser J, Maier W, Kozel D, Henigsberg N, Barreto M, Placentino A, Dernovsek MZ, Schulze TG, Kalember P, Zobel A, Czerski PM, Larsen ER, Souery D, Giovannini C, Gray JM, Lewis CM, Farmer A, Aitchison KJ, McGuffin P, Craig I: Genetic predictors of response to antidepressants in the GENDEP project. Pharmacogenomics J 2009; 9:225–233

32. Smith DF, Jakobsen S: Molecular tools for assessing human depression by positron emission tomography. Eur Neuropsychopharmacol 2009; 19:611–628

33. Ruhe HG, Mason NS, Schene AH: Mood is indirectly related to serotonin, norepinephrine and dopamine levels in humans: a meta-analysis of monoamine depletion studies. Mol Psychiatry 2007; 12:331–359

34. Muglia P, Tozzi F, Galwey NW, Francks C, Upmanyu R, Kong XQ, Antoniades A, Domenici E, Perry J, Rothen S, Vandeleur CL, Mooser V, Waeber G, Vollenweider P, Preisig M, Lucae S, Muller-Myhsok B, Holsboer F, Middleton LT, Roses AD: Genome-wide association study of recurrent major depressive disorder in two European case-control cohorts. Mol Psychiatry 2008; 15:589–601

35. Risch N, Herrell R, Lehner T, Liang KY, Eaves L, Hoh J, Griem A, Kovacs M, Ott J, Merikangas KR: Interaction between the serotonin transporter gene (5-HTTLPR), stressful life events, and risk of depression: a meta-analysis. JAMA 2009; 301:2462–2471

36. Nestler EJ, Barrot M, DiLeone RJ, Eisch AJ, Gold SJ, Monteggia LM: Neurobiology of depression. Neuron 2002; 34:13–25

37. Zarate CA Jr, Singh JB, Carlson PJ, Brutsche NE, Ameli R, Luckenbaugh DA, Charney DS, Manji HK: A randomized trial of an N-methyl-D-aspartate antagonist in treatment-resistant major depression. Arch Gen Psychiatry 2006; 63:856–864

38. Cryan JF, Slattery DA: Animal models of mood disorders: recent developments. Curr Opin Psychiatry 2007; 20:1–7

39. Kendler KS, Karkowski LM, Prescott CA: Causal relationship between stressful life events and the onset of major depression. Am J Psychiatry 1999; 156:837–841

40. Sloman L: A new comprehensive evolutionary model of depression and anxiety. J Affect Disord 2008; 106:219–228

41. Nesse RM: Is depression an adaptation? Arch Gen Psychiatry 2000; 57:14–20

42. Watson PJ, Andrews PW: Toward a revised evolutionary adaptationist analysis of depression: the social navigation hypothesis. J Affect Disord 2002; 72:1–14

43. Berton O, Covington HE 3rd, Ebner K, Tsankova NM, Carle TL, Ulery P, Bhonsle A, Barrot M, Krishnan V, Singewald GM, Singewald N, Birnbaum S, Neve RL, Nestler EJ: Induction of ΔFosB in the periaqueductal gray by stress promotes active coping responses. Neuron 2007; 55:289–300

44. Berton O, McClung CA, Dileone RJ, Krishnan V, Renthal W, Russo SJ, Graham D, Tsankova NM, Bolanos CA, Rios M, Monteggia LM, Self DW, Nestler EJ: Essential role of BDNF in the mesolimbic dopamine pathway in social defeat stress. Science 2006; 311:864–868

45. Lutter M, Krishnan V, Russo SJ, Jung S, McClung CA, Nestler EJ: Orexin signaling mediates the antidepressant-like effect of calorie restriction. J Neurosci 2008; 28:3071–3075

46. Lutter M, Sakata I, Osborne-Lawrence S, Rovinsky SA, Anderson JG, Jung S, Birnbaum S, Yanagisawa M, Elmquist JK, Nestler EJ, Zigman JM: The orexigenic hormone ghrelin defends against depressive symptoms of chronic stress. Nat Neurosci 2008; 11:752–753

47. Tsankova NM, Berton O, Renthal W, Kumar A, Neve RL, Nestler EJ: Sustained hippocampal chromatin regulation in a mouse model of depression and antidepressant action. Nat Neurosci 2006; 9:519–525

48. Wilkinson MB, Xiao G, Kumar A, LaPlant Q, Renthal W, Sikder D, Kodadek TJ, Nestler EJ: Imipramine treatment and resiliency exhibit similar chromatin regulation in the mouse nucleus accumbens in depression models. J Neurosci 2009; 29:7820–7832

49. Renthal W, Maze I, Krishnan V, Covington HE 3rd, Xiao G, Kumar A, Russo SJ, Graham A, Tsankova N, Kippin TE, Kerstetter KA, Neve RL, Haggarty SJ, McKinsey TA, Bassel-Duby R, Olson EN, Nestler EJ: Histone deacetylase 5 epigenetically controls behavioral adaptations to chronic emotional stimuli. Neuron 2007; 56:517–529

50. Anstrom KK, Miczek KA, Budygin EA: Increased phasic dopamine signaling in the mesolimbic pathway during social defeat in rats. Neuroscience 2009; 161:3–12

51. Chuang JC, Krishnan V, Yu HG, Mason B, Cui H, Wilkinson MB, Zigman JM, Elmquist JK, Nestler EJ, Lutter M: A beta3-adrenergic-leptin-melanocortin circuit regulates behavioral and metabolic changes induced by chronic stress. Biol Psychiatry 2010; 67:1075–1082

52. Vialou V, Robison AJ, Laplant QC, Covington HE 3rd, Dietz DM, Ohnishi YN, Mouzon E, Rush AJ 3rd, Watts EL, Wallace DL, Iniguez SD, Ohnishi YH, Steiner MA, Warren BL, Krishnan V, Bolanos CA, Neve RL, Ghose S, Berton O, Tamminga CA, Nestler

EJ: ΔFosB in brain reward circuits mediates resilience to stress and antidepressant responses. Nat Neurosci 2010; 13:745–752

53. Coryell MW, Wunsch AM, Haenfl er JM, Allen JE, Schnizler M, Ziemann AE, Cook MN, Dunning JP, Price MP, Rainier JD, Liu Z, Light AR, Langbehn DR, Wemmie JA: Acid-sensing ion channel-1a in the amygdala, a novel therapeutic target in depression-related behavior. J Neurosci 2009; 29:5381–5388

54. Ziemann AE, Allen JE, Dahdaleh NS, Drebot II, Coryell MW, Wunsch AM, Lynch CM, Faraci FM, Howard MA 3rd, Welsh MJ, Wemmie JA: The amygdala is a chemosensor that detects carbon dioxide and acidosis to elicit fear behavior. Cell 2009; 139:1012–1021

55. Heurteaux C, Lucas G, Guy N, El Yacoubi M, Thummler S, Peng XD, Noble F, Blondeau N, Widmann C, Borsotto M, Gobbi G, Vaugeois JM, Debonnel G, Lazdunski M: Deletion of the background potassium channel TREK-1 results in a depression-resistant phenotype. Nat Neurosci 2006; 9:1134–1141

56. Mazella J, Petrault O, Lucas G, Deval E, Beraud-Dufour S, Gandin C, El-Yacoubi M, Widmann C, Guyon A, Chevet E, Taouji S, Conductier G, Corinus A, Coppola T, Gobbi G, Nahon JL, Heurteaux C, Borsotto M: Spadin, a sortilin-derived peptide, targeting rodent TREK-1 channels: a new concept in the antidepressant drug design. PLoS Biol 2010; 8(4):e1000355

57. Kempermann G: The neurogenic reserve hypothesis: what is adult hippocampal neurogenesis good for? Trends Neurosci 2008; 31:163–169

58. Sahay A, Hen R: Adult hippocampal neurogenesis in depression. Nat Neurosci 2007; 10:1110–1115

59. Eisch AJ, Cameron HA, Encinas JM, Meltzer LA, Ming GL, Overstreet-Wadiche LS: Adult neurogenesis, mental health, and mental illness: hope or hype? J Neurosci 2008; 28:11785–11791

60. Airan RD, Meltzer LA, Roy M, Gong Y, Chen H, Deisseroth K: High-speed imaging reveals neurophysiological links to behavior in an animal model of depression. Science 2007; 317:819–823

61. Santarelli L, Saxe M, Gross C, Surget A, Battaglia F, Dulawa S, Weisstaub N, Lee J, Duman R, Arancio O, Belzung C, Hen R: Requirement of hippocampal neurogenesis for the behavioral effects of antidepressants. Science 2003; 301:805–809

62. Surget A, Saxe M, Leman S, Ibarguen-Vargas Y, Chalon S, Griebel G, Hen R, Belzung C: Drug-dependent requirement of hippocampal neurogenesis in a model of depression and of antidepressant reversal. Biol Psychiatry 2008; 64:293–301

63. Couillard-Despres S, Wuertinger C, Kandasamy M, Caioni M, Stadler K, Aigner R, Bogdahn U, Aigner L: Ageing abolishes the effects of fl uoxetine on neurogenesis. Mol Psychiatry 2009; 14:856–864

64. David DJ, Samuels BA, Rainer Q, Wang JW, Marsteller D, Mendez I, Drew M, Craig DA, Guiard BP, Guilloux JP, Artymyshyn RP, Gardier AM, Gerald C, Antonijevic IA, Leonardo ED, Hen R: Neurogenesis-dependent and -independent effects of fluoxetine in an animal model of anxiety/depression. Neuron 2009; 62:479–493

65. Tfilin M, Sudai E, Merenlender A, Gispan I, Yadid G, Turgeman G: Mesenchymal stem cells increase hippocampal neurogenesis and counteract depressive-like behavior. Mol Psychiatry 2009; Oct 27 [Epub ahead of print]

66. Lagace DC, Donovan MH, Decarolis NA, Farnbach LA, Malhotra S, Berton O, Nestler EJ, Krishnan V, Eisch AJ: Adult hippocampal neurogenesis is functionally important for stress-induced social avoidance. Proc Natl Acad Sci USA 2010; 107:4436–4441

67. Pittenger C, Duman RS: Stress, depression, and neuroplasticity: a convergence of mechanisms. Neuropsychopharmacology 2008; 33:88–109

68. Li Y, Luikart BW, Birnbaum S, Chen J, Kwon CH, Kernie SG, Bassel-Duby R, Parada LF: TrkB regulates hippocampal neurogenesis and governs sensitivity to antidepressive treatment. Neuron 2008; 59:399–412

69. Monteggia LM, Luikart B, Barrot M, Theobold D, Malkovska I, Nef S, Parada LF, Nestler EJ: Brain-derived neurotrophic factor conditional knockouts show gender differences in depression-related behaviors. Biol Psychiatry 2007; 61:187–197

70. Taliaz D, Stall N, Dar DE, Zangen A: Knockdown of brain-derived neurotrophic factor in specific brain sites precipitates behaviors associated with depression and reduces neurogenesis. Mol Psychiatry 2010; 15:80–92

71. Govindarajan A, Rao BS, Nair D, Trinh M, Mawjee N, Tonegawa S, Chattarji S: Transgenic brain-derived neurotrophic factor expression causes both anxiogenic and antidepressant effects. Proc Natl Acad Sci USA 2006; 103:13208–13213

72. Shirayama Y, Chen AC, Nakagawa S, Russell DS, Duman RS: Brain-derived neurotrophic factor produces antidepressant effects in behavioral models of depression. J Neurosci 2002; 22:3251–3261

73. Hoshaw BA, Malberg JE, Lucki I: Central administration of IGF-I and BDNF leads to long-lasting antidepressant-like effects. Brain Res 2005; 1037:204–208

74. Kato M, Serretti A: Review and meta-analysis of antidepressant pharmacogenetic findings in major depressive disorder. Mol Psychiatry 2010; 15:473–500

75. Verhagen M, van der Meij A, van Deurzen PA, Janzing JG, Arias-Vasquez A, Buitelaar JK, Franke B: Meta-analysis of the BDNF Val66Met polymorphism in major depressive disorder: effects of gender and ethnicity. Mol Psychiatry 2010; 15:260–271

76. Kaplitt MG, Feigin A, Tang C, Fitzsimons HL, Mattis P, Lawlor PA, Bland RJ, Young D, Strybing K, Eidelberg D, During MJ: Safety and tolerability of gene therapy with an adeno-associated virus (AAV) borne GAD gene for Parkinson's disease: an open label, phase I trial. Lancet 2007; 369:2097–2105

77. Croll SD, Chesnutt CR, Greene NA, Lindsay RM, Wiegand SJ: Peptide immunoreactivity in aged rat cortex and hippocampus as a function of memory and BDNF infusion. Pharmacol Biochem Behav 1999; 64:625–635

78. Sniderhan LF, Garcia-Bates TM, Burgart M, Bernstein SH, Phipps RP, Maggirwar SB: Neurotrophin signaling through tropomyosin receptor kinases contributes to survival and proliferation of non-Hodgkin lymphoma. Exp Hematol 2009; 37:1295–1309

79. Okamoto H, Voleti B, Banasr M, Sarhan M, Duric V, Girgenti MJ, Dileone RJ, Newton SS, Duman RS: Wnt2 expression and signaling is increased by different classes of antidepressant treatments. Biol Psychiatry 2010; June 4 [Epub ahead of print]

80. Caspi A, Moffitt TE: Gene-environment interactions in psychiatry: joining forces with neuroscience. Nat Rev Neurosci 2006; 7:583–590

81. Mill J, Petronis A: Molecular studies of major depressive disorder: the epigenetic perspective. Mol Psychiatry 2007; 12:799–814

82. Tsankova N, Renthal W, Kumar A, Nestler EJ: Epigenetic regulation in psychiatric disorders. Nat Rev Neurosci 2007; 8:355–367

83. Sharma S, Kelly TK, Jones PA: Epigenetics in cancer. Carcinogenesis 2010; 31:27–36

84. McGowan PO, Meaney MJ, Szyf M: Diet and the epigenetic (re)programming of phenotypic differences in behavior. Brain Res 2008; 1237:12–24

85. Murgatroyd C, Patchev AV, Wu Y, Micale V, Bockmuhl Y, Fischer D, Holsboer F, Wotjak CT, Almeida OF, Spengler D: Dynamic DNA methylation programs persistent adverse effects of early-life stress. Nat Neurosci 2009; 12:1559–1566

86. Renthal W, Nestler EJ: Epigenetic mechanisms in drug addiction. Trends Mol Med 2008; 14:341–350

87. Akbarian S, Huang HS: Epigenetic regulation in human brain—focus on histone lysine methylation. Biol Psychiatry 2009; 65:198–203

88. Nestler EJ, Carlezon WA Jr: The mesolimbic dopamine reward circuit in depression. Biol Psychiatry 2006; 59:1151–1159

89. Schultz W: Getting formal with dopamine and reward. Neuron 2002; 36:241–263

90. Dremencov E, El Mansari M, Blier P: Effects of sustained serotonin reuptake inhibition on the firing of dopamine neurons in the rat ventral tegmental area. J Psychiatry Neurosci 2009; 34:223–229

91. Tidey JW, Miczek KA: Social defeat stress selectively alters mesocorticolimbic dopamine release: an in vivo microdialysis study. Brain Res 1996; 721:140–149

92. Nelson JC, Papakostas GI: Atypical antipsychotic augmentation in major depressive disorder: a meta-analysis of placebo-controlled randomized trials. Am J Psychiatry 2009; 166:980–991

93. Brady KT, Sinha R: Co-occurring mental and substance use disorders: the neurobiological effects of chronic stress. Am J Psychiatry 2005; 162:1483–1493

94. Graham DL, Edwards S, Bachtell RK, DiLeone RJ, Rios M, Self DW: Dynamic BDNF activity in nucleus accumbens with cocaine use increases self-administration and relapse. Nat Neurosci 2007; 10:1029–1037

95. Wallace DL, Han MH, Graham DL, Green TA, Vialou V, Iniguez SD, Cao JL, Kirk A, Chakravarty S, Kumar A, Krishnan V, Neve RL, Cooper DC, Bolanos CA, Barrot M, McClung CA, Nestler EJ: CREB regulation of nucleus accumbens excitability mediates social isolation-induced behavioral deficits. Nat Neurosci 2009; 12:200–209

96. Wacker J, Dillon DG, Pizzagalli DA: The role of the nucleus accumbens and rostral anterior cingulate cortex in anhedonia: integration of resting EEG, fMRI, and volumetric techniques. Neuroimage 2009; 46:327–337

97. Smoski MJ, Felder J, Bizzell J, Green SR, Ernst M, Lynch TR, Dichter GS: fMRI of alterations in reward selection, anticipation, and feedback in major depressive disorder. J Affect Disord 2009; 118:69–78

98. Pizzagalli DA, Holmes AJ, Dillon DG, Goetz EL, Birk JL, Bogdan R, Dougherty DD, Iosifescu DV, Rauch SL, Fava M: Reduced caudate and nucleus accumbens response to rewards in unmedicated individuals with major depressive disorder. Am J Psychiatry 2009; 166:702–710

99. McCracken CB, Grace AA: Nucleus accumbens deep brain stimulation produces region-specific alterations in local field potential oscillations and evoked responses in vivo. J Neurosci 2009; 29:5354–5363

100. Golden SH: A review of the evidence for a neuroendocrine link between stress, depression and diabetes mellitus. Curr Diabetes Rev 2007; 3:252–259

101. McEwen BS: Physiology and neurobiology of stress and adaptation: central role of the brain. Physiol Rev 2007; 87:873–904

102. Pace TW, Miller AH: Cytokines and glucocorticoid receptor signaling: relevance to major depression. Ann NY Acad Sci 2009; 1179:86–105

103. Nemeroff CB, Widerlov E, Bissette G, Walleus H, Karlsson I, Eklund K, Kilts CD, Loosen PT, Vale W: Elevated concentrations of CSF corticotropin-releasing factor-like immunoreactivity in depressed patients. Science 1984; 226:1342–1344

104. Keller J, Flores B, Gomez RG, Solvason HB, Kenna H, Williams GH, Schatzberg AF: Cortisol circadian rhythm alterations in psychotic major depression. Biol Psychiatry 2006; 60:275–281

105. Gourley SL, Wu FJ, Kiraly DD, Ploski JE, Kedves AT, Duman RS, Taylor JR: Regionally specific regulation of ERK MAP kinase in a model of antidepressant-sensitive chronic depression. Biol Psychiatry 2008; 63:353–359

106. Brown ES: Effects of glucocorticoids on mood, memory, and the hippocampus: treatment and preventive therapy. Ann NY Acad Sci 2009; 1179:41–55

107. Simpson GM, El Sheshai A, Loza N, Kingsbury SJ, Fayek M, Rady A, Fawzy W: An 8-week open-label trial of a 6-day course of mifepristone for the treatment of psychotic depression. J Clin Psychiatry 2005; 66:598–602

108. Berton O, Nestler EJ: New approaches to antidepressant drug discovery: beyond monoamines. Nat Rev Neurosci 2006; 7:137–151

109. Holsboer F, Ising M: Central CRH system in depression and anxiety—evidence from clinical studies with CRH1 receptor antagonists. Eur J Pharmacol 2008; 583:350–357

110. Rakofsky JJ, Holtzheimer PE, Nemeroff CB: Emerging targets for antidepressant therapies. Curr Opin Chem Biol 2009; 13:291–302

111. Brouwer JP, Appelhof BC, Hoogendijk WJ, Huyser J, Endert E, Zuketto C, Schene AH, Tijssen JG, Van Dyck R, Wiersinga WM, Fliers E: Thyroid and adrenal axis in major depression: a controlled study in outpatients. Eur J Endocrinol 2005; 152:185–191

112. Vreeburg SA, Hoogendijk WJ, van Pelt J, Derijk RH, Verhagen JC, van Dyck R, Smit JH, Zitman FG, Penninx BW: Major depressive disorder and hypothalamic-pituitary-adrenal axis activity: results from a large cohort study. Arch Gen Psychiatry 2009; 66: 617–626

113. Stewart JW, Quitkin FM, McGrath PJ, Klein DF: Defining the boundaries of atypical depression: evidence from the HPA axis supports course of illness distinctions. J Affect Disord 2005; 86:161–167

114. Yehuda R: Status of glucocorticoid alterations in post-traumatic stress disorder. Ann NY Acad Sci 2009; 1179:56–69

115. Boyle MP, Brewer JA, Funatsu M, Wozniak DF, Tsien JZ, Izumi Y, Muglia LJ: Acquired deficit of forebrain glucocorticoid receptor produces depression-like changes in adrenal axis regulation and behavior. Proc Natl Acad Sci USA 2005; 102:473–478

116. Wei Q, Lu XY, Liu L, Schafer G, Shieh KR, Burke S, Robinson TE, Watson SJ, Seasholtz AF, Akil H: Glucocorticoid receptor overexpression in forebrain: a mouse model of increased emotional lability. Proc Natl Acad Sci USA 2004; 101:11851–11856

117. Dowlati Y, Herrmann N, Swardfager W, Liu H, Sham L, Reim EK, Lanctôt KL: A meta-analysis of cytokines in major depression. Biol Psychiatry 2010; 67:446–457

118. Miller AH, Maletic V, Raison CL: Inflammation and its discontents: the role of cytokines in the pathophysiology of major depression. Biol Psychiatry 2009; 65:732–741

119. Dunn AJ, Swiergiel AH, de Beaurepaire R: Cytokines as mediators of depression: what can we learn from animal studies? Neurosci Biobehav Rev 2005; 29:891–909

120. Koo JW, Russo SJ, Ferguson D, Nestler EJ, Duman RS: Nuclear factor-κb is a critical mediator of stress-impaired neurogenesis and depressive behavior. Proc Natl Acad Sci USA 2010; 107:2669–2674

121. Osterlund MK: Underlying mechanisms mediating the antidepressant effects of estrogens. Biochim Biophys Acta 2009; Nov 10 [Epub ahead of print]

122. Covington HE 3rd, Vialou V, Nestler EJ: From synapse to nucleus: novel targets for treating depression. Neuropharmacology 2010; 58:683–693

123. Goel N, Bale TL: Examining the intersection of sex and stress in modelling neuropsychiatric disorders. J Neuroendocrinol 2009; 21:415–420

124. LaPlant Q, Chakravarty S, Vialou V, Mukherjee S, Koo JW, Kalahasti G, Bradbury KR, Taylor SV, Maze I, Kumar A, Graham A, Birnbaum SG, Krishnan V, Truong HT, Neve RL, Nestler EJ, Russo SJ: Role of nuclear factor κb in ovarian hormone-

mediated stress hypersensitivity in female mice. Biol Psychiatry 2009; 65:874–880

125. Arnold AP, Chen X: What does the "four core genotypes" mouse model tell us about sex differences in the brain and other tissues? Front Neuroendocrinol 2009; 30:1–9

126. Quinn JJ, Hitchcott PK, Umeda EA, Arnold AP, Taylor JR: Sex chromosome complement regulates habit formation. Nat Neurosci 2007; 10:1398–1400

127. Lutter M, Nestler EJ: Homeostatic and hedonic signals interact in the regulation of food intake. J Nutr 2009; 139:629–632

128. Kishi T, Elmquist JK: Body weight is regulated by the brain: a link between feeding and emotion. Mol Psychiatry 2005; 10:132–146

129. Chaki S, Hirota S, Funakoshi T, Suzuki Y, Suetake S, Okubo T, Ishii T, Nakazato A, Okuyama S: Anxiolytic-like and antidepressant-like activities of MCL0129 (1-[(S)-2-(4-fluorophenyl)-2-(4-isopropylpiperadin-1-yl)ethyl]-4-[4-(2-methoxynaphthalen-1-yl)butyl]piperazine), a novel and potent nonpeptide antagonist of the melanocortin-4 receptor. J Pharmacol Exp Ther 2003; 304:818–826

130. Hommel JD, Trinko R, Sears RM, Georgescu D, Liu ZW, Gao XB, Thurmon JJ, Marinelli M, DiLeone RJ: Leptin receptor signaling in midbrain dopamine neurons regulates feeding. Neuron 2006; 51:801–810

131. Zigman JM, Elmquist JK: Minireview: from anorexia to obesity—the yin and yang of body weight control. Endocrinology 2003; 144:3749–3756

132. Lu XY, Kim CS, Frazer A, Zhang W: Leptin: a potential novel antidepressant. Proc Natl Acad Sci USA 2006; 103:1593–1598

133. Garza JC, Guo M, Zhang W, Lu XY: Leptin increases adult hippocampal neurogenesis in vivo and in vitro. J Biol Chem 2008; 283:18238–18247

134. Moon M, Kim S, Hwang L, Park S: Ghrelin regulates hippocampal neurogenesis in adult mice. Endocr J 2009; 56:525–531

135. Diano S, Farr SA, Benoit SC, McNay EC, da Silva I, Horvath B, Gaskin FS, Nonaka N, Jaeger LB, Banks WA, Morley JE, Pinto S, Sherwin RS, Xu L, Yamada KA, Sleeman MW, Tschop MH, Horvath TL: Ghrelin controls hippocampal spine synapse density and memory performance. Nat Neurosci 2006; 9:381–388

136. Oomura Y, Hori N, Shiraishi T, Fukunaga K, Takeda H, Tsuji M, Matsumiya T, Ishibashi M, Aou S, Li XL, Kohno D, Uramura K, Sougawa H, Yada T, Wayner MJ, Sasaki K: Leptin facilitates learning and memory performance and enhances hippocampal CA1 long-term potentiation and CaMK II phosphorylation in rats. Peptides 2006; 27:2738–2749

137. Abizaid A, Liu ZW, Andrews ZB, Shanabrough M, Borok E, Elsworth JD, Roth RH, Sleeman MW, Picciotto MR, Tschop MH, Gao XB, Horvath TL: Ghrelin modulates the activity and synaptic input organization of midbrain dopamine neurons while promoting appetite. J Clin Invest 2006; 116:3229–3239

138. Fulton S, Pissios P, Manchon RP, Stiles L, Frank L, Pothos EN, Maratos-Flier E, Flier JS: Leptin regulation of the mesoaccumbens dopamine pathway. Neuron 2006; 51:811–822

139. Luppino FS, de Wit LM, Bouvy PF, Stijnen T, Cuijpers P, Penninx BW, Zitman FG: Overweight, obesity, and depression: a systematic review and meta-analysis of longitudinal studies. Arch Gen Psychiatry 2010; 67:220–229

Paul E. Holtzheimer, M.D.

Advances in the Management of Treatment-Resistant Depression

Abstract: Treatment-resistant depression (TRD) is a prevalent, disabling, and costly condition affecting 1%–4% of the U.S. population. Current approaches to managing TRD include medication augmentation (with lithium, thyroid hormone, buspirone, atypical antipsychotics, or various antidepressant medications), psychotherapy, and ECT. Advances in understanding the neurobiology of mood regulation and depression have led to a number of new potential approaches to managing TRD, including medications with novel mechanisms of action and focal brain stimulation techniques. This review will define and discuss the epidemiology of TRD, review the current approaches to its management, and then provide an overview of several developing interventions.

TREATMENT-RESISTANT DEPRESSION: DEFINITION AND EPIDEMIOLOGY

Major depressive disorder is a widespread and costly illness, with a 1-year U.S. prevalence of about 7% (1). A variety of antidepressant treatments are available, but many patients fail to achieve sustained symptomatic remission. Continued depressive symptoms are associated with ongoing functional impairment (2), increased usage of health care resources (3), a greater risk of suicide (4–6), and overall increased mortality, especially associated with cardiovascular disease (7–10).

Despite the growing recognition of the public health importance of treatment-resistant depression (TRD), a consensus definition for this condition does not exist. Various approaches to stages of treatment resistance have been developed, including the Thase-Rush (11), Massachu-

setts General Hospital (12), and Maudsley systems (13). It has been conservatively estimated that >10% of depressed patients will not respond to multiple, adequate interventions (including medications, psychotherapy, and ECT) (14), and data from a large, community-based sequential treatment study (STAR*D) suggest that up to 33% of patients may fail to achieve full symptomatic remission despite multiple medication attempts (15). Studies of TRD have varied widely in the operational criteria used, but failure of at least two antidepressant treatments (of adequate dose and duration) from two distinct classes is one of the most consistent definitions in the literature (16). This definition also has predictive validity. In STAR*D, remission rates with the first two treatments were quite similar (36.8% in the first level and 30.6% in the second) but decreased significantly after a failure of two treatments (13.7% in the third level and 13.0% in the fourth) (15).

Considering these various definitions of TRD, the estimated prevalence ranges from 10% to 60% of all depressed patients (12, 14, 15), resulting in a U.S. prevalence of about 1%–4%, equal to or greater than the prevalence of schizophrenia, obsessive-compulsive disorder (OCD), or Alzheimer's dementia. And, for those patients who do eventually respond after multiple treatments, relapse is quite high (up to 80%) (17–19), emphasizing the fact that better strategies are needed to both treat and prevent depressive episodes.

CME Disclosure

Paul E. Holtzheimer, M.D. Assistant Professor, Department of Psychiatry and Behavioral Sciences, Emory University School of Medicine, Atlanta, GA

Dr. Holtzheimer has received grant funding from the Dana Foundation, Greenwall Foundation, NARSAD, NIMH (grant K23-MH077869), National Institutes of Health Loan Repayment Program, Northstar, Inc., Stanley Medical Research Institute, and Woodruff Foundation; he has received consulting fees from AvaCat Consulting, St. Jude Medical Neuromodulation, and Oppenheimer & Co.

Address correspondence to Paul E. Holtzheimer, M.D., 101 Woodruff Circle, Suite 4000, Atlanta, GA 30322; e-mail: pholtzh@emory.edu.

Reprinted with permission from FOCUS Fall 2010; 8(4):488–500.

Table 1. Common, Evidence-Based Medication Augmentation Approaches for TRD

Approach	Highest Level of Support	Comments
Lithium	Several placebo-controlled RCTs	Best data are from studies using TCAs or MAOIs; limited data with newer antidepressant medications
Thyroid hormone (T₃)	Several placebo-controlled RCTs	Best data are from studies using TCAs; limited data with newer antidepressant medications
Buspirone	Two placebo-controlled RCTs	One RCT was positive for patients with severe depression (but was not positive overall), the other was negative
Atypical antipsychotics	Several placebo-controlled RCTs for various agents	
Additional antidepressants		
Bupropion	Open-label studies	Most common approach in clinical practice
Mirtazapine	One placebo-controlled RCT	
TCA + SSRI/SNRI	Open-label studies	

RCT, randomized controlled trial.

CURRENT APPROACHES FOR MANAGING TRD

ESTABLISHING THE CORRECT DIAGNOSIS

When a patient presents with TRD, the first step is to confirm the primary diagnosis, assess for the presence of psychiatric and medical comorbidity, and verify the adequacy of prior treatments through a careful patient interview (with collateral information if available) and review of medical records (20). More than 10% of patients with the initial diagnosis of major depression may ultimately meet the criteria for bipolar disorder (21) and may require a modified treatment approach. Psychiatric comorbidity is common in depression and TRD (primarily anxiety, personality, and substance use disorders) (22, 23), and failure to achieve remission may be associated with inadequate treatment of these other conditions. Similarly, certain comorbid medical illnesses (e.g., sleep apnea, anemia, thyroid disease, hypogonadism, and others), as well as nonpsychiatric medications (e.g., corticosteroids, interferon alfa, and chemotherapy), may be associated with symptoms and side effects that overlap with those of depression. Finally, many patients with depression labeled as "treatment-resistant" may not have actually achieved adequate doses of prior medications for a sufficient duration (12, 14), such that a first step in management often includes increasing and potentially maximizing dose and duration of a current or prior treatment.

MEDICATION AUGMENTATION

For patients with documented treatment resistance to one or more medications, augmentation is a typical approach. Accepted augmentation agents for TRD include lithium, thyroid hormone, buspi-

rone, and atypical antipsychotics. Combining antidepressant medications is also quite common. Table 1 provides a summary of these approaches, including the highest level of support for each.

Lithium. Lithium augmentation (typically at doses ≥600 mg/day) currently has the most extensive evidence base with reported response rates between 40% and 50% (in depression studies, response is typically defined as a decrease in depression severity of at least 50% compared with baseline) (24). However, it should be noted that the majority of these studies combined lithium with a tricyclic antidepressant (TCA) or monoamine oxidase inhibitor (MAOI). The efficacy of lithium augmentation of newer antidepressants, especially selective serotonin reuptake inhibitors (SSRIs), is less clear (25). It is notable that lithium probably acts in part through modulation of the serotonin neurotransmitter system (26), such that it may be less mechanistically distinct from many newer medications compared with the older agents. In STAR*D, lithium was added after two failed treatment attempts that included bupropion, citalopram plus bupropion, citalopram plus buspirone, sertraline, or venlafaxine (27). Lithium augmentation was compared with triiodothyronine (T₃) augmentation (results for T₃ are described below). Lithium augmentation was associated with a 16% remission rate and a 16% response rate; 23% of patients dropped out due to side effects.

Thyroid hormone. Augmentation with 25–50 μg of T₃ also has an extensive database in medication-refractory depression (again with most studies adding this agent to a TCA). One meta-analysis found mixed results but generally confirmed a statistically significant advantage for T₃ augmentation of TCAs, with an overall response rate of 57% (a 23% improvement over placebo) (28). Another meta-analysis identified a statistically significant benefit for T_3 in accelerating the response to TCAs (29). In STAR*D, patients were randomly assigned to augmentation with either T_3 or lithium after two failed treatments (see above for details). T_3 augmentation was associated with a 25% remission rate and a 23% response rate (response was defined using a different scale than that used to define remission; in addition, it is possible that some patients achieved remission without having a 50% decrease in depression severity because of a partial response in the previous STAR*D levels); 10% of patients dropped out due to side effects. The numerical advantage of T3 over lithium augmentation was not statistically significant.

Buspirone. Buspirone augmentation (at doses ranging from 10 to 60 mg/day) has a mixed database supporting antidepressant efficacy (largely comprising open-label studies). One placebo-controlled trial (N=119) found no statistically significant benefit for buspirone augmentation in patients not responding to an SSRI (30). A second placebo-controlled trial (N=102) also found no overall augmentation benefit for buspirone but did identify statistically significantly greater antidepressant effects in patients with severe depression (31). Buspirone augmentation was used in the second level of STAR*D (for patients not achieving remission with citalopram) and compared with bupropion augmentation. Remission rates were virtually identical with the two agents (roughly 30%), although bupropion was associated with a greater reduction in self-rated depression severity and a lower dropout rate due to side effects.

Atypical antipsychotics. Atypical antipsychotic medications have previously shown benefit as augmentation agents for a number of SSRI-resistant nonpsychotic anxiety disorders (32–36). A recent meta-analysis of placebo-controlled trials found that atypical antipsychotic augmentation of an antidepressant medication was associated with statistically significantly greater response and remission rates, with a pooled response rate of 44% compared with 30% for placebo (37). Discontinuation due to side effects was greater for the antipsychotics compared with placebo. Aripiprazole is currently U.S. Food and Drug Administration (FDA)-approved for the treatment of depression not responding to an SSRI or a serotonin-norepinephrine reuptake inhibitor (SNRI). Quetiapine monotherapy and the combination agent olanzapine/fluoxetine have each received FDA approval for the treatment of bipolar depression.

Combining antidepressants. The most common combination of antidepressants is the addition of bupropion to an SSRI or SNRI (38, 39), despite a limited database with no placebo-controlled studies (40). As described above, bupropion augmentation of citalopram had a remission rate similar to that of buspirone augmentation in STAR*D, although there was some evidence for greater antidepressant effectiveness of bupropion overall. The efficacy of adding mirtazapine to an SSRI/SNRI is supported by a small database including at least one placebo-controlled trial (41, 42). The combination of an SSRI/SNRI with a TCA is somewhat supported by a limited dataset (43–46).

PSYCHOTHERAPY

Psychotherapy is a mainstay in the treatment of depression, and it is generally accepted that structured, evidence-based psychotherapies such as behavioral activation, cognitive behavior therapy, and interpersonal psychotherapy are as effective as antidepressant medications, even in moderate and severe depression (47–50). These therapies may also be effective in medication-resistant depression (48, 51, 52). Short-term psychodynamic therapies have also shown benefit for depression (53–56). The combination of psychotherapy with an antidepressant medication may be more effective than medication alone (49, 54, 57). Finally, psychotherapy may help prevent relapse, possibly to a greater degree than continued pharmacotherapy (58, 59). One challenge in managing patients with psychotherapy is that efficacy probably correlates with therapist skill and expertise (50), and some patients may not have ready or affordable access to an appropriate psychotherapist.

ECT

ECT was introduced in 1938 as a treatment for "schizophrenia" (60), yet has proved to be the most effective acute treatment for a major depressive episode (61, 62), with remission rates of more than 40%, even in patients with TRD (63–65). The efficacy of ECT has been validated in a number of open and blinded controlled trials, including comparisons with medication, sham ECT, and transcranial magnetic stimulation (62, 66–68). Cognitive side effects, especially retrograde amnesia, are common with ECT, and may be persistent (61, 69, 70). In addition, despite its acute efficacy, depressive relapse after a successful ECT course is still common, even when continuation ECT (ECT treatments delivered at an increasing time interval beyond the acute course) or optimal medication management is used (18, 63). Despite these limitations, ECT remains the best validated acute treatment for a major depressive episode, even when standard medication and psychotherapeutic interventions have not been effective.

ABLATIVE SURGERY

The first antidepressant medications were developed in the 1950s (71–73). Before this, treatments for patients with severe depression unresponsive to ECT were limited and often invasive [such as the prefrontal leucotomy (74)]. After the advent of pharmacotherapy for depression, neurosurgery remained an option for a small group of patients with severe and treatment-resistant depression, facilitated by the development of stereotactic neurosurgical techniques that allowed more focal ablation (75, 76). Ablative procedures in use today include capsulotomy (a lesion in the anterior limb of the internal capsule), cingulotomy (a lesion in the dorsal anterior cingulate), subcaudate tractotomy (a lesion in thalamocortical white matter tracts inferior to the anterior striatum), and limbic leucotomy (which combines a subcaudate tractotomy with a cingulotomy) (77). In TRD, the efficacy for these procedures in open-label, naturalistic studies has been judged to be between 22% and 75% (78, 79); side effects include epilepsy, cognitive abnormalities, and personality changes (78–80).

ADVANCES IN THE MANAGEMENT OF TRD

Two main approaches have defined the search for improved strategies for managing depression and TRD. The first has focused on development of novel medications. Although some of these continue to rely on modulation of monoaminergic neurotransmitter systems, the majority are based on targets in neuromodulatory systems beyond the monoamines. The second approach has focused on development and refinement of focal brain stimulation techniques, in which a focal electrical current is introduced in neural tissue with the goal of modulating activity locally and within a broader network of connected brain regions. This review will focus on medications and brain stimulation approaches for which published clinical data are available (see Table 2 for a summary).

NOVEL PHARMACOLOGICAL TARGETS

Dopamine agonists. Dopamine receptor agonists (pramipexole and ropinirole) are accepted treatments for Parkinson's disease (81). Data in TRD are limited, although two placebo-controlled trials in treatment-resistant bipolar depression (82, 83) and two open-label studies in treatment-resistant unipolar depression support potential efficacy (84, 85). A long-term (48-week) extension of an open-label study of pramipexole in unipolar TRD showed that 36% of patients achieving remission relapsed; the absence of a comparison group limits the interpretation of this finding (86). Larger, placebo-controlled trials of both pramipexole and ropinirole as augmentation agents in TRD have been initiated and/or completed (http://www.clinicaltrials.gov), but results have not been published.

Modulators of hypothalamic-pituitary-adrenal axis function. It is well-recognized that emotional or physical stress predisposes an individual to developing depression. Corticotrophin-releasing factor (CRF), a neuropeptide produced in the hypothalamus and released after a stressful event to initiate the stress hormone cascade, has been implicated in the pathophysiology of depression, largely through its actions at the CRF-1 receptor (87–90). Several CRF-1 receptor antagonists possess anxiolytic- and antidepressant-like effects in animal models (88). However, the early clinical data on these agents are mixed (91, 92), although several agents are currently in phase II/III studies (93).

Another strategy for modulating the hypothalamic-pituitary-adrenal axis involves interfering with the synthesis or action of glucocorticoids. Several medications (e.g., ketoconazole, aminoglutethimide, and metyrapone) decrease cortisol synthesis and have demonstrated antidepressant effects, although poor tolerability has hampered use and further development of these agents (94). The glucocorticoid 2 receptor antagonist mifepristone has shown antidepressant efficacy for chronic depression in a single case series (95), and overall clinical efficacy for psychotic depression in one open (96) and one blinded placebo-controlled study (97). In the latter, effects were greater for psychotic than depressive symptoms.

Substance P (NK-1) antagonists. Neurokinins are neuropeptides known to help mediate the neural processing of pain. The neurokinin substance P has been associated with the mammalian response to stressful stimuli (98, 99), and blocking its action can decrease the physiological and behavioral reactions to stress (100, 101). Substance P has also been implicated in the stress response in patients with major depression (102), and successful antidepressant treatment has been associated with decreased serum substance P levels (103). Agents that block a major substance P receptor (NK-1) have shown antidepressant-like effects in animal models. One NK-1 receptor antagonist, aprepitant, demonstrated antidepressant efficacy in a placebo-controlled study (100), but these results were not confirmed in a larger, phase III trial (104). Antidepressant effects have been seen with two other agents in early pilot studies (105, 106), but these findings await replication.

Glutamatergic modulation. Glutamate is the primary excitatory neurotransmitter in the brain that binds to both ionotropic [*N*-methyl-D-aspartate (NMDA), α-amino-3-hydroxy-5-methyl-4-isoxazolepropionic acid, and kainate) and metabotropic (G protein-coupled) receptors. Glutamatergic function is implicated in the neurobiology of depression (107–110). NMDA antagonists have shown antidepressant-like properties in animal studies (111, 112). Amantadine, an orally administered NMDA receptor antagonist, has show antidepressant-like effects as an augmentation agent in preclinical and clinical studies (113).

More recently, placebo-controlled trials have demonstrated very rapid (within a few hours) and significant antidepressant effects with a single intravenous infusion of ketamine in patients with treatment-resistant unipolar (114) and bipolar (115) depression. Unfortunately, these effects were time-limited, and depressive relapse occurred within days to weeks. An open-label study found that six repeated ketamine infusions were safe and generally well-tolerated in a group of 10 patients with TRD (116). Of the nine patients who received repeated infusions, all responded and eight achieved remission. One patient remained generally well for more than 3 months, but the other eight relapsed within 2 months (with a mean time to relapse of 19 days).

The antidepressant effects of ketamine may be mediated by a family history of alcoholism as suggested in an open-label study (117). Further, although memantine, an orally administered NMDA antagonist, did not have statistically significant antidepressant effects in a double-blind, placebo-controlled trial (118), it did show antidepressant effects equivalent to those of escitalopram in patients with major depression and alcohol dependence (119).

Riluzole is a medication with a complex and largely unknown mechanism of action that may involve inhibition of glutamate release. Open-label studies in treatment-resistant unipolar and bipolar depression suggest antidepressant efficacy for riluzole (120–122). However, riluzole failed to prevent relapse after successful antidepressant treatment with ketamine (123).

Scopolamine. Based on a database suggesting a role for the cholinergic system in the neurobiology of depression and antidepressant treatment, the antimuscarinic agent scopolamine was tested and demonstrated rapid (within days) antidepressant effects in a series of small, placebo-controlled trials (124, 125). No data on relapse were presented in these reports, so the duration of these effects is unknown.

S-Adenosylmethionine. *S*-Adenosylmethionine (SAMe) is a molecule involved in the transfer of methyl groups across a variety of biological substrates. A number of controlled studies have demonstrated antidepressant effects for intravenous or intramuscular SAMe (126). A recent double-blind, placebo-controlled trial of oral SAMe augmentation in patients not responding to an SSRI showed statistically significant antidepressant effects (127).

FOCAL BRAIN STIMULATION

The emergence of focal brain stimulation therapies over the past few decades has been jointly facilitated by major advances in neuroimaging and the technical ability to acutely and chronically stimulate a discrete neural target. Neuroimaging studies have helped map out a network of brain regions involved in the pathophysiology of depression and the neurobiological mechanisms of various treatments (128, 129); this work has helped postulate critical nodes within this network that might reasonably serve as targets for direct modulation. Such focal neuromodulation is now possible via noninvasive acute stimulation techniques [e.g., transcranial magnetic stimulation (TMS) and transcranial DC stimulation (tDCS)] as well as methods that allow for chronic stimulation but require surgery [e.g., vagus nerve stimulation (VNS), direct cortical stimulation (DCS), and deep brain stimulation (DBS)]. Two of these procedures (VNS and TMS) are currently approved by the FDA for the treatment of depression.

VNS. VNS involves stimulating the vagus nerve via an electrode that is surgically attached to the nerve where it courses through the neck. A subcutaneously implanted pulse generator (IPG) controls stimulation and serves as the power supply for the system. Common treatment parameters include chronic but intermittent stimulation (e.g., 30 seconds on every 5 minutes). In 1997, VNS was approved by the FDA for the treatment of medication-resistant epilepsy. Observations of positive mood effects in some patients with epilepsy led to testing in medication-resistant depression. A double-blind, sham-controlled trial (on versus off stimulation) showed no statistically significant antidepressant effects for 10 weeks of active VNS, with a response of 15% for active VNS versus a 10% response rate with sham VNS (130). However, open-label data suggest increasing antidepressant efficacy over a year of stimulation [in combination with

Table 2. Developing Treatment Options for TRD

Approach	Highest Level of Support	Comments
Dopamine agonists	Two placebo-controlled RCTs	
CRF-1 receptor antagonists	Open-label data	One negative placebo-controlled RCT has been published
Glucocorticoid receptor antagonists	One placebo-controlled RCT for mifepristone	Study was done in patients with psychotic depression; benefits were greater for psychotic than depressive symptoms
Substance P receptor antagonists	Two placebo-controlled RCTs for aprepitant Open-label data for 2 other agents	The smaller RCT was positive, but the larger phase III study was negative
Ketamine	Two placebo-controlled RCTs	Effects are acute (within a few hours), but relapse generally occurs within a few days
Riluzole	Open-label studies	
Scopolamine	Two placebo-controlled RCTs	
SAMe	One placebo-controlled RCT	
VNS	Three long-term open-label studies	A 10-week sham-controlled RCT was negative; data from one long-term open-label study were compared with those from a nonrandomized, treatment-as-usual group followed for a similar period of time
TMS	Several sham-controlled RCTs	Data from a large, industry-sponsored RCT suggest no statistically significant antidepressant effect for TMS in patients in whom more than one adequate antidepressant medication has failed
MST	Open-label comparisons to ECT	One study suggested greater antidepressant efficacy for ECT over MST
tDCS	Three sham-controlled RCTs	Two of the three RCTs were positive; one was negative
DCS	One open-label study	
DBS	One open-label study for each of 3 targets (SCC, VC/VS, and NAcc) Single case reports for 2 other targets (ITP and habenula)	

RCT, randomized controlled trial; SCC, subcallosal cingulate; VC/VS, ventral capsule/ventral striatum; NAcc, nucleus accumbens; ITP, inferior thalamic peduncle.

treatment-as-usual (TAU)] in patients in whom between two and six adequate treatments in the current episode have failed, with reported response rates of 27%–53% and remission rates of 16%–33% (131–133). Response and remission rates appear to either remain stable or may continue to increase with 2 years of stimulation (134, 135).

In a nonrandomized comparison with patients with TRD receiving only TAU, 1-year response rates were statistically significantly higher in the VNS + TAU group (27% versus 13%). In addition, VNS + TAU only showed a 23%–35% relapse rate over an additional year of stimulation (136) compared with a 62% relapse rate in the TAU-only group over an equivalent time period (137). However, a European study suggested that only 44% of patients receiving VNS sustain a response over an additional year of stimulation (133).

Risks of VNS surgery are minor, and adverse effects associated with acute and chronic stimulation include

Figure 1. A Proposed General Algorithm for Approaching and Managing a Patient with TRD. EEG, Electroencephalography.

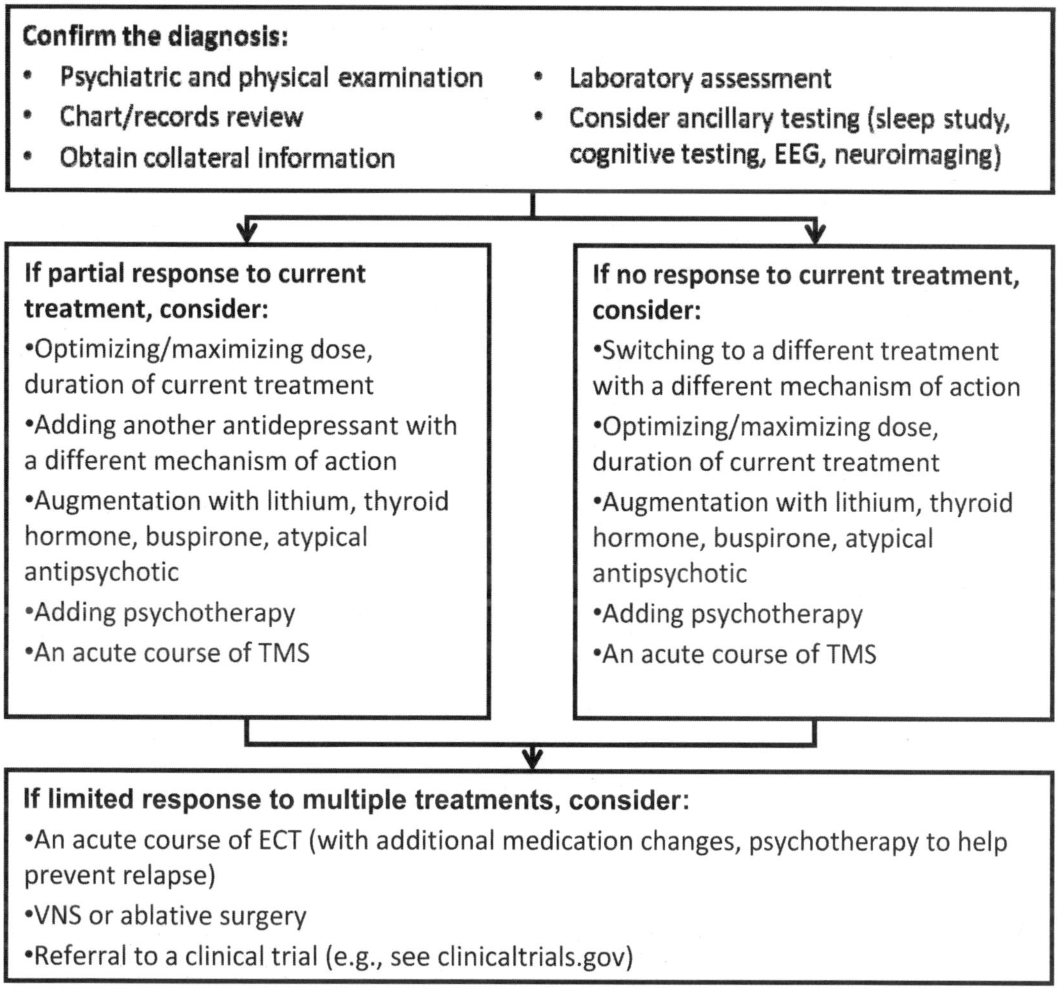

Confirm the diagnosis:

- Psychiatric and physical examination
- Chart/records review
- Obtain collateral information
- Laboratory assessment
- Consider ancillary testing (sleep study, cognitive testing, EEG, neuroimaging)

If partial response to current treatment, consider:

- Optimizing/maximizing dose, duration of current treatment
- Adding another antidepressant with a different mechanism of action
- Augmentation with lithium, thyroid hormone, buspirone, atypical antipsychotic
- Adding psychotherapy
- An acute course of TMS

If no response to current treatment, consider:

- Switching to a different treatment with a different mechanism of action
- Optimizing/maximizing dose, duration of current treatment
- Augmentation with lithium, thyroid hormone, buspirone, atypical antipsychotic
- Adding psychotherapy
- An acute course of TMS

If limited response to multiple treatments, consider:

- An acute course of ECT (with additional medication changes, psychotherapy to help prevent relapse)
- VNS or ablative surgery
- Referral to a clinical trial (e.g., see clinicaltrials.gov)

voice changes, coughing, and difficulty swallowing. In general, VNS appears to be cognitively safe, although stimulation intensity may be associated with some modest cognitive impairments (80, 138). The published data suggest that more than 80% of patients receiving VNS choose to continue stimulation even in the absence of an antidepressant response, suggesting that the treatment is generally well-tolerated.

TMS. TMS uses an electromagnetic coil placed on the head to generate a depolarizing electrical current in the underlying cortex. Repetitive TMS (rTMS) delivers a train of stimuli at a set frequency, with "high-frequency" denoting ≥ 5 Hz stimulation and "low-frequency" denoting ≤ 1 Hz stimulation. A series of stimulation trains are given during each treatment session, and a typical treatment course involves daily sessions (each lasting about 1 hour) for 3–6 weeks. Pa-

tients are awake during treatment, and no anesthesia is required.

The types of rTMS most commonly studied for the treatment of depression include high-frequency rTMS (generally 5–20 Hz) applied to the left dorsolateral prefrontal cortex (DLPFC) and low-frequency rTMS (generally 1 Hz) applied to the right DLPFC. Safety and efficacy have been demonstrated for both approaches through a number of relatively small open-label and sham-controlled studies (139–144). Although effect sizes in favor of active rTMS have been moderately strong, absolute response rates have been relatively low (generally between 20% and 40% in sham-controlled studies).

Higher stimulation intensity and total number of pulses delivered (i.e., longer treatment sessions and more sessions over time) are associated with better antidepressant effects (145). High-frequency rTMS seems to be less effective in psychotic versus nonpsychotic depressed patients (67) and those with a longer versus shorter (<5 years) duration of the current episode (146). One study suggests lower efficacy in patients with late-life depression (147), although it is noted that this study probably did not use optimal treatment parameters, and the efficacy of rTMS may be lower if stimulation intensity is not adjusted upward to account for prefrontal cortical atrophy (148, 149), which was not done in this study of older patients.

Two multicenter, randomized, sham-controlled studies have helped clarify the safety and efficacy of rTMS as a monotherapy for medication-resistant depression. In an industry-sponsored study of medication-free patients who had not responded to at least one antidepressant medication, 4–6 weeks of high-frequency left DLPFC rTMS was associated with statistically significant antidepressant effects compared to sham rTMS, including higher response (24% versus 12%) and remission rates (14% versus 6%) after 6 weeks of treatment (150). However, a secondary analysis showed that the difference in antidepressant efficacy between active and sham rTMS was only statistically significant in those patients in whom no more than one medication (of adequate dose and duration) had failed in the current episode (151). A four-site National Institute of Mental Health-funded study using stimulation parameters and eligibility criteria similar to the industry-sponsored study also showed statistically significant antidepressant effects for active rTMS with remission rates similar to those in the industry study (152). These data also suggested that rTMS was more effective in patients with a lower degree of medication resistance. The long-term efficacy of rTMS is largely unknown, with studies suggesting relapse rates similar to those seen after ECT (153, 154). Repeated rTMS courses may be beneficial in helping to maintain benefit over time (155).

Although rTMS can result in seizures, this is highly unlikely when stimulation parameters are maintained within suggested safety guidelines (156). Common side effects of rTMS include pain at the site of stimulation and headaches, although most patients tolerate treatments very well (150, 152). There are no cognitive side effects associated with rTMS for depression (80). A potential disadvantage of rTMS as currently administered is the need for daily treatments over several weeks. However, in a recent open-label study testing accelerated rTMS (in which 15 treatment sessions were delivered over 2 days in an inpatient setting) (157), response and remission rates immediately after treatment were 43% and 29%, respectively, and were largely maintained over the next 6 weeks; side effects

were similar to and no more severe than those seen with daily rTMS.

Magnetic seizure therapy. More focal ECT administration is associated with fewer cognitive side effects but equivalent efficacy compared with less focal techniques (158, 159). Based on this finding, it was hypothesized that if seizures could be generated using very focal stimulation (i.e., with TMS), then efficacy approaching that of ECT could be achieved with an even better cognitive side effect profile. Similar to ECT, magnetic seizure therapy (MST) is performed under general anesthesia and involves the serial induction of seizures over several weeks. Preliminary data suggest that MST has antidepressant effects and may result in fewer cognitive side effects than ECT (160–162). Larger trials are currently underway.

tDCS. tDCS is a noninvasive technique that modulates cortical excitatory tone (rather than causing neuronal depolarization) via a weak electrical current generated by two scalp electrodes. Five sessions of tDCS applied to the left DLPFC have shown mixed antidepressant efficacy in sham-controlled studies with one study finding a statistically significant antidepressant benefit (163) but another failing to replicate this (164). A third sham-controlled study using 10 sessions demonstrated antidepressant efficacy for active tDCS (165). In general, tDCS is very well-tolerated with no known cognitive side effects.

DCS. Direct cortical stimulation involves electrical stimulation of the cortex via one or more electrodes surgically placed in either the epidural or subdural space. Similar to VNS, stimulation is driven by an IPG connected to the electrodes via subcutaneous wires. In a small pilot study of DCS of the medial and lateral prefrontal cortices, three of five patients with TRD achieved remission after 7 months of chronic, intermittent stimulation (in these patients at least four adequate treatments had failed in the current episode) (166). DCS was very well tolerated, although one patient required explantation due to a scalp infection.

DBS. DBS is achieved by placing a thin electrode through a burr hole in the skull into a specific brain region using imaging-guided stereotactic neurosurgical techniques. Electrodes can be placed in essentially any brain region and can be implanted unilaterally or bilaterally. Each electrode typically contains several distinct contacts that can be used to provide monopolar or bipolar stimulation. As with VNS and DCS, the electrodes are connected via subcutaneous wires to an IPG that controls stimulation.

DBS is an established treatment for patients with severe, treatment-resistant Parkinson's disease, essential tremor, and dystonia. DBS has largely replaced ablative surgery in these conditions because it can be adjusted to achieve maximal benefit with a minimum of side effects and can be turned off or completely removed in the case of severe, unwanted side effects. DBS of the anterior internal capsule [as a potential replacement for capsulotomy; this target is also referred to as the ventral capsule/ventral striatum (VC/VS)] has shown potential safety and efficacy for patients with severe treatment-refractory OCD based on a multicenter open-label case series of 26 patients (167). This intervention is now FDA-approved via a Humanitarian Device Exemption. DBS of the subthalamic nucleus has also shown efficacy for OCD in a 6-month sham-controlled study (168).

Based on a converging neuroanatomical database suggesting a critical role for Brodmann area 25 in a neural network involved in depression and antidepressant response, Mayberg and colleagues (169, 170) demonstrated that open-label subcallosal cingulate DBS was associated with antidepressant effects in a cohort of 20 patients with severe TRD in whom at least four treatments had failed in the current episode. After 6 months of chronic stimulation, 60% of patients achieved response and 35% achieved remission; these effects were largely maintained over an additional 6 months with 72% of 6-month responders still meeting the response criteria at 12 months (and three additional patients achieving response by 12 months). Adverse events related to the procedure included skin infection (leading to explantation in two patients) and perioperative pain/headache related to surgery. There were no negative effects associated with acute or chronic DBS, and no negative cognitive effects (171).

In studies of VC/VS DBS for OCD, it was noted that many patients experienced significant improvement in comorbid depression (167), leading to testing of VC/VS DBS for TRD without comorbid OCD. After 6 months of chronic stimulation in 15 patients with TRD enrolled in a three-center open-label pilot study, 40% of patients achieved response and 27% achieved remission (172). At the last follow-up (an average of 24 ± 15 months after onset of stimulation, with a range of 6–51 months), there was a 53% response rate and a 33% remission rate. Adverse effects related to surgery and/or the device included perioperative pain and a DBS electrode break. Adverse effects of stimulation included hypomania, anxiety, perseverative speech, autonomic symptoms, and involuntary facial movements; these were mostly reversible with a stimulation parameter change. No cognitive side effects were described.

The most ventral aspect of the VC/VS DBS target includes the nucleus accumbens, a region implicated in reward processing. This region was targeted for DBS in a cohort of 10 patients with TRD in an open-label pilot study, with 50% of patients achieving an antidepressant response after 6 months of chronic stimulation (173). Case reports have described potential antidepressant efficacy of DBS of the inferior thalamic peduncle (which contains thalamocortical projection fibers) (174) and the habenula (which is involved in modulation of monoaminergic neurotransmission) (175).

SUMMARY AND CONCLUSIONS

TRD is a prevalent and disabling condition with few evidence-based treatments available. Several medication augmentation or combination strategies currently exist, but the supporting database is limited and overall response and remission rates are relatively low in patients with TRD. Psychotherapy has shown significant potential as a treatment for depression and TRD but it is relatively understudied, and patient access can be limited. ECT is highly effective, even in TRD, for getting a patient out of a depressed episode, but relapse rates are high. A general algorithm for approaching the patient with TRD is given in Figure 1.

Advances in the management of TRD include the development of a number of novel pharmacological agents, many of which target systems outside the monoamines, as well as several focal neuromodulation techniques. Overall, there is optimism that these strategies will lead to antidepressant treatments to help achieve and sustain remission in a greater number of depressed patients. However, progress to date has been limited: despite encouraging preliminary results, none of the novel drugs are yet established for clinical use; the two FDA-approved brain stimulation therapies (VNS and TMS) are associated with relatively low response and remission rates, and neither has shown efficacy in those patients with the most extreme forms of treatment-resistant depression (i.e., more than six treatment failures in the current episode); and data on the remaining brain stimulation approaches are far too preliminary to draw meaningful conclusions regarding safety and efficacy. Still, the efforts of the past decade herald a new era of antidepressant treatment development, and it is highly likely that this work will eventually result in new and more powerful antidepressant therapies.

REFERENCES

1. Kessler RC, Chiu WT, Demler O, Merikangas KR, Walters EE: Prevalence, severity, and comorbidity of 12-month DSM-IV disorders in the National Comorbidity Survey Replication. Arch Gen Psychiatry 2005; 62:617–627
2. Miller IW, Keitner GI, Schatzberg AF, Klein DN, Thase ME, Rush AJ, Markowitz JC, Schlager DS, Kornstein SG, Davis SM, Harrison WM, Keller MB: The treatment of chronic depression, part 3: psychosocial

functioning before and after treatment with sertraline or imipramine. J Clin Psychiatry 1998; 59:608–619

3. Crown WH, Finkelstein S, Berndt ER, Ling D, Poret AW, Rush AJ, Russell JM: The impact of treatment-resistant depression on health care utilization and costs. J Clin Psychiatry 2002; 63:963–971

4. Nelsen MR, Dunner DL: Clinical and differential diagnostic aspects of treatment-resistant depression. J Psychiatr Res 1995; 29:43–50

5. Papakostas GI, Petersen T, Pava J, Masson E, Worthington JJ 3rd, Alpert JE, Fava M, Nierenberg AA: Hopelessness and suicidal ideation in outpatients with treatment-resistant depression: prevalence and impact on treatment outcome. J Nerv Ment Dis 2003; 191:444–449

6. Fawcett J, Harris SG: Suicide in treatment-refractory depression, in Treatment-Resistant Mood Disorders. New York, NY, Cambridge University Press, 2001, pp 479–488

7. Everson SA, Roberts RE, Goldberg DE, Kaplan GA: Depressive symptoms and increased risk of stroke mortality over a 29-year period. Arch Intern Med 1998; 158:1133–1138

8. Penninx BW, Beekman AT, Honig A, Deeg DJ, Schoevers RA, van Eijk JT, van Tilburg W: Depression and cardiac mortality: results from a community-based longitudinal study. Arch Gen Psychiatry 2001; 58:221–227

9. Carney RM, Freedland KE: Treatment-resistant depression and mortality after acute coronary syndrome. Am J Psychiatry 2009; 166:410–417

10. Murphy JM, Monson RR, Olivier DC, Sobol AM, Leighton AH: Affective disorders and mortality. A general population study. Arch Gen Psychiatry 1987; 44:473–480

11. Thase M, Rush A: When at first you don't succeed: sequential strategies for antidepressant non-responders. J Clin Psychiatry 1997; 58(suppl 13):23–29

12. Fava M: Diagnosis and definition of treatment-resistant depression. Biol Psychiatry 2003; 53:649–659

13. Fekadu A, Wooderson S, Donaldson C, Markopoulou K, Masterson B, Poon L, Cleare AJ: A multidimensional tool to quantify treatment resistance in depression: The Maudsley staging method. J Clin Psychiatry 2009; 70:177–184

14. Nierenberg AA, Amsterdam JD: Treatment-resistant depression: definition and treatment approaches. J Clin Psychiatry 1990; 51(suppl):39–47; discussion 48–50

15. Rush AJ, Trivedi MH, Wisniewski SR, Nierenberg AA, Stewart JW, Warden D, Niederehe G, Thase ME, Lavori PW, Lebowitz BD, McGrath PJ, Rosenbaum JF, Sackeim HA, Kupfer DJ, Luther J, Fava M: Acute and longer-term outcomes in depressed outpatients requiring one or several treatment steps: a STAR*D report. Am J Psychiatry 2006; 163:1905–1917

16. Berlim MT, Turecki G: What is the meaning of treatment resistant/refractory major depression (TRD)? A systematic review of current randomized trials. Eur Neuropsychopharmacol 2007; 17:696–707

17. Fekadu A, Wooderson SC, Markopoulo K, Donaldson C, Papadopoulos A, Cleare AJ: What happens to patients with treatment-resistant depression? A systematic review of medium to long term outcome studies. J Affect Disord 2009; 116:4–11

18. Sackeim HA, Haskett RF, Mulsant BH, Thase ME, Mann JJ, Pettinati HM, Greenberg RM, Crowe RR, Cooper TB, Prudic J: Continuation pharmacotherapy in the prevention of relapse following electroconvulsive therapy: a randomized controlled trial. JAMA 2001; 285:1299–1307

19. Rasmussen KG, Mueller M, Rummans TA, Husain MM, Petrides G, Knapp RG, Fink M, Sampson SM, Bailine SH, Kellner CH: Is baseline medication resistance associated with potential for relapse after successful remission of a depressive episode with ECT? Data from the Consortium for Research on Electroconvulsive Therapy (CORE). J Clin Psychiatry 2009; 70:232–237

20. Berlim MT, Fleck MP, Turecki G: Current trends in the assessment and somatic treatment of resistant/refractory major depression: an overview. Ann Med 2008; 40:149–159

21. Akiskal HS, Maser JD, Zeller PJ, Endicott J, Coryell W, Keller M, Warshaw M, Clayton P, Goodwin F: Switching from 'unipolar' to bipolar II. An 11-year prospective study of clinical and temperamental predictors in 559 patients. Arch Gen Psychiatry 1995; 52:114–123

22. Souery D, Oswald P, Massat I, Bailer U, Bollen J, Demyttenaere K, Kasper S, Lecrubier Y, Montgomery S, Serretti A, Zohar J, Mendlewicz J, Group for the Study of Resistant Depression: Clinical factors associated with treatment resistance in major depressive disorder: results from a European multicenter study. J Clin Psychiatry 2007; 68:1062–1070

23. Kessler RC, Berglund P, Demler O, Jin R, Koretz D, Merikangas KR, Rush AJ, Walters EE, Wang PS, National Comorbidity Survey Replication: The epidemiology of major depressive disorder: results from the National Comorbidity Survey Replication (NCS-R). JAMA 2003; 289:3095–3105

24. Bauer M, Forsthoff A, Baethge C, Adli M, Berghöfer A, Döpfmer S, Bschor T: Lithium augmentation therapy in refractory depression-update 2002. Eur Arch Psychiatry Clin Neurosci 2003; 253:132–139

25. Fava M, Rush AJ, Trivedi MH, Nierenberg AA, Thase ME, Sackeim HA, Quitkin FM, Wisniewski S, Lavori PW, Rosenbaum JF, Kupfer DJ: Background and rationale for the sequenced treatment alternatives to relieve depression (STAR*D) study. Psychiatr Clin North Am 2003; 26:457–494, x

26. Chenu F, Bourin M: Potentiation of antidepressant-like activity with lithium: mechanism involved. Curr Drug Targets 2006; 7:159–163

27. Nierenberg AA, Fava M, Trivedi MH, Wisniewski SR, Thase ME, McGrath PJ, Alpert JE, Warden D, Luther JF, Niederehe G, Lebowitz B, Shores-Wilson K, Rush AJ: A comparison of lithium and T_3. Augmentation following two failed medication treatments for depression: A STAR*D report. Am J Psychiatry 2006; 163:1519–1530; quiz 1665

28. Aronson R, Offman HJ, Joffe RT, Naylor CD: Triiodothyronine augmentation in the treatment of refractory depression. A meta-analysis. Arch Gen Psychiatry 1996; 53:842–848

29. Altshuler LL, Bauer M, Frye MA, Gitlin MJ, Mintz J, Szuba MP, Leight KL, Whybrow PC: Does thyroid supplementation accelerate tricyclic antidepressant response? A review and meta-analysis of the literature. Am J Psychiatry 2001; 158:1617–1622

30. Landén M, Björling G, Agren H, Fahlén T: A randomized, double-blind, placebo-controlled trial of buspirone in combination with an SSRI in patients with treatment-refractory depression. J Clin Psychiatry 1998; 59:664–668

31. Appelberg BG, Syvälahti EK, Koskinen TE, Mehtonen OP, Muhonen TT, Naukkarinen HH: Patients with severe depression may benefit from buspirone augmentation of selective serotonin reuptake inhibitors: results from a placebo-controlled, randomized, double-blind, placebo wash-in study. J Clin Psychiatry 2001; 62:448–452

32. Bystritsky A, Ackerman DL, Rosen RM, Vapnik T, Gorbis E, Maidment KM, Saxena S: Augmentation of serotonin reuptake inhibitors in refractory obsessive-compulsive disorder using adjunctive olanzapine: a placebo-controlled trial. J Clin Psychiatry 2004; 65:565–568

33. Bartzokis G, Lu PH, Turner J, Mintz J, Saunders CS: Adjunctive risperidone in the treatment of chronic combat-related posttraumatic stress disorder. Biol Psychiatry 2005; 57:474–479

34. Stein MB, Kline NA, Matloff JL: Adjunctive olanzapine for SSRI-resistant combat-related PTSD: a double-blind, placebo-controlled study. Am J Psychiatry 2002; 159:1777–1779

35. Pollack MH, Simon NM, Zalta AK, Worthington JJ, Hoge EA, Mick E, Kinrys G, Oppenheimer J: Olanzapine augmentation of fluoxetine for refractory generalized anxiety disorder: a placebo controlled study. Biol Psychiatry 2006; 59:211–215

36. Brawman-Mintzer O, Knapp RG, Nietert PJ: Adjunctive risperidone in generalized anxiety disorder: a double-blind, placebo-controlled study. J Clin Psychiatry 2005; 66:1321–1325

37. Nelson JC, Papakostas GI: Atypical antipsychotic augmentation in major depressive disorder: a meta-analysis of placebo-controlled randomized trials. Am J Psychiatry 2009; 166:980–991

38. Mischoulon D, Nierenberg AA, Kizilbash L, Rosenbaum JF, Fava M: Strategies for managing depression refractory to selective serotonin reuptake inhibitor treatment: a survey of clinicians. Can J Psychiatry 2000; 45:476–481

39. Fredman SJ, Fava M, Kienke AS, White CN, Nierenberg AA, Rosenbaum JF: Partial response, nonresponse, and relapse with selective serotonin reuptake inhibitors in major depression: a survey of current "next-step" practices. J Clin Psychiatry 2000; 61:403–408

40. Zisook S, Rush AJ, Haight BR, Clines DC, Rockett CB: Use of bupropion in combination with serotonin reuptake inhibitors. Biol Psychiatry 2006; 59:203–210

41. Papakostas GI: Managing partial response or nonresponse: switching, augmentation, and combination strategies for major depressive disorder. J Clin Psychiatry 2009; 70(suppl 6):16–25

42. Carpenter LL, Yasmin S, Price LH: A double-blind, placebo-controlled study of antidepressant augmentation with mirtazapine. Biol Psychiatry 2002; 51:183–188

43. Gillman PK: Tricyclic antidepressant pharmacology and therapeutic drug interactions updated. Br J Pharmacol 2007; 151:737–748

44. Gómez Gómez JM, Teixidó Perramón C: Combined treatment with venlafaxine and tricyclic antidepressants in depressed patients who had partial response to clomipramine or imipramine: initial findings. J Clin Psychiatry 2000; 61:285–289

45. Amsterdam JD, García-España F, Rosenzweig M: Clomipramine augmentation in treatment-resistant depression. Depress Anxiety 1997; 5:84–90

46. Fava M, Rosenbaum JF, McGrath PJ, Stewart JW, Amsterdam JD, Quitkin FM: Lithium and tricyclic augmentation of fluoxetine treatment for resistant major depression: a double-blind, controlled study. Am J Psychiatry 1994; 151:1372–1374

47. Gloaguen V, Cottraux J, Cucherat M, Blackburn IM: A meta-analysis of

the effects of cognitive therapy in depressed patients. J Affect Disord 1998; 49:59–72

48. Thase ME, Friedman ES, Biggs MM, Wisniewski SR, Trivedi MH, Luther JF, Fava M, Nierenberg AA, McGrath PJ, Warden D, Niederehe G, Hollon SD, Rush AJ: Cognitive therapy versus medication in augmentation and switch strategies as second-step treatments: a STAR*D report. Am J Psychiatry 2007; 164:739–752

49. Keller MB, McCullough JP, Klein DN, Arnow B, Dunner DL, Gelenberg AJ, Markowitz JC, Nemeroff CB, Russell JM, Thase ME, Trivedi MH, Zajecka J: A comparison of nefazodone, the cognitive behavioral-analysis system of psychotherapy, and their combination for the treatment of chronic depression. N Engl J Med 2000; 342:1462–1470

50. DeRubeis RJ, Hollon SD, Amsterdam JD, Shelton RC, Young PR, Salomon RM, O'Reardon JP, Lovett ML, Gladis MM, Brown LL, Gallop R: Cognitive therapy vs medications in the treatment of moderate to severe depression. Arch Gen Psychiatry 2005; 62:409–416

51. Eisendrath SJ, Delucchi K, Bitner R, Fenimore P, Smit M, McLane M: Mindfulness-based cognitive therapy for treatment-resistant depression: a pilot study. Psychother Psychosom 2008; 77:319–320

52. Fava GA, Savron G, Grandi S, Rafanelli C: Cognitive-behavioral management of drug-resistant major depressive disorder. J Clin Psychiatry 1997; 58:278–282, quiz 283–274

53. Bressi C, Porcellana M, Marinaccio PM, Nocito EP, Magri L: Short-term psychodynamic psychotherapy versus treatment as usual for depressive and anxiety disorders: a randomized clinical trial of efficacy. J Nerv Ment Dis 2010; 198:647–652

54. de Maat S, Dekker J, Schoevers R, van Aalst G, Gijsbers-van Wijk C, Hendriksen M, Kool S, Peen J, Van R, de Jonghe F: Short psychodynamic supportive psychotherapy, antidepressants, and their combination in the treatment of major depression: a mega-analysis based on three randomized clinical trials. Depress Anxiety 2008; 25:565–574

55. Driessen E, Cuijpers P, de Maat SC, Abbass AA, de Jonghe F, Dekker JJ: The efficacy of short-term psychodynamic psychotherapy for depression: a meta-analysis. Clin Psychol Rev 2010; 30:25–36

56. Salminen JK, Karlsson H, Hietala J, Kajander J, Aalto S, Markkula J, Rasi-Hakala H, Toikka T: Short-term psychodynamic psychotherapy and fluoxetine in major depressive disorder: a randomized comparative study. Psychother Psychosom 2008; 77:351–357

57. Cuijpers P, Dekker J, Hollon SD, Andersson G: Adding psychotherapy to pharmacotherapy in the treatment of depressive disorders in adults: a meta-analysis. J Clin Psychiatry 2009; 70:1219–1229

58. Hollon SD, DeRubeis RJ, Shelton RC, Amsterdam JD, Salomon RM, O'Reardon JP, Lovett ML, Young PR, Haman KL, Freeman BB, Gallop R: Prevention of relapse following cognitive therapy vs medications in moderate to severe depression. Arch Gen Psychiatry 2005; 62:417–422

59. Fava GA, Ruini C, Rafanelli C, Finos L, Conti S, Grandi S: Six-year outcome of cognitive behavior therapy for prevention of recurrent depression. Am J Psychiatry 2004; 161:1872–1876

60. Bini L: Experimental researches on epileptic attacks induced by the electric current. Am J Psychiatry 1938; 94:172–174

61. Fink M: Convulsive therapy: a review of the first 55 years. J Affect Disord 2001; 63:1–15

62. The UK ECT Review Group: Efficacy and safety of electroconvulsive therapy in depressive disorders: a systematic review and meta-analysis. Lancet 2003; 361:799–808

63. Kellner CH, Knapp RG, Petrides G, Rummans TA, Husain MM, Rasmussen K, Mueller M, Bernstein HJ, O'Connor K, Smith G, Biggs M, Bailine SH, Malur C, Yim E, McClintock S, Sampson S, Fink M: Continuation electroconvulsive therapy vs pharmacotherapy for relapse prevention in major depression: a multisite study from the Consortium for Research in Electroconvulsive Therapy (CORE). Arch Gen Psychiatry 2006; 63:1337–1344

64. Sackeim HA, Dillingham EM, Prudic J, Cooper T, McCall WV, Rosenquist P, Isenberg K, Garcia K, Mulsant BH, Haskett RF: Effect of concomitant pharmacotherapy on electroconvulsive therapy outcomes: short-term efficacy and adverse effects. Arch Gen Psychiatry 2009; 66:729–737

65. Prudic J, Haskett RF, Mulsant B, Malone KM, Pettinati HM, Stephens S, Greenberg R, Rifas SL, Sackeim HA: Resistance to antidepressant medications and short-term clinical response to ECT. Am J Psychiatry 1996; 153:985–992

66. Kho KH, van Vreeswijk MF, Simpson S, Zwinderman AH: A meta-analysis of electroconvulsive therapy efficacy in depression. J ECT 2003; 19:139–147

67. Grunhaus L, Dannon PN, Schreiber S, Dolberg OH, Amiaz R, Ziv R, Lefkifker E: Repetitive transcranial magnetic stimulation is as effective as electroconvulsive therapy in the treatment of nondelusional major depressive disorder: an open study. Biol Psychiatry 2000; 47:314–324

68. Grunhaus L, Schreiber S, Dolberg OT, Polak D, Dannon PN: A randomized controlled comparison of electroconvulsive therapy and repetitive

transcranial magnetic stimulation in severe and resistant nonpsychotic major depression. Biol Psychiatry 2003; 53:324–331

69. Lisanby SH, Maddox JH, Prudic J, Devanand DP, Sackeim HA: The effects of electroconvulsive therapy on memory of autobiographical and public events. Arch Gen Psychiatry 2000; 57:581–590

70. Sackeim HA, Prudic J, Fuller R, Keilp J, Lavori PW, Olfson M: The cognitive effects of electroconvulsive therapy in community settings. Neuropsychopharmacology 2007; 32:244–254

71. Kuhn R: The treatment of depressive states with G 22355 (imipramine hydrochloride). Am J Psychiatry 1958; 115:459–464

72. Bailey SD, Bucci L, Gosline E, Kline NS, Park IH, Rochlin D, Saunders JC, Vaisberg M: Comparison of iproniazid with other amine oxidase inhibitors, including W-1544, JB-516, RO 4–1018, and RO 5–0700. Ann NY Acad Sci 1959; 80:652–668

73. Kiloh LG, Child JP, Latner G: A controlled trial of iproniazid in the treatment of endogenous depression. J Ment Sci 1960; 106:1139–1144

74. Jasper HH: A historical perspective. The rise and fall of prefrontal lobotomy. Adv Neurol 1995; 66:97–114

75. Hariz MI, Blomstedt P, Zrinzo L: Deep brain stimulation between 1947 and 1987: the untold story. Neurosurg Focus 2010; 29:E1

76. Sachdev P, Sachdev J: Sixty years of psychosurgery: its present status and its future. Aust NZ J Psychiatry 1997; 31:457–464

77. Marino Júnior R, Cosgrove GR: Neurosurgical treatment of neuropsychiatric illness. Psychiatr Clin North Am 1997; 20:933–943

78. Sachdev PS, Sachdev J: Long-term outcome of neurosurgery for the treatment of resistant depression. J Neuropsychiatry Clin Neurosci 2005; 17:478–485

79. Shields DC, Asaad W, Eskandar EN, Jain FA, Cosgrove GR, Flaherty AW, Cassem EH, Price BH, Rauch SL, Dougherty DD: Prospective assessment of stereotactic ablative surgery for intractable major depression. Biol Psychiatry 2008; 64:449–454

80. Moreines JL, McClintock SM, Holtzheimer PE: Neuropsychologic effects of neuromodulation techniques for treatment-resistant depression: a review. Brain Stimul (In press)

81. Clarke CE, Guttman M: Dopamine agonist monotherapy in Parkinson's disease. Lancet 2002; 360:1767–1769

82. Zarate CA Jr, Payne JL, Singh J, Quiroz JA, Luckenbaugh DA, Denicoff KD, Charney DS, Manji HK: Pramipexole for bipolar II depression: a placebo-controlled proof of concept study. Biol Psychiatry 2004; 56:54–60

83. Goldberg JF, Burdick KE, Endick CJ: Preliminary randomized, double-blind, placebo-controlled trial of pramipexole added to mood stabilizers for treatment-resistant bipolar depression. Am J Psychiatry 2004; 161:564–566

84. Lattanzi L, Dell'Osso L, Cassano P, Pini S, Rucci P, Houck PR, Gemignani A, Battistini G, Bassi A, Abelli M, Cassano GB: Pramipexole in treatment-resistant depression: a 16-week naturalistic study. Bipolar Disord 2002; 4:307–314

85. Cassano P, Lattanzi L, Fava M, Navari S, Battistini G, Abelli M, Cassano GB: Ropinirole in treatment-resistant depression: a 16-week pilot study. Can J Psychiatry 2005; 50:357–360

86. Cassano P, Lattanzi L, Soldani F, Navari S, Battistini G, Gemignani A, Cassano GB: Pramipexole in treatment-resistant depression: an extended follow-up. Depress Anxiety 2004; 20:131–138

87. Arborelius L, Owens MJ, Plotsky PM, Nemeroff CB: The role of corticotropin-releasing factor in depression and anxiety disorders. J Endocrinol 1999; 160:1–12

88. Gutman DA, Owens MJ, Nemeroff CB: Corticotropin-releasing factor receptor and glucocorticoid receptor antagonists: new approaches to antidepressant treatment, in Current and Future Developments in Psychopharmacology. Edited by Benecke NI. Amsterdam, 2005, pp 133–158

89. Holsboer F: Corticotropin-releasing hormone modulators and depression. Curr Opin Investig Drugs 2003; 4:46–50

90. Nemeroff CB: Recent advances in the neurobiology of depression. Psychopharmacol Bull 2002; 36(suppl 2):6–23

91. Zobel AW, Nickel T, Künzel HE, Ackl N, Sonntag A, Ising M, Holsboer F: Effects of the high-affinity corticotropin-releasing hormone receptor 1 antagonist R121919 in major depression: the first 20 patients treated. J Psychiatr Res 2000; 34:171–181

92. Binneman B, Feltner D, Kolluri S, Shi Y, Qiu R, Stiger T: A 6-week randomized, placebo-controlled trial of CP-316,311 (a selective CRH1 antagonist) in the treatment of major depression. Am J Psychiatry 2008; 165:617–620

93. Zorrilla EP, Koob GF: Progress in corticotropin-releasing factor-1 antagonist development. Drug Discov Today 2010; 15:371–383

94. Wolkowitz OM, Reus VI: Treatment of depression with antiglucocorticoid drugs. Psychosom Med 1999; 61:698–711

95. Murphy BE, Filipini D, Ghadirian AM: Possible use of glucocorticoid receptor antagonists in the treatment of major depression: preliminary results using RU 486. J Psychiatry Neurosci 1993; 18:209–213

96. Belanoff JK, Flores BH, Kalezhan M, Sund B, Schatzberg AF: Rapid reversal of psychotic depression using mifepristone. J Clin Psychopharmacol 2001; 21:516–521

97. DeBattista C, Belanoff J, Glass S, Khan A, Horne RL, Blasey C, Carpenter LL, Alva G: Mifepristone versus placebo in the treatment of psychosis in patients with psychotic major depression. Biol Psychiatry 2006; 60:1343–1349

98. Culman J, Unger T: Central tachykinins: mediators of defence reaction and stress reactions. Can J Physiol Pharmacol 1995; 73:885–891

99. Helke CJ, Krause JE, Mantyh PW, Couture R, Bannon MJ: Diversity in mammalian tachykinin peptidergic neurons: multiple peptides, receptors, and regulatory mechanisms. FASEB J 1990; 4:1606–1615

100. Kramer MS, Cutler N, Feighner J, Shrivastava R, Carman J, Sramek JJ, Reines SA, Liu G, Snavely D, Wyatt-Knowles E, Hale JJ, Mills SG, MacCoss M, Swain CJ, Harrison T, Hill RG, Hefti F, Scolnick EM, Cascieri MA, Chicchi GG, Sadowski S, Williams AR, Hewson L, Smith D, Carlson EJ, Hargreaves RJ, Rupniak NM: Distinct mechanism for antidepressant activity by blockade of central substance P receptors. Science 1998; 281:1640–1645

101. Culman J, Klee S, Ohlendorf C, Unger T: Effect of tachykinin receptor inhibition in the brain on cardiovascular and behavioral responses to stress. J Pharmacol Exp Ther 1997; 280:238–246

102. Geracioti TD Jr, Carpenter LL, Owens MJ, Baker DG, Ekhator NN, Horn PS, Strawn JR, Sanacora G, Kinkead B, Price LH, Nemeroff CB: Elevated cerebrospinal fluid substance p concentrations in posttraumatic stress disorder and major depression. Am J Psychiatry 2006; 163:637–643

103. Bondy B, Baghai TC, Minov C, Schüle C, Schwarz MJ, Zwanzger P, Rupprecht R, Möller HJ: Substance P serum levels are increased in major depression: preliminary results. Biol Psychiatry 2003; 53:538–542

104. Keller M, Montgomery S, Ball W, Morrison M, Snavely D, Liu G, Hargreaves R, Hietala J, Lines C, Beebe K, Reines S: Lack of efficacy of the substance p (neurokinin1 receptor) antagonist aprepitant in the treatment of major depressive disorder. Biol Psychiatry 2006; 59:216–223

105. Kramer MS, Winokur A, Kelsey J, Preskorn SH, Rothschild AJ, Snavely D, Ghosh K, Ball WA, Reines SA, Munjack D, Apter JT, Cunningham L, Kling M, Bari M, Getson A, Lee Y: Demonstration of the efficacy and safety of a novel substance P (NK1) receptor antagonist in major depression. Neuropsychopharmacology 2004; 29:385–392

106. Herpfer I, Lieb K: Substance P receptor antagonists in psychiatry: rationale for development and therapeutic potential. CNS Drugs 2005; 19:275–293

107. Paul IA, Skolnick P: Glutamate and depression: clinical and preclinical studies. Ann NY Acad Sci 2003; 1003:250–272

108. Zarate CA Jr, Du J, Quiroz J, Gray NA, Denicoff KD, Singh J, Charney DS, Manji HK: Regulation of cellular plasticity cascades in the pathophysiology and treatment of mood disorders: role of the glutamatergic system. Ann NY Acad Sci 2003; 1003:273–291

109. McEwen BS, Seeman T: Protective and damaging effects of mediators of stress. Elaborating and testing the concepts of allostasis and allostatic load. Ann NY Acad Sci 1999; 896:30–47

110. Sapolsky RM: The possibility of neurotoxicity in the hippocampus in major depression: a primer on neuron death. Biol Psychiatry 2000; 48:755–765

111. Rogóz Z, Skuza G, Maj J, Danysz W: Synergistic effect of uncompetitive NMDA receptor antagonists and antidepressant drugs in the forced swimming test in rats. Neuropharmacology 2002; 42:1024–1030

112. Rogóz Z, Skuza G, Kuśmider M, Wójcikowski J, Kot M, Daniel WA: Synergistic effect of imipramine and amantadine in the forced swimming test in rats. Behavioral and pharmacokinetic studies. Pol J Pharmacol 2004; 56:179–185

113. Stryjer R, Strous RD, Shaked G, Bar F, Feldman B, Kotler M, Polak L, Rosenzcwaig S, Weizman A: Amantadine as augmentation therapy in the management of treatment-resistant depression. Int Clin Psychopharmacol 2003; 18:93–96

114. Zarate CA Jr, Singh JB, Carlson PJ, Brutsche NE, Ameli R, Luckenbaugh DA, Charney DS, Manji HK: A randomized trial of an N-methyl-D-aspartate antagonist in treatment-resistant major depression. Arch Gen Psychiatry 2006; 63:856–864

115. Diazgranados N, Ibrahim L, Brutsche NE, Newberg A, Kronstein P, Khalife S, Kammerer WA, Quezado Z, Luckenbaugh DA, Salvadore G, Machado-Vieira R, Manji HK, Zarate CA Jr: A randomized add-on trial of an N-methyl-D-aspartate antagonist in treatment-resistant bipolar depression. Arch Gen Psychiatry 2010; 67:793–802

116. aan het Rot M, Collins KA, Murrough JW, Perez AM, Reich DL, Charney DS, Mathew SJ: Safety and efficacy of repeated-dose intravenous ketamine for treatment-resistant depression. Biol Psychiatry 2010; 67:139–145

117. Phelps LE, Brutsche N, Moral JR, Luckenbaugh DA, Manji HK, Zarate CA Jr: Family history of alcohol dependence and initial antidepressant response to an N-methyl-D-aspartate antagonist. Biol Psychiatry 2009; 65:181–184

118. Zarate CA Jr, Singh JB, Quiroz JA, De Jesus G, Denicoff KK, Luckenbaugh DA, Manji HK, Charney DS: A double-blind, placebo-controlled study of memantine in the treatment of major depression. Am J Psychiatry 2006; 163:153–155

119. Muhonen LH, Lönnqvist J, Juva K, Alho H: Double-blind, randomized comparison of memantine and escitalopram for the treatment of major depressive disorder comorbid with alcohol dependence. J Clin Psychiatry 2008; 69:392–399

120. Sanacora G, Kendell SF, Levin Y, Simen AA, Fenton LR, Coric V, Krystal JH: Preliminary evidence of riluzole efficacy in antidepressant-treated patients with residual depressive symptoms. Biol Psychiatry 2007; 61:822–825

121. Zarate CA Jr, Payne JL, Quiroz J, Sporn J, Denicoff KK, Luckenbaugh D, Charney DS, Manji HK: An open-label trial of riluzole in patients with treatment-resistant major depression. Am J Psychiatry 2004; 161:171–174

122. Zarate CA Jr, Quiroz JA, Singh JB, Denicoff KD, De Jesus G, Luckenbaugh DA, Charney DS, Manji HK: An open-label trial of the glutamate-modulating agent riluzole in combination with lithium for the treatment of bipolar depression. Biol Psychiatry 2005; 57:430–432

123. Mathew SJ, Murrough JW, aan het Rot M, Collins KA, Reich DL, Charney DS: Riluzole for relapse prevention following intravenous ketamine in treatment-resistant depression: a pilot randomized, placebo-controlled continuation trial. Int J Neuropsychopharmacol 2010; 13:71–82

124. Furey ML, Drevets WC: Antidepressant efficacy of the antimuscarinic drug scopolamine: a randomized, placebo-controlled clinical trial. Arch Gen Psychiatry 2006; 63:1121–1129

125. Drevets WC, Furey ML: Replication of scopolamine's antidepressant efficacy in major depression: a randomized, placebo-controlled clinical trial. Biol Psychiatry 2010; 67:432–438

126. Papakostas GI: Evidence for S-adenosyl-L-methionine (SAM-e) for the treatment of major depressive disorder. J Clin Psychiatry 2009; 70(suppl 5):18–22

127. Papakostas GI, Mischoulon D, Shyu I, Alpert JE, Fava M: S-Adenosyl methionine (SAMe) augmentation of serotonin reuptake inhibitors for antidepressant nonresponders with major depressive disorder: a double-blind, randomized clinical trial. Am J Psychiatry 2010; 167:942–948

128. Mayberg HS: Targeted electrode-based modulation of neural circuits for depression. J Clin Invest 2009; 119:717–725

129. Price JL, Drevets WC: Neurocircuitry of mood disorders. Neuropsychopharmacology 2010; 35:192–216

130. Rush AJ, Marangell LB, Sackeim HA, George MS, Brannan SK, Davis SM, Howland R, Kling MA, Rittberg BR, Burke WJ, Rapaport MH, Zajecka J, Nierenberg AA, Husain MM, Ginsberg D, Cooke RG: Vagus nerve stimulation for treatment-resistant depression: a randomized, controlled acute phase trial. Biol Psychiatry 2005; 58:347–354

131. Sackeim HA, Rush AJ, George MS, Marangell LB, Husain MM, Nahas Z, Johnson CR, Seidman S, Giller C, Haines S, Simpson RK Jr, Goodman RR: Vagus nerve stimulation (VNS) for treatment-resistant depression: efficacy, side effects, and predictors of outcome. Neuropsychopharmacology 2001; 25:713–728

132. Marangell LB, Rush AJ, George MS, Sackeim HA, Johnson CR, Husain MM, Nahas Z, Lisanby SH: Vagus nerve stimulation (VNS) for major depressive episodes: one year outcomes. Biol Psychiatry 2002; 51:280–287

133. Schlaepfer TE, Frick C, Zobel A, Maier W, Heuser I, Bajbouj M, O'Keane V, Corcoran C, Adolfsson R, Trimble M, Rau H, Hoff HJ, Padberg F, Müller-Siecheneder F, Audenaert K, Van den Abbeele D, Matthews K, Christmas D, Stanga Z, Hasdemir M: Vagus nerve stimulation for depression: efficacy and safety in a European study. Psychol Med 2008; 38:651–661

134. Nahas Z, Marangell LB, Husain MM, Rush AJ, Sackeim HA, Lisanby SH, Martinez JM, George MS: Two-year outcome of vagus nerve stimulation (VNS) for treatment of major depressive episodes. J Clin Psychiatry 2005; 66:1097–1104

135. Bajbouj M, Merkl A, Schlaepfer TE, Frick C, Zobel A, Maier W, O'Keane V, Corcoran C, Adolfsson R, Trimble M, Rau H, Hoff HJ, Padberg F, Müller-Siecheneder F, Audenaert K, van den Abbeele D, Matthews K, Christmas D, Eljamel S, Heuser I: Two-year outcome of vagus nerve stimulation in treatment-resistant depression. J Clin Psychopharmacol 2010; 30:273–281

136. Sackeim HA, Brannan SK, Rush AJ, George MS, Marangell LB, Allen J: Durability of antidepressant response to vagus nerve stimulation (VNS). Int J Neuropsychopharmacol 2007; 10:817–826

137. Dunner DL, Rush AJ, Russell JM, Burke M, Woodard S, Wingard P, Allen J: Prospective, long-term, multicenter study of the naturalistic outcomes of patients with treatment-resistant depression. J Clin Psychiatry 2006; 67:688–695

138. Helmstaedter C, Hoppe C, Elger CE: Memory alterations during acute high-intensity vagus nerve stimulation. Epilepsy Res 2001; 47:37–42

139. Holtzheimer PE 3rd, Russo J, Avery DH: A meta-analysis of repetitive transcranial magnetic stimulation in the treatment of depression. Psychopharmacol Bull 2001; 35:149–169

140. Burt T, Lisanby SH, Sackeim HA: Neuropsychiatric applications of transcranial magnetic stimulation: a meta analysis. Int J Neuropsychopharmacol 2002; 5:73–103

141. Kozel FA, George MS: Meta-analysis of left prefrontal repetitive transcranial magnetic stimulation (rTMS) to treat depression. J Psychiatr Pract 2002; 8:270–275

142. Martin JL, Barbanoj MJ, Schlaepfer TE, Thompson E, Pérez V, Kulisevsky J: Repetitive transcranial magnetic stimulation for the treatment of depression. Systematic review and meta-analysis. Br J Psychiatry 2003; 182:480–491

143. Schutter DJ: Quantitative review of the efficacy of slow-frequency magnetic brain stimulation in major depressive disorder. Psychol Med 2010; 40:1789–1795

144. Fitzgerald PB, Brown TL, Marston NA, Daskalakis ZJ, De Castella A, Kulkarni J: Transcranial magnetic stimulation in the treatment of depression: a double-blind, placebo-controlled trial. Arch Gen Psychiatry 2003; 60:1002–1008

145. Gershon AA, Dannon PN, Grunhaus L: Transcranial magnetic stimulation in the treatment of depression. Am J Psychiatry 2003; 160:835–845

146. Holtzheimer PE 3rd, Russo J, Claypoole KH, Roy-Byrne P, Avery DH: Shorter duration of depressive episode may predict response to repetitive transcranial magnetic stimulation. Depress Anxiety 2004; 19:24–30

147. Manes F, Jorge R, Morcuende M, Yamada T, Paradiso S, Robinson RG: A controlled study of repetitive transcranial magnetic stimulation as a treatment of depression in the elderly. Int Psychogeriatr 2001; 13:225–231

148. Nahas Z, Teneback CC, Kozel A, Speer AM, DeBrux C, Molloy M, Stallings L, Spicer KM, Arana G, Bohning DE, Risch SC, George MS: Brain effects of TMS delivered over prefrontal cortex in depressed adults: role of stimulation frequency and coil-cortex distance. J Neuropsychiatry Clin Neurosci 2001; 13:459–470

149. Kozel FA, Nahas Z, deBrux C, Molloy M, Lorberbaum JP, Bohning D, Risch SC, George MS: How coil-cortex distance relates to age, motor threshold, and antidepressant response to repetitive transcranial magnetic stimulation. J Neuropsychiatry Clin Neurosci 2000; 12:376–384

150. O'Reardon JP, Solvason HB, Janicak PG, Sampson S, Isenberg KE, Nahas Z, McDonald WM, Avery D, Fitzgerald PB, Loo C, Demitrack MA, George MS, Sackeim HA: Efficacy and safety of transcranial magnetic stimulation in the acute treatment of major depression: a multisite randomized controlled trial. Biol Psychiatry 2007; 62:1208–1216

151. Lisanby SH, Husain MM, Rosenquist PB, Maixner D, Gutierrez R, Krystal A, Gilmer W, Marangell LB, Aaronson S, Daskalakis ZJ, Canterbury R, Richelson E, Sackeim HA, George MS: Daily left prefrontal repetitive transcranial magnetic stimulation in the acute treatment of major depression: clinical predictors of outcome in a multisite, randomized controlled clinical trial. Neuropsychopharmacology 2009; 34:522–534

152. George MS, Lisanby SH, Avery D, McDonald WM, Durkalski V, Pavlicova M, Anderson B, Nahas Z, Bulow P, Zarkowski P, Holtzheimer PE 3rd, Schwartz T, Sackeim HA: Daily left prefrontal transcranial magnetic stimulation therapy for major depressive disorder: a sham-controlled randomized trial. Arch Gen Psychiatry 2010; 67:507–516

153. Avery DH, Holtzheimer PE 3rd, Fawaz W, Russo J, Neumaier J, Dunner DL, Haynor DR, Claypoole KH, Wajdik C, Roy-Byrne P: A controlled study of repetitive transcranial magnetic stimulation in medication-resistant major depression. Biol Psychiatry 2006; 59:187–194

154. Dannon PN, Dolberg OT, Schreiber S, Grunhaus L: Three and six-month outcome following courses of either ECT or rTMS in a population of severely depressed individuals—preliminary report. Biol Psychiatry 2002; 51:687–690

155. Demirtas-Tatlidede A, Mechanic-Hamilton D, Press DZ, Pearlman C, Stern WM, Thall M, Pascual-Leone A: An open-label, prospective study of repetitive transcranial magnetic stimulation (rTMS) in the long-term treatment of refractory depression: reproducibility and duration of the antidepressant effect in medication-free patients. J Clin Psychiatry 2008; 69:930–934

156. Wassermann EM: Risk and safety of repetitive transcranial magnetic stimulation: report and suggested guidelines from the International Workshop on the Safety of Repetitive Transcranial Magnetic Stimulation, June 5–7, 1996. Electroencephalogr Clin Neurophysiol 1998; 108:1–16

157. Holtzheimer PE 3rd, McDonald WM, Mufti M, Kelley ME, Quinn S, Corso G, Epstein CM: Accelerated repetitive transcranial magnetic stimulation for treatment-resistant depression. Depress Anxiety 2010; 27:960–963

158. Lisanby SH: Electroconvulsive therapy for depression. N Engl J Med 2007; 357:1939–1945

159. Sackeim HA, Prudic J, Nobler MS, Fitzsimons L, Lisanby SH, Payne N, Berman RM, Brakemeier EL, Perera T, Devanand DP: Effects of pulse width and electrode placement on the efficacy and cognitive effects of electroconvulsive therapy. Brain Stimul 2008; 1:71–83

160. Lisanby SH, Luber B, Schlaepfer TE, Sackeim HA: Safety and feasibility of magnetic seizure therapy (MST) in major depression: randomized within-subject comparison with electroconvulsive therapy. Neuropsychopharmacology 2003; 28:1852–1865

161. Kosel M, Frick C, Lisanby SH, Fisch HU, Schlaepfer TE: Magnetic seizure therapy improves mood in refractory major depression. Neuropsychopharmacology 2003; 28:2045–2048

162. White PF, Amos Q, Zhang Y, Stool L, Husain MM, Thornton L, Downing M, McClintock S, and Lisanby SH: Anesthetic considerations for magnetic seizure therapy: a novel therapy for severe depression. Anesth Analg 2006; 103:76–80, table of contents

163. Fregni F, Boggio PS, Nitsche MA, Marcolin MA, Rigonatti SP, Pascual-Leone A: Treatment of major depression with transcranial direct current stimulation. Bipolar Disord 2006; 8:203–204

164. Loo CK, Sachdev P, Martin D, Pigot M, Alonzo A, Malhi GS, Lagopoulos J, Mitchell P: A double-blind, sham-controlled trial of transcranial direct current stimulation for the treatment of depression. Int J Neuropsychopharmacol 2010; 13:61–69

165. Boggio PS, Rigonatti SP, Ribeiro RB, Myczkowski ML, Nitsche MA, Pascual-Leone A, Fregni F: A randomized, double-blind clinical trial on the efficacy of cortical direct current stimulation for the treatment of major depression. Int J Neuropsychopharmacol 2008; 11:249–254

166. Nahas Z, Anderson BS, Borckardt J, Arana AB, George MS, Reeves ST, Takacs I: Bilateral epidural prefrontal cortical stimulation for treatment-resistant depression. Biol Psychiatry 2010; 67:101–109

167. Greenberg BD, Gabriels LA, Malone DA Jr, Rezai AR, Friehs GM, Okun MS, Shapira NA, Foote KD, Cosyns PR, Kubu CS, Malloy PF, Salloway SP, Giftakis JE, Rise MT, Machado AG, Baker KB, Stypulkowski PH, Goodman WK, Rasmussen SA, Nuttin BJ: Deep brain stimulation of the ventral internal capsule/ventral striatum for obsessive-compulsive disorder: worldwide experience. Mol Psychiatry 2010; 15:64–79

168. Mallet L, Polosan M, Jaafari N, Baup N, Welter ML, Fontaine D, du Montcel ST, Yelnik J, Chéreau I, Arbus C, Raoul S, Aouizerate B, Damier P, Chabardès S, Czernecki V, Ardouin C, Krebs MO, Bardinet E, Chaynes P, Burbaud P, Cornu P, Derost P, Bougerol T, Bataille B, Mattei V, Dormont D, Devaux B, Vérin M, Houeto JL, Pollak P, Benabid AL, Agid Y, Krack P, Millet B, Pelissolo A, STOC Study Group: Subthalamic nucleus stimulation in severe obsessive-compulsive disorder. N Engl J Med 2008; 359:2121–2134

169. Mayberg HS, Lozano AM, Voon V, McNeely HE, Seminowicz D, Hamani C, Schwalb JM, Kennedy SH: Deep brain stimulation for treatment-resistant depression. Neuron 2005; 45:651–660

170. Lozano AM, Mayberg HS, Giacobbe P, Hamani C, Craddock RC, Kennedy SH: Subcallosal cingulate gyrus deep brain stimulation for treatment-resistant depression. Biol Psychiatry 2008; 64:461–467

171. McNeely HE, Mayberg HS, Lozano AM, Kennedy SH: Neuropsychological impact of Cg25 deep brain stimulation for treatment-resistant depression: preliminary results over 12 months. J Nerv Ment Dis 2008; 196:405–410

172. Malone DA Jr, Dougherty DD, Rezai AR, Carpenter LL, Friehs GM, Eskandar EN, Rauch SL, Rasmussen SA, Machado AG, Kubu CS, Tyrka AR, Price LH, Stypulkowski PH, Giftakis JE, Rise MT, Malloy PF, Salloway SP, Greenberg BD: Deep brain stimulation of the ventral capsule/ventral striatum for treatment-resistant depression. Biol Psychiatry 2009; 65:267–275

173. Bewernick BH, Hurlemann R, Matusch A, Kayser S, Grubert C, Hadrysiewicz B, Axmacher N, Lemke M, Cooper-Mahkorn D, Cohen MX, Brockmann H, Lenartz D, Sturm V, Schlaepfer TE: Nucleus accumbens deep brain stimulation decreases ratings of depression and anxiety in treatment-resistant depression. Biol Psychiatry 2010; 67:110–116

174. Jimenez F, Velasco F, Salin-Pascual R, Hernandez JA, Velasco M, Criales JL and Nicolini H: A patient with a resistant major depression disorder treated with deep brain stimulation in the inferior thalamic peduncle. Neurosurgery 2005; 57:585–593

175. Sartorius A, Kiening KL, Kirsch P, von Gall CC, Haberkorn U, Unterberg AW, Henn FA and Meyer-Lindenberg A: Remission of major depression under deep brain stimulation of the lateral habenula in a therapy-refractory patient. Biol Psychiatry 2010; 67:e9–e11

What Did STAR*D Teach Us? Results From a Large-Scale, Practical, Clinical Trial for Patients With Depression

Bradley N. Gaynes, M.D., M.P.H.
Diane Warden, Ph.D., M.B.A.
Madhukar H. Trivedi, M.D.
Stephen R. Wisniewski, Ph.D.
Maurizio Fava, M.D.
A. John Rush, M.D.

The authors provide an overview of the Sequenced Treatment Alternatives to Relieve Depression (STAR*D) study (www.star-d.org), a large-scale practical clinical trial to determine which of several treatments are the most effective "next-steps" for patients with major depressive disorder whose symptoms do not remit or who cannot tolerate an initial treatment and, if needed, ensuing treatments. Entry criteria were broadly defined and inclusive, and patients were enrolled from psychiatric and primary care clinics. All participants began on citalopram and were managed by clinic physicians, who followed an algorithm-guided acute-phase treatment through five visits over 12 weeks. At the end of each sequence, patients whose depression had not fully remitted were eligible for subsequent randomized trials in a sequence of up to three clinical trials. In general, remission rates in the study clinics were lower than expected, suggesting the need for several steps to achieve remission for most patients. There was no clear medication "winner" for patients whose depression did not remit after one or more aggressive medication trials. Both switching and augmenting appeared to be reasonable options when an initial antidepressant treatment failed, although these two strategies could not be directly compared. Further, the likelihood of remission after two vigorous medication trials substantially decreased, and remission would likely require more complicated medication regimens for which the existing evidence base is quite thin. STAR*D demonstrated that inclusion of more real-world patients in clinical trials is both feasible and informative. Policy implications of the findings, as well as the study's limitations, are discussed. (*Psychiatric Services* 60:1439–1445, 2009)

*Dr. Gaynes is affiliated with the Department of Psychiatry, University of North Carolina School of Medicine, CB #7160, Chapel Hill, NC 27599 (e-mail: bgaynes@med.unc.edu). Dr. Warden, Dr. Trivedi, and Dr. Rush are with the Department of Psychiatry, University of Texas Southwestern Medical Center at Dallas. Currently Dr. Rush is also with the Duke–National University of Singapore. Dr. Wisniewski is with the Epidemiology Data Center, Graduate School of Public Health, University of Pittsburgh. Dr. Fava is with the Depression Clinical and Research Program, Massachusetts General Hospital, Harvard Medical School, Boston. This article is part of a special section on the STAR*D trial (Sequenced Treatment Alternatives to Relieve Depression) and the implications of its findings for practice and policy. Grayson S. Norquist, M.D., M.S.P.H., served as guest editor of the special section.*

Reprinted with permission from Psych Serv 60:1439–1445, 2009.

Depression affects one in eight persons in the United States (1) and is projected to become the second leading cause of disability in the world by the year 2020 (2). However, generalizable evidence from clinical trials to inform treatment selection and sequencing is quite limited. Most clinical trial participants are recruited by advertisement rather than from representative practice settings. Eligibility criteria often exclude persons who have coexisting general medical or psychiatric disorders or who are taking medication other than antidepressants (3,4). Those with chronic depression or current suicidal ideation are also excluded (1,5). Consequently, the available "evidence" from clinical trials involves a largely "pure," uncomplicated population of depressed patients that is rarely seen by most practicing clinicians (6).

In addition, the care delivered in these efficacy trials, which involves using interviewer-administered measures and frequent and time-intensive follow-up interviews, blinding patients and physicians to treatment, and employing fixed dosing strategies, does not reflect what is and can be done in real-world practices. The available evidence may not translate to the care provided by practicing psychiatrists and primary care physicians (7). Further, the bulk of the evidence base is for patients who have yet to experience treatment failure in their current episode of depression, even though only about a third of patients achieve remission after a single treatment (8). Management of most patients after one or more failed treatments is not evidence based.

To address these knowledge deficits, the Sequenced Treatment Alternatives to Relieve Depression (STAR*D) study (www.star-d.org), a large-scale clinical trial funded by the National Institutes of Health, aimed to develop and evaluate feasible treatment strategies to improve clinical outcomes for more representative, "real-world" outpatients with one or more prior failed treatments. The study created its own prospectively defined sample of treatment-resistant patients from a pool of patients currently experiencing a major depressive episode for subsequent inclusion in a series of up to five prospective treatments. Specifically, STAR*D aimed to determine which of several treatments are the most effective "next-step" treatments for patients whose symptoms do not remit or who cannot tolerate the initial treatment and, if needed, ensuing treatments. This article provides an

overview of the design, methods, and results of STAR*D, with attention to the implications and limitations of the trial.

The rationale and design of STAR*D
Design
The rationale and design of the study have been fully described elsewhere (3,4,9). STAR*D is the largest prospective clinical trial of major depressive disorder ever conducted. It was a multicenter, nationwide association of 14 university-based regional centers, which oversaw a total of 23 participating psychiatric clinics and 18 primary care clinics. Enrollment began in 2000, with follow-up completed in 2004. All enrolled patients began on a single selective serotonin reuptake inhibitor (SSRI) (citalopram) and were managed by clinic physicians, who followed an algorithm-guided acute phase treatment through five visits over a 12-week course. Dosing was aggressive and focused on maximizing the tolerable dose; if patients who were tolerating a medication had not achieved remission (that is, complete recovery from the depressive epi-

sode) by any of the critical decision points (weeks 4, 6, and 9), the algorithm recommended increasing the dose. Patients whose depression did not remit after this initial treatment were able to participate in a sequence of up to three randomized clinical trials or levels. For example, at the end of level 1, patients whose depression had not fully recovered were eligible to participate in level 2 (Figure 1).

Treatment assignments were made using an equipoise stratified randomized design (10). To reflect treatment decisions in clinical practice, patients were allowed to choose among acceptable options (for example, to switch to a different treatment or augment the current treatment with an additional treatment). Participants could opt out of certain strategies as long as there were at least two possible options to which they might be randomly assigned.

Participants
Study entry criteria were broadly defined and inclusive. Patients had to have nonpsychotic major depressive disorder identified by clinicians and confirmed with a symptom checklist based on *DSM-IV-TR* (11), for which antidepressant treatment is recommended. Patients, whose ages ranged from 18 to 75, had to score of ≥14 on the 17-item Hamilton Rating Scale for Depression (HAM-D) (12) and could not have a primary diagnosis of bipolar disorder, obsessive-compulsive disorder, or an eating disorder or have a history of a seizure disorder. A total of 4,041 patients were enrolled in the first level of treatment, making STAR*D the largest prospective clinical trial of depression ever conducted.

Setting
Both primary and specialty care sites that provided care to public- and private-sector patients were selected on the basis of having sufficient numbers of patients, sufficient numbers of clinicians, sufficient administrative support, and sufficient numbers of patients from racial-ethnic minority groups to ensure that the study population would mirror the U.S. census data and that results would be widely generalizable. The median number of

Figure 1

STAR*D treatment levels

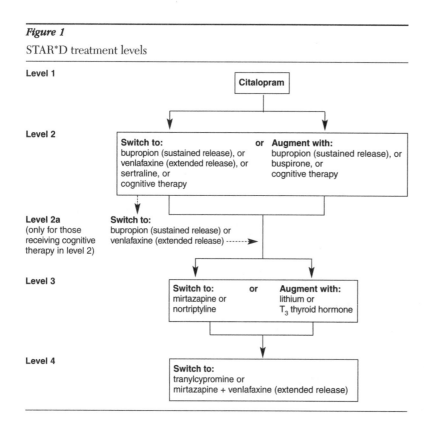

clinicians was 14 at the 18 primary care sites and 12 at the 23 specialty sites. Three-quarters of the facilities were privately owned, and approximately two-thirds were freestanding (not hospital based).

Measures

The primary research outcome was the standard definition of remission as measured by the HAM-D (13). Assessments were conducted by treatment-blinded raters at exit from each treatment level. A secondary instrument, the 16-item Quick Inventory of Depressive Symptomatology–Self-Report (QIDS-SR), was administered at each clinic visit, and remission was measured as a score of ≤5. Because the QIDS-SR was most often successfully collected at a time point closer to when a patient exited a level, the QIDS-SR provided more frequent assessment points during the acute phase and may have been a slightly better reflection of actual remission. The group of patients who improved but whose symptoms did not completely remit was defined as those who showed a ≥50% reduction in QIDS-SR score from baseline to the last assessment in the level.

Intervention

A systematic approach to treatment called measurement-based care was used that can be easily implemented in busy primary care or psychiatric settings (14,15). Measurement-based care involves the routine use of symptom and side-effect measurement, with guidance on when and how to modify medication dosages at critical decision points.

STAR*D results

Level 1 outcomes

A total of 2,876 individuals with analyzable data completed level 1 treatment. Measurement-based care was feasible and led to an average citalopram dosage of greater than 40 mg per day, indicating that high-quality care was delivered in these real-world settings. Remission rates were 27% as measured by HAM-D and 33% as measured by QIDS-SR, and response rates were 47% as measured by QIDS-SR. For those whose symptoms remitted, the mean time to re-

mission was approximately 47 days. Factors that increased the chance of remission included being Caucasian, female, and employed and having more years of education and income. Factors associated with lower remission rates were greater chronicity of the current episode, more concurrent psychiatric disorders (especially anxiety disorders or drug abuse), greater degree of general medical comorbidity, and lower levels of functioning and quality of life at baseline.

On average, patients required nearly seven weeks of measurement-based care to achieve remission. Notably, approximately half of the patients who ultimately remitted did so after six weeks, and 40% of those who achieved remission required eight or more weeks to do so (15).

Level 2 outcomes

After consideration of patient preference, 727 patients were randomly assigned to the switch strategy option in level 2. Nearly one-quarter of patients achieved remission when switched to measurement-based care–guided treatment with sertraline (a "within class" SSRI switch), venlafaxine-XR (a serotonin-norepinephrine reuptake inhibitor), or bupropion-SR (a norepinephrine and dopamine reuptake inhibitor) (16). Remission rates for bupropion-SR (21% by HAM-D and 26% by QIDS-SR), sertraline (18% and 27%), and venlafaxine-XR (25% for both) were neither statistically nor clinically different by either measure. Mean daily dosage at the final visit for bupropion-SR was 282.7 mg, for sertraline it was 135.5 mg, and for venlafaxine-XR was it 193.6 mg. Of note, the dosage of venlafaxine was less likely to approach the protocol-recommended maximum than that of either of the other two drugs. The overall side effect burden and the rate of serious adverse events did not differ significantly among the three medications.

Moderators of remission were also studied but offered little help in the selection of antidepressants after an initial treatment failure. Neither clinical symptom patterns (including anxious, atypical, and melancholic features) nor standard demographic

measures were of clear value in recommending any particular medication for a second step treatment (17).

Augmentation strategy. After consideration of patient preference, 565 patients were randomly assigned to the augmentation strategy option in level 2. Augmentation of citalopram with bupropion-SR or buspirone led to similar rates of remission as measured by the HAM-D (30% and 30%, respectively) and by the QIDS-SR (39% and 33%, respectively) (18). However, on an alternative outcome measure, bupropion-SR was associated with a greater total reduction in QIDS-SR scores than buspirone (25% compared with 17%, p<.04). Mean daily dosages at the end of level 2 were 267.5 mg of bupropion-SR and 40.9 mg of buspirone. Of note, augmentation with bupropion-SR was slightly better tolerated than buspirone (intolerable for 13% compared with 21% for buspirone, p<.001). Overall, these results indicate that the choice of either augmentation agent did not produce substantial clinical differences in efficacy.

The data collected did not allow direct comparison of the benefits of switching versus augmenting. Patient preferences were a part of the equipoise randomization strategy, and most patients preferred either augmentation or switching at level 2 (19). Consequently, patient groups were not equivalent at the point of randomization at the beginning of level 2; the augmentation group at level 2 was somewhat less depressed than the group that switched.

Cognitive therapy. Of those for whom cognitive therapy was acceptable, 182 patients were randomly assigned either to the cognitive therapy switch option or to augmentation of citalopram with cognitive therapy. Remission rates did not differ between those who switched to cognitive therapy (31%) and those who switched medications (31% and 27% remission, respectively) nor were there differences in response or time to remission or response (20). Switching to cognitive therapy was better tolerated than switching to a different antidepressant. Augmentation results were also similar. Remission rates did not differ between augmentation with cognitive therapy and augmentation with medication (31% and 33% remission). Response rates and tolerability were also similar. However, augmentation of citalopram with medication was more rapidly effective than augmentation with cognitive therapy (40 days compared with 55 days, p<.022).

Level 3

Switch strategy. A total of 235 patients switched medications in level 3. For those whose symptoms did not remit after two antidepressant medication trials, the likelihood of recovery did not differ significantly between patients who switched to mirtazapine and those who switched to nortriptyline (21). Remission rates for mirtazapine (mean exit dosage of 42.1 mg per day) were 12% as measured by the HAM-D and 8% by the QIDS-SR. The rates for nortriptyline (mean exit dosage of 96.8 mg per day) were 20% and 12%, respectively. QIDS-SR response rates were also similar (13% for mirtazapine and 17% for nortriptyline). Further, tolerability or side-effect burden did not differ significantly between the two treatments.

Consequently, after two consecutive unsuccessful antidepressant trials, a change in pharmacologic mechanism did not affect the likelihood of remission. Also, switching to a third antidepressant single-agent treatment resulted in lower remission rates than in the first two levels.

Augmentation strategy. Medication augmentation was employed for 142 patients in level 3. Similarly, after two

Figure 2

Cumulative remission rate by STAR*D treatment level

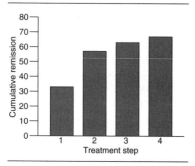

failed antidepressant medication treatments (levels 1 and 2), augmentation with a second agent at level 3 was less effective than augmentation at level 2 (22). Remission rates for lithium augmentation (mean exit dosage of 859.9 mg per day) were 16% as measured by the HAM-D and 13% by the QIDS-SR. For T_3 thyroid hormone augmentation (mean exit dosage of 45.2 micrograms per day) the rates were 25% for both measures. QIDS-SR response rates were 16% for lithium augmentation and 23% for T_3 augmentation. Although these treatment rates did not differ statistically, T_3 was less frequently associated with side effects (p=.045) and with treatment discontinuation because of side effects (23% discontinued compared with 10%, p=.027). When a clinician is considering an augmentation trial, T_3 may have advantages over lithium in effectiveness and tolerability. Further, T_3 offers the advantages of ease of use and no need for blood level monitoring.

Level 4

The switch strategy was employed for 109 patients in level 4. Patients who reached level 4 had failed three aggressive, consecutive, antidepressant trials and had a highly treatment-resistant depressive illness. Remission rates for the combination of mirtazapine (mean dosage of 35.7 mg per day) and venlafaxine-XR (mean dosage of 210.3 mg per day) were 14% as measured by the HAM-D and 16% by the QIDS-SR. For the monoamine oxidase inhibitor tranylcypromine (mean dosage of 36.9 mg per day), rates were 7% by the HAM-D and 14% by the QIDS-SR (23). Response rates as measured by the QIDS-SR were 24% with the combination and 12% with tranylcypromine. Neither remission nor response rates differed significantly between the combination and tranylcypromine. However, the combination was associated with greater symptomatic improvement and less attrition because of side effects. This comparison is limited by the lower likelihood of an adequate dosage and adequate duration of treatment for patients taking tranylcypromine. Overall, even though clinical out-

comes were similar for both groups, the lower likelihood of attrition because of side effect burden and the absence of dietary and concomitant drug restrictions suggest that the combination has some advantages.

Cumulative remission rate and long-term follow-up

Over the course of the four levels of treatment, the theoretical cumulative remission rate was 67% (see Figure 2). Remission was more likely to occur during the first two treatment levels (20%–30%) than during levels 3 and 4 (10%–20%).

Patients with a clinically meaningful response, preferably remission, in any of the four levels could enter into a 12-month naturalistic follow-up phase. Those who had required more treatment levels had higher relapse rates during this phase (24). Also, patients in remission at any level had a better prognosis than those who merely responded, which again provides support for using remission as the preferred aim of treatment.

STAR*D limitations

Although the selection of certain study design elements successfully addressed some primary concerns, such as generalizability and feasibility in real-world practice, the selection came with some clear tradeoffs. First, because patient preference was built into the randomization strategy and patients clearly demonstrated distinct preferences (with the vast majority electing either the switch or augmentation strategies), differences in depressive severity at entrance to the next level and small samples precluded direct comparison of switching and augmenting strategies. Indeed, those who switched to a new medication had more severe illness than those who received augmentation or cognitive therapy.

Thus, if a patient did not achieve remission after treatment in levels 1 and 2, we do not know whether switching medications or augmenting with a second medication led to a better outcome. Similarly, even if a patient had a partial response, STAR*D could not evaluate whether augmentation would have led to a better outcome than switching.

Second, fewer patients than expected selected cognitive therapy, which prevented a more comprehensive assessment of its role. The lower rate of selection of cognitive therapy was likely attributable to the requirement that study participants accept medication (citalopram) as the initial treatment (level 1 entry), which may have biased selection toward individuals who preferred medication. Other likely factors were additional copayments for cognitive therapy or the need to visit an additional provider at another site.

Third, level 1 did not include either a placebo or usual-care control group, which may limit conclusions about remission rates for an initial antidepressant trial. For example, the remission rates approximate what might be expected in eight-week placebo-controlled clinical trials, although such standard efficacy trials do not enroll the diverse population that STAR*D did, which may suggest higher placebo response rates in the traditional trials. However, inclusion of a placebo arm is likely to lead to inclusion of a sample that can limit generalizability of findings, and the aim of STAR*D was not to determine whether treatment is more effective than placebo but rather to show how effective it can be in a representative, community population.

Fourth, the study did not require dosage changes; instead, it used measurement-based care to guide treatment, which reflects use of guidelines in real-world practice. As a result, the trials of STAR*D medications may have been at a lower-than-recommended dosages, as may have happened for some patients who received venlafaxine-XR and tranylcypromine. A difference in the likelihood of having an antidepressant trial at a therapeutic dosage limits the direct comparison of effectiveness of the medications. For example, comparison of venlafaxine at a low-to-moderate dosage and sertraline at a dosage closer to the therapeutic level might unfairly favor a sertraline outcome.

Fifth, the results provide data on the average proportion of patients who are likely to respond to a particular medication or treatment strategy.

However, the results do not tell us which patients will respond to which treatments.

Further limitations unrelated to the STAR*D design also can restrict its applicability to current treatments. Since the study was designed approximately a decade ago, not all currently available and employed treatment options were examined. For example, augmentation strategies did not include second-generation antipsychotics, mood stabilizers, or psychostimulants.

Implications of STAR*D findings

STAR*D has key features that define it as an effectiveness trial (25). Design elements such as broadly inclusive selection criteria and enrollment of patients from primary and specialty settings and with multiple concurrent medical and psychiatric illnesses give STAR*D results high external validity. Comparison of STAR*D participants with the U.S. population highlights the generalizability. The racial-ethnic composition of the enrolled participants approximates that of the U.S. population on the basis of data from the 2000 Census, and the distribution of depressive severity seen in STAR*D participants is consistent with the spectrum reported by Kessler and colleagues (1) in a nationally representative sample (10% mild, 38% moderate, 39% severe, and 13% very severe). Both facts suggest that the sample was representative of depressed patients in the United States. Further, the participants' ability to choose which clinic to attend and what treatments were acceptable alternatives mirrors what happens in routine clinical practice, which also enhances the generalizability of these results.

Clinical implications

The primary implications of the STAR*D findings are summarized below.

♦ Remission rates in these representative clinics, in general, were lower than expected on the basis of clinical efficacy trials of antidepressants, which typically report remission rates of 35% to 40% (9), suggesting the need for several steps to achieve remission for most patients.

♦ There is no clear medication

"winner" for patients whose depression does not remit after one or more aggressive medication trials.

♦ Both switching and augmenting are reasonable options for patients after an initial antidepressant treatment has failed.

♦ It may take longer to reach remission than expected, and thus medication trials of at least eight weeks with at least moderately aggressive dosing may be necessary.

♦ Cognitive therapy is a well-tolerated treatment option for patients when an antidepressant treatment fails, and the outcomes patients achieve appear equivalent to those they would have achieved with the trial of a new medication. At the same time, it should be noted that augmentation of citalopram with medication was more rapidly effective than augmentation with cognitive therapy.

♦ Pharmacologic differences between psychotropic medications do not translate into meaningful clinical differences, although tolerability differs.

♦ Neither standard sociodemographic measures nor the symptom patterns that were measured in STAR*D (including anxious, atypical, and melancholic features) predicted a differential benefit from the available switch options at level 2, suggesting that the common practice of selecting treatments based on symptom patterns has little empirical support (17).

♦ The likelihood of remission after two vigorous medication trials substantially decreases, and remission likely requires more complicated medication regimens for which the existing evidence base is quite thin. Thus an empirically supported definition for treatment-resistant depression seems to be two antidepressant failures.

♦ No statistically significant difference in outcome was found between patients treated in primary care and psychiatric settings when measurement-based care was used in level 1 (26) or level 2 (17). Thus primary care physicians, who manage the majority of depressed patients, can be reasonable providers of depression care for at least the first two treatment steps.

♦ The finding that about two-thirds of patients may be expected to reach remission with up to four treatment attempts is encouraging for this disabling illness. Continued treatment attempts, even beyond a second treatment failure, do yield results for some patients.

♦ Longer-term outcomes supported remission as the preferred goal of treatment. During the naturalistic follow-up phase, lower relapse rates were found among participants who entered follow-up in remission than for those who were not (27).

♦ An important predictor of relapse was greater axis I or III comorbidity. The greater the number of acute treatment steps required from before entry to follow-up (that is, the greater the degree of treatment resistance), the greater the risk of relapse (27).

Policy implications

STAR*D policy implications are summarized below.

♦ Inclusion of more real-world patients in clinical trials is both feasible and informative. For example, of the group of participants enrolled as a result of the broadly inclusive selection criteria used by STAR*D, only one-fourth would have been enrolled in a standard phase III clinical trial. Results of STAR*'D suggest that broader phase III inclusion criteria would increase generalizability of results to real-world practice, which might reduce placebo response and remission rates (reducing the risk of failed trials) but with some increased risk of adverse events (6).

♦ The choice of medications for formularies must be carefully considered. Because there was no antidepressant "winner" and the chance of remission did not clearly differ by medication choice, some may argue that formularies can be restricted because of antidepressant equivalence. However, some findings would argue for a broader formulary. For example, antidepressant medications differed in the likelihood of particular side effects, and at this time tolerance cannot be readily predicted. Further, given the multiple treatment steps needed for most participants, availability of a large armamentarium of treatments seems prudent, especially given our inability to predict who will respond to what medication. Finally,

given the similar likelihood of response to treatments at level 1 and 2 (some of which have generic formulations) and the inability to predict who will respond better to a particular treatment, available generic antidepressants seem reasonable choices for these first two medication trials.

♦ Measurement-based care—that is, using brief, easy-to-administer instruments to monitor depression severity and side effects, following an evidence-based treatment algorithm, making decisions at key time points, and having remission as a goal of treatment—is a feasible strategy that can be adapted in real-world practice settings—both psychiatric and primary care settings (14,15).

♦ Referral guidelines can incorporate the findings that most patients with depressive illness can be adequately treated in primary care for at least two antidepressant trials when measurement-based care is used, thereby reducing the rate of premature referral to psychiatric clinics.

♦ The large number of patients with either recurrent major depressive disorder or with chronic major depressive episodes (>75% in this study), the fact that only about half the patients reached remission after two treatments, and the poor long-term outcomes for patients when two or more acute treatments failed all suggest the need for more evidence to guide the effective treatment of treatment-resistant depression.

Conclusions

STAR*D was a seminal, large-scale, practical clinical trial that provided a great deal of data for clinicians, researchers, and policy makers. The findings are still being actively discussed, analyzed, and disseminated, and the acute-treatment data set is now available in the public domain to allow further analysis. The research infrastructure, which continues as the Depression Trials Network (www.DTN.com), has completed enrollment for two separate clinical trials whose design was guided, in part, by the findings of STAR*D.

Acknowledgments and disclosures

This project was funded by the National Institute of Mental Health (NIMH) under contract N01MH90003 to the University of Texas Southwestern Medical Center at Dallas. The content of this publication does not necessarily reflect the views or policies of the U.S. Department of Health and Human Services nor does mention of trade names, commercial products, or organizations imply endorsement by the U.S. government. NIMH approved the design of the overall study and reviewed its conduct but performed no role in the collection, management, and interpretation of the data analyzed for this report or in the preparation, review, or approval of the manuscript.

Dr. Gaynes has received grants and research support from Bristol-Myers Squibb and Novartis and has served as an advisor for Bristol-Myers Squibb. Dr. Warden has owned stock in Pfizer in the past year. Dr. Trivedi has received consulting fees from AstraZeneca, Bristol-Myers Squibb, Cephalon, Inc., Eli Lilly and Company, Evotec, Fabre-Kramer Pharmaceuticals, Forest Pharmaceuticals, GlaxoSmithKline, Janssen, Johnson and Johnson, Medtronic, Neuronetics, Otsuka Pharmaceuticals, Pfizer, Shire, and Wyeth-Ayerst Laboratories. He has received research support from Targacept. Dr. Wisniewski has received consultant fees from Cyberonics Inc. The other authors report no competing interests.

References

1. Kessler RC, Berglund P, Demler O, et al: The epidemiology of major depressive disorder: results from the National Comorbidity Survey Replication (NCS-R). JAMA 289:3095–3105, 2003

2. Murray CJ, Lopez AD: Global mortality, disability, and the contribution of risk factors: Global Burden of Disease Study. Lancet 349:1436–1442, 1997

3. Gaynes B, Davis L, Rush A, et al: The aims and design of the Sequenced Treatment Alternatives to Relieve Depression (STAR*D) study. Primary Psychiatry 12:36–41, 2005

4. Rush A, Fava M, Wisniewski S, et al: Sequenced Treatment Alternatives to Relieve Depression (STAR*D): rationale and design. Controlled Clinical Trials 25:119–142, 2004

5. Zimmerman M, Chelminski I, Posternak MA: Generalizability of antidepressant efficacy trials: differences between depressed psychiatric outpatients who would or would not qualify for an efficacy trial. American Journal of Psychiatry 162:1370–1372, 2005

6. Wisniewski SR, Rush AJ, Nierenberg AA, et al: Can Phase III trial results of antidepressant medications be generalized to clinical practice? A STAR*D report. American Journal of Psychiatry 166:599–607, 2009

7. Rothwell PM: External validity of randomised controlled trials: to whom do the results of this trial apply? Lancet. 365:82–93, 2005

8. Fava M, Davidson KG: Definition and epidemiology of treatment-resistant depression. Psychiatric Clinics of North America 19:179–200, 1996

9. Fava M, Rush A, Trivedi M, et al: Background and rationale for the Sequenced Treatment Alternatives to Relieve Depression (STAR*D) study. Psychiatric Clinics of North America 26:457–494, 2003

10. Lavori P, Rush A, Wisniewski S, et al: Strengthening clinical effectiveness trials: equipoise-stratified randomization. Biological Psychiatry 50:792–801, 2001

11. Diagnostic and Statistical Manual of Mental Disorders, Fourth Edition, Text Revision. Washington, DC, American Psychiatric Association, 2000

12. Hamilton M: A rating scale for depression. Journal of Neurologic and Neurosurgical Psychiatry 23:56–61, 1960

13. Hamilton M: Development of a rating scale for primary depressive illness. British Journal of Social and Clinical Psychology 6:278–296, 1967

14. Trivedi MH, Rush AJ, Gaynes BN, et al: Maximizing the adequacy of medication treatment in controlled trials and clinical practice: STAR*D measurement-based care. Neuropsychopharmacology 32:2479–2489, 2007

15. Trivedi MH, Rush AJ, Wisniewski SR, et al: Evaluation of outcomes with citalopram for depression using measurement-based care in STAR*D: implications for clinical practice. American Journal of Psychiatry 163:28–40, 2006

16. Rush AJ, Trivedi MH, Wisniewski SR, et al: Bupropion-SR, sertraline, or venlafaxine-XR after failure of SSRIs for depression. New England Journal of Medicine 354:1231–1242, 2006

17. Rush AJ, Wisniewski SR, Warden D, et al: Selecting among second-step antidepressant medication monotherapies: predictive value of clinical, demographic, or first-step treatment features. Archives of General Psychiatry 65:870–880, 2008

18. Trivedi MH, Fava M, Wisniewski SR, et al: Medication augmentation after the failure of SSRIs for depression. New England Journal of Medicine 354:1243–1252, 2006

19. Wisniewski SR, Fava M, Trivedi MH, et al: Acceptability of second-step treatments to depressed outpatients: a STAR*D report. American Journal of Psychiatry 164:753–760, 2007

20. Thase ME, Friedman ES, Biggs MM, et al: Cognitive therapy versus medication in augmentation and switch strategies as second-step treatments: a STAR*D report. American Journal of Psychiatry 164:739–752, 2007

21. Fava M, Rush AJ, Wisniewski SR, et al: A comparison of mirtazapine and nortriptyline following two consecutive failed medication treatments for depressed outpatients: a STAR*D report. American Journal of Psychiatry 163:1161–1172, 2006

22. Nierenberg AA, Fava M, Trivedi MH, et al: A comparison of lithium and T(3) augmentation following two failed medication treatments for depression: a STAR*D report. American Journal of Psychiatry 163:1519–1530, 2006

23. McGrath PJ, Stewart JW, Fava M, et al: Tranylcypromine versus venlafaxine plus mirtazapine following three failed antidepressant medication trials for depression: a STAR*D report. American Journal of Psychiatry 163:1531–1541, 2006

24. Rush AJ, Trivedi MH, Wisniewski SR, et al: Acute and longer-term outcomes in depressed outpatients requiring one or several treatment steps: a STAR*D report. American Journal of Psychiatry 163:1905–1917, 2006

25. Gartlehner G, Hansen RA, Nissman D, et al: A simple and valid tool distinguished efficacy from effectiveness studies. Journal of Clinical Epidemiology 59:1040–1048, 2006

26. Gaynes BN, Rush AJ, Trivedi MH, et al: Primary versus specialty care outcomes for depressed outpatients managed with measurement-based care: results from STAR*D. Journal of General Internal Medicine 23:551–560, 2008

27. Rush AJ: STAR*D: what have we learned? American Journal of Psychiatry 164:201–204, 2007

The Evolution of the Cognitive Model of Depression and Its Neurobiological Correlates

Aaron T. Beck, M.D.

Although the cognitive model of depression has evolved appreciably since its first formulation over 40 years ago, the potential interaction of genetic, neurochemical, and cognitive factors has only recently been demonstrated. Combining findings from behavioral genetics and cognitive neuroscience with the accumulated research on the cognitive model opens new opportunities for integrated research. Drawing on advances in cognitive, personality, and social psychology as well as clinical observations, expansions of the original cognitive model have incorporated in successive stages automatic thoughts, cognitive distortions, dysfunctional beliefs, and information-processing biases. The developmental model identified early traumatic experiences and the formation of dysfunctional beliefs as predisposing events and congruent stressors in later life as precipitating factors. It is now possible to sketch out possible genetic and neurochemical pathways that interact with or are parallel to cognitive variables. A hypersensitive amygdala is associated with both a genetic polymorphism and a pattern of negative cognitive biases and dysfunctional beliefs, all of which constitute risk factors for depression. Further, the combination of a hyperactive amygdala and hypoactive prefrontal regions is associated with diminished cognitive appraisal and the occurrence of depression. Genetic polymorphisms also are involved in the overreaction to the stress and the hypercortisolemia in the development of depression—probably mediated by cognitive distortions. I suggest that comprehensive study of the psychological as well as biological correlates of depression can provide a new understanding of this debilitating disorder.

(Am J Psychiatry 2008; 165:969–977)

I was privileged to start my research on depression at a time when the modern era of systematic clinical and biological research was just getting underway. Consequently, the field for new investigations was wide open. The climate at the time was friendly for such research. The National Institute of Mental Health had only recently been funding research and providing salary support for full-time clinical investigators. The Group for Advancement of Psychiatry, under the leadership of pioneers like David Hamburg, was providing guidelines as well as the impetus for clinical research.

Caught up with the contagion of the times, I was prompted to start something on my own. I was particularly intrigued by the paradox of depression. This disorder appeared to violate the time-honored canons of human nature: the self-preservation instinct, the maternal instinct, the sexual instinct, and the pleasure principle. All of these normal human yearnings were dulled or reversed. Even vital biological functions like eating or sleeping were attenuated. The leading causal theory of depression at the time was the notion of inverted hostility. This seemed a reasonable, logical explanation if translated into a need to suffer. The need to punish one's self could account for the loss of pleasure, loss of libido, self-criticism, and suicidal wishes and would be triggered by guilt. I was drawn to conducting clinical research in depression because the field was wide open—and besides, I had a testable hypothesis.

Cross-Sectional Model of Depression

I decided at first to make a foray into the "deepest" level: the dreams of depressed patients. I expected to find signs of more hostility in the dream content of depressed patients than nondepressed patients, but they actually showed less hostility. I did observe, however, that the dreams of depressed patients contained the themes of loss, defeat, rejection, and abandonment, and the dreamer was represented as defective or diseased. At first I assumed the idea that the negative themes in the dream content expressed the need to punish one's self (or "masochism"), but I was soon disabused of this notion. When encouraged to express hostility, my patients became more, not less, depressed. Further, in experiments, they reacted positively to success experiences and positive reinforcement when the "masochism" hypothesis predicted the opposite (summarized in Beck [1]).

Some revealing observations helped to provide the basis for the subsequent cognitive model of depression. I noted that the dream content contained the same themes as the patients' conscious cognitions—their negative self-evaluations, expectancies, and memories—but in an exaggerated, more dramatic form. The depressive cognitions contained errors or distortions in the interpretations (or misinterpretations) of experience. What finally clinched the new model (for me) was our research finding that when the patients reappraised and corrected their misinterpretations, their depression started to lift and—in 10 or 12 sessions—would remit (2).

Thus, I undertook the challenge of attempting to integrate the different psychological pieces of the puzzle of depression. The end product was a comprehensive cognitive model of depression. At the surface, readily accessible level was the *negativity* in the patients' self-reports, including their dreams and their negative interpretations of their experiences. These variables seemed to account for the manifestations of depression, such as hopelessness, loss of motivation, self-criticism, and suicidal wishes. The next level appeared to be a *systematic cognitive bias* in information processing leading to selective attention to negative aspects of experiences, negative interpretations, and blocking of positive events and memories. These findings raised the question: "What is producing the negative bias?" On the basis of clinical observations supported by research, I concluded that when depressed, patients had highly charged *dysfunctional attitudes* or beliefs about themselves that hijacked the information processing and produced the negative cognitive bias, which led to the symptoms of depression (1, 3, 4).

A large number of studies have demonstrated that depressed patients have dysfunctional attitudes, show a systematic negative attentional and recall bias in laboratory experiments, and report cognitive distortions (selective abstraction, overgeneralizing, personalization, and interpretational biases [4]). Dysfunctional attitudes, measured by the Dysfunctional Attitudes Scale (5), are represented by beliefs such as "If I fail at something, it means I'm a total failure." During a full-blown episode of depression, the hypersalient dysfunctional attitudes lead into absolute negative beliefs about the self, their personal world, and the future ("I am a failure"). I suggested that these dysfunctional attitudes are embedded within cognitive structures, or schemas, in the meaning assignment system and thus have structural qualities, such as stability and density as well as thresholds and levels of activation. The degree of salience (or "energy") of the schemas depends on the intensity of a negative experience and the threshold for activation at a given time (successive stressful experiences, for example, can lower the threshold [1]).

When the schemas are activated by an event or series of events, they skew the information processing system, which then directs attentional resources to negative stimuli and translates a specific experience into a distorted negative interpretation. The hypersalience of these negative schemas leads not only to a global negative perception of reality but also to the other symptoms of depression, such as sadness, hopelessness, loss of motivation, and regressive behaviors such as social withdrawal and in-

activity. These symptoms are also subjected to negative evaluation ("My poor functioning is a burden on my family" and "My loss of motivation shows how lazy I am"). Thus, the depressive constellation consists of a continuous feedback loop with negative interpretations and attentional biases with the subjective and behavioral symptoms reinforcing each other.

Developmental Model of Depression

Cognitive Vulnerability

What developmental event or events might lead to the formation of dysfunctional attitudes and how these events might relate to later stressful events leading to the precipitation of depression was another piece of the puzzle. In our earlier studies, we found that severely depressed patients were more likely than moderately or mildly depressed patients to have experienced parental loss in childhood (6). We speculated that such a loss would sensitize an individual to a significant loss at a later time in adolescence or adulthood, thus precipitating depression. Brij Sethi, a member of our group, showed that the combination of a loss in childhood with an analogous loss in adulthood led to depression in a significant number of depressed patients (7). The meaning of the early events (such as "If I lose an important person, I am helpless") is transformed into a durable attitude, which may be activated by a similar experience at a later time. A recent *prospective* study observed that early life stress sensitizes individuals to later negative events through impact on cognitive vulnerability leading to depression (8).

The accumulated research findings have supported the original cognitive vulnerability model derived from clinical observations (4). As shown in Figure 1, early adverse events foster negative attitudes and biases about the self, which are integrated into the cognitive organization in the form of schemas; the schemas become activated by later adverse events impinging on the specific cognitive vulnerability and lead to the systematic negative bias at the core of depression (1, 9).

Much of the early research by others on the cognitive model overlooked the role of stress in activating previously latent dysfunctional schemas. Scher and colleagues (10) provided a comprehensive review of the diathesis-stress formulation based on prospective studies and priming methodologies to test the cognitive model.

Although the original cognitive model proposed that severe life events (e.g., death of a loved one or loss of a job) were the usual precipitants of depression (1), more recent research has suggested that milder stressful life events provide an alternate pathway to depression in vulnerable individuals (11, 12). Moreover, the triggering events of successive episodes of depression become progressively milder, suggesting a "kindling" effect (13, 14).

Cognitive vulnerability to the experience of depressive symptoms following stress has been reported in children, adolescents, and adults (10, 12, 15). For example, students showing cognitive vulnerability were more likely to become depressed following negative outcomes on college applications than were students not showing cognitive vulnerability (12, 16). It should be noted that these studies generally described minor depressive episodes rather than full-blown major depression.

What relevance do dysfunctional attitudes have to the vulnerability to *recurrence* of depression? Segal and colleagues (17) showed that the muted dysfunctional attitudes of recovered depressed patients could be primed by a negative mood induction procedure. Furthermore, the extent to which the mood induction activated the dysfunctional attitudes during the nondepressed period predicted future relapse and recurrence. This activation of the dysfunctional attitudes was more likely to occur with patients who had received pharmacotherapy than those receiving cognitive therapy. The prospective and priming studies thus indicated that dysfunctional attitudes could be regarded as a *cognitive vulnerability* factor for depression.

A more recent refinement of the cognitive vulnerability model has added the concept of *cognitive reactivity*, expressed clinically as fluctuations in patients' negative attitudes about themselves in response to daily events (18). Cognitive reactivity has been demonstrated experimentally by a variety of priming interventions (or "mood interventions") such as sad music, imaging of sad autobiographical memories, social rejection film clip, or contrived failure. Following these priming interventions, clinically vulnerable subjects report more dysfunctional attitudes, negative cognitive biases, and erosion of normal positive biases than do other subjects (10). Clinical vulnerability was defined in terms of high-risk variables (e.g., a personal or family history of depression).

Studies have shown that the presence of cognitive reactivity before a stressful life event predicts the onset of depressive episodes (10). The importance of the meaning assigned to a stressful event as a crucial component of cognitive reactivity was borne out by the finding (19) that the daily negative appraisals of daily stressors predicted daily depressive symptoms. The addition of the concept of cognitive reactivity to the cognitive model suggested that the predisposition to depression may be observable in the *daily* cognitive-emotional reactions of the depression-prone individual (18). However, the model left unanswered why certain individuals were more reactive to daily events (or were more likely to develop dysfunctional attitudes and cognitive biases) than others.

As indicated previously, the experience of episodes of depressive symptoms is different from the total immersion of the personality in a full-blown major depression. Severe depression is characterized not only by a broad range of intense symptoms but also "endogenous" features, such as relative insensitivity to external events. To account for the complex characteristics of the fully expressed depression, I proposed an expanded cognitive model (4, 20). I presented the concept of the *mode*, a network of cognitive, affective, motivational, behavioral, and physiological schemas, to account for the profound retardation, anhedonia, and sleep and appetite disturbance, as well as the cognitive aberrations. The activation of this mode (network) produces the various phenomena of depression.

In the formation of the mode, the connections among the various negatively oriented schemas become strengthened over time in response to negatively interpreted events. Successive symptom-producing events or a major depressogenic event locks these connections into place. In a sense, the cognitive schemas serve as the hub and the other schemas as nodes with continuous communication among them. A major stressful event or events symbolizing a loss of some type trigger the cognitive schemas that activate the other (affective, motivational, etc.) schemas. When fully activated, the mode becomes relatively autonomous and is no longer as reactive to external stimuli; that is, positive events do not reduce the negative thinking or mood. Attentional resources are disproportionately allocated from the external environment to internal experiences such as negative cognitions and sadness, manifested clinically as rumination. Also, resources are withdrawn from adaptive schemas such as coping and problem solving. The mode presumably would correspond to a complex neural network, including multiple relevant brain regions that are activated or deactivated during depression.

The negatively biased cognitive schemas function as *automatic* information processors. The biased automatic processing is rapid, involuntary, and sparing of resources. The dominance of this system (efficient but maladaptive) in depression could account for the negative attentional and interpretational bias. In contrast, the role of the cognitive control system (consisting of executive functions, problem solving, and reappraisal) is attenuated during depression. The operation of this system is deliberate, reflective, and effortful (resource demanding), can be reactivated in therapy, and, thus, can be used to appraise the depressive misinterpretations and dampen the salience of the depressive mode.

The concept of the two forms of processing can be traced back to Freud's model of primary and secondary processes (21) and has been reformulated many times since (22). Recently, Beevers (23) suggested a similar formulation of a two-factor processing in depression. He proposed that cognitive vulnerability to depression occurs when negatively biased associative processing is uncorrected by reflective processing.

The expanded cognitive model includes the following progression in the development of depression: adverse early life experiences contribute to the formation of dysfunctional attitudes incorporated within cognitive structures, labeled cognitive schemas (cognitive vulnerability). When activated by daily life events, the schemas produce an attentional bias, negatively biased interpretations, and mild depressive symptoms (cognitive reactivity).

FIGURE 1. A Developmental Model of Depression Based on Vulnerability Diathesis and Stressful Life Events

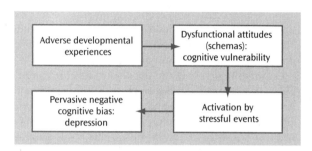

After repeated activation, the negative schemas become organized into a depressive mode, which also includes affective, behavioral, and motivational schemas (cognitive vulnerability). Accumulated negative events or a severe adverse event impacts on the mode and makes it hypersalient. The hypersalient mode takes control of the information processing, reflected by increased negative appraisals and rumination. The cognitive control of emotionally significant appraisals is attenuated and, thus, reappraisal of negative interpretations is limited. The culmination of these processes is clinical depression. Crick and Dodge (24) point out that with repeated activation, maladaptive information-processing patterns become routinized and resistant to change. Thus, cognitive schemas, after repeated activation before and during depressive episodes, become more salient and more ingrained over time, consistent with the "kindling" phenomenon.

Although supportive evidence for this model was meager in early years, support for the fundamental hypotheses has accumulated over the past 40 years. In 1999, David A. Clark and I (4) reviewed over 1,000 publications relevant to the cognitive model of depression and found substantial research support for the various facets of the cognitive theory. Several more recent reviews have provided additional research support (10, 12, 15, 25).

As the cognitive model of depression buttressed by years of systematic research has grown to maturity, it seems timely and appropriate to compare it with the burgeoning findings in neurogenetics and neuroimaging.

Biological Correlates of the Cognitive Model

Genetic Vulnerability

I still had an unsolved problem: how can we account for the observation that only a proportion of individuals subjected to child abuse, other adverse events, and major traumatic experiences become depressed? Many of us had speculated about the existence of a "blue gene," but the technology for identifying it had not been available. Also, although there was considerable support for the cognitive model of depression at the psychological and clinical levels (4), there were minimal data from neurophysiological

studies to correlate with these findings. It was not until this century that these problems could be addressed, as a result of investigations by researchers in behavioral genetics and cognitive neuroscience. The spectacular technological advances in genetics and functional neuroimaging have enabled researchers to demonstrate that genetic variations and their impact on neural functioning play a major role in the hyperreactivity to negative experiences leading to depression. A number of studies have provided a structure for understanding the relationships between life events, neural dysregulation, cognitive processes, and depression. This research has also provided a preliminary basis for formulating the neurobiological correlates of such psychological constructs as cognitive vulnerability, cognitive reactivity, and cognitive biases.

These advances have facilitated a breakthrough in understanding the relationship between cognitive, biological, and experiential factors in the development of depression. The genetic and neurobiological findings illuminated some probable causal pathways to depression as well as suggesting biological correlates of the cognitive model. The pioneering paper by Caspi and colleagues (26) suggested that individuals possessing either one or two copies of the short variant of the 5-HTTLPR (serotonin transporter) gene, which is not transcriptionally as effective as the long form, experienced higher levels of depression and suicidality following a recent life stressor. The study by Caspi and colleagues (26) has since been supported by a large number of other studies (27).

The types of stressful life events moderated by the 5-HTTLPR gene varied considerably in these studies, ranging from mild stressors to a single, large traumatic event. Also, in some studies, adverse experiences, for example, abuse in childhood (28), appear to represent a distal predisposition to depression, whereas in others, 5-HTTLPR genotype moderates the depressogenic effects of more proximal events (11). Studies of *both* predispositional (biological and psychological) and precipitating events would provide a test of this aspect of the cognitive model. Kilpatrick and colleagues (29) found that carriers of the low-expression variant of the short-form 5-HTTLPR polymorphism were prone to develop major depression and postdisaster posttraumatic stress disorder under conditions of high exposure to hurricanes *and* low social support. Kaufman and colleagues (28) have also found evidence that social support buffers against depressive reactions to stressful experiences among genetically vulnerable individuals. Although questions have been raised regarding the generalizability of the 5-HTTLPR findings (e.g., 30), they are useful to illustrate parallels between biological and psychological concepts. The more exhaustive analyses would include other variants such as the CREB and COMT genes (31, 32).

Investigators have also found that the brain-derived neurotrophic factor genotype interacted with the 5-HTTLPR gene to predict depression in children (28) and older adults (33). Of interest, variants of the brain-derived neurotrophic factor predicted ruminations and depression differently in adolescent girls and their mothers (34). Specifically, Hilt and colleagues (34) found that girls with the *Val/Val* genotype had higher rumination scores and exhibited more symptoms of depression than girls with the *Val/Met* genotype. In contrast, mothers with *adult*-onset depression and the *Val/Met* genotype exhibited more symptoms of depression and rumination. Of interest, mothers with *childhood*-onset depression were more likely to have the *Val/Val* genotype. Kaufman and colleagues (28) found that in maltreated children, depressive severity was predicted in part by an interaction of the 5-HTTLPR (short allele) with the brain-derived neurotrophic factor (*Val/Met*) genotype, particularly among children with low social support. A variant of the HTR-2A gene has been found to potentiate the effect of maternal nurturance in mitigating the experience of depressive symptoms in children (35). As research proceeds in this area, it seems likely that a variety of other gene-gene and gene-environment interactions will be discovered. In general, the established relationships between environmental events, biological predisposition, and depression appear to run parallel to the findings of the cognitive model regarding environmental events, cognitive factors, and depression.

Genetic Diathesis and Cognitive Bias

While the genetic studies have pointed to the innate biological vulnerability to stress leading to depression, the relation of biological to cognitive vulnerability needed to be clarified. The gene-by-environment findings for depression have prompted an interest in uncovering their relationships to cognitive variables. A variety of experimental procedures have been used to test for cognitive bias in individuals at genetic risk for depression. The negative attentional, recall, and interpretative biases are generally elicited by mood induction procedures, such as viewing sad movie clips or imagining sad experiences (36). Genetic antecedents for these observed cognitive biases have been identified. A number of studies indicate that negative cognitive processing and negative cognitions are associated with the presence of the 5-HTTLPR short allele (37–40). Of particular relevance to possible cognitive predisposition, Hayden and colleagues (40) found that nondepressed children homozygous for the short allele showed greater negative processing on a self-referential encoding task following a negative mood induction than did children with other genotypes. Thus, the accumulating evidence suggests the genetic predisposition to depression is associated with biases in the processing of information.

Neurophysiological and Cognitive Factors/Bias

What *neurophysiological processes* are related to the cognitive biases? Multiple findings have tied amygdala hyperactivity to depression (41, 42). However, the findings need to be considered within a broader framework, including many brain regions implicated in depression (43, 44). A specific line of inquiry has tied the 5-HTTLPR variant to activation in brain regions critical for processing negative stimuli. Hyperreactivity of the amygdala in the short 5-HTTLPR variant carriers is associated with increased sensitivity to negative stimuli (45) and leads to negative bias in the processing or interpretation of emotional stimuli (46, 47). Since the amygdala is involved in the evaluation and storage of emotionally charged events (48), its hyperreactivity to negative stimuli in predisposed individuals would appear to represent a neurophysiological correlate of cognitive bias.

The systematic bias in information processing in depression is reflected not only in selective attention and exaggerated reaction to negative stimuli (49, 50) but also in the *expectancy* of aversive events (51). Abler and colleagues (51) found that the anticipation of noxious stimuli produced excessive amygdala activation in genetically prone individuals. Further, there is evidence that the 5-HTTLPR gene interacted with children's attentional and inferential biases to predict depressive symptoms; inferential bias alone predicts lifetime diagnosis of depression among carriers of the 5-HTTLPR short allele, but not among those homozygous for the long allele (unpublished work by Gibb BE, Benas JS, Grassia M, McGeary J and unpublished work by Gibb BE, Uhrlass DJ, Grassia M, McGeary J).

The pathway from genetic and cognitive predisposition to depression may be clarified by studies of the impact of stress on neural functioning. Gotlib and colleagues (52) have found that carriers of the short-form serotonin transporter gene (5-HTTLPR) show elevated cortisol response, cognitive biases, and activation of the amygdala during a mood repair procedure. Adverse circumstances engage the hypothalamic-pituitary-adrenal (HPA) axis, which leads to the secretion of excessive "stress hormones" such as cortisol (52). Presumably, the continual secretion of cortisol culminates in the hypercortisolemia characteristic of most depressed individuals (1, 53).

Several converging findings suggest that the cognitive appraisal of a stressor plays a role in the evocation of cortisol response and the generation of depressive symptoms. In a review of relevant literature, Dickerson and Kemeny (54), for example, noted consistent findings that experimental manipulations appraised as threat of social rejection produced an elevated cortisol response. These results, combined with the findings by Hankin and colleagues (19) on the negative cognitive responses to daily stressful events leading to depressive symptoms, suggest a pathway to depressive symptoms: stress→ distorted appraisal→ engagement of the HPA axis→ cortisol→ depressive symptoms. Of course, there are undoubtedly feedback loops involving both psychological and biological variables.

A further elaboration of this hypothesis is suggested by Gotlib (unpublished work by Gotlib IH), who proposed a

FIGURE 2. A Developmental Model of Depression Based on Anomalous Genes[a]

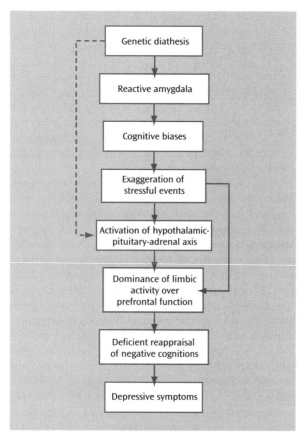

Genetic diathesis

↓

Reactive amygdala

↓

Cognitive biases

↓

Exaggeration of stressful events

↓

Activation of hypothalamic-pituitary-adrenal axis

↓

Dominance of limbic activity over prefrontal function

↓

Deficient reappraisal of negative cognitions

↓

Depressive symptoms

[a] Multiple interactions are not shown. Genetic pathways leading to reduced prefrontal activity have not been determined as yet. Increased limbic activity overrides prefrontal control.

reciprocal model involving the dysregulated HPA axis (in response to specific stressors) leading to increased cortisol secretion, which affects the serotonergic system. He also proposes a more complex theory that involves the impact of increased cortisol secretion on the short form of the 5-HTTLPR gene, leading to an alteration in the transmission of serotonin and, consequently, negative feedback to the HPA axis and increased cortisol secretion.

Gotlib's theory can be amplified to take into account research findings demonstrating interactions between measures of cognitive reactivity and serotonin. Studies have shown that increases or decreases in serotonin activity are related to self-assessment of dysfunctional attitudes or cognitive reactivity. Meyer and colleagues (55) reported that acute tryptophan depletion of serotonin increases dysfunctional attitudes, while Booij and colleagues (56) found that depletion of serotonin increased cognitive reactivity. The finding that individuals with the short variant of the 5-HTTLPR gene show depressive symptoms after experimental depletion of serotonin provides evidence of the association of genomic with neurochemical vulnera-

bility. Finally, Meyer and colleagues (57) reported increased dysfunctional attitudes in depressed patients with low intracellular serotonin. Thus, the preliminary evidence suggests linkages between cognitive vulnerability and genetic vulnerability expressed as a hyperreactive serotonergic system.

Recent neurophysiological research is pertinent to another aspect of the expanded cognitive model, mainly the formulation that during depression of the cognitive control system, top-down processing is dysregulated while the bottom-up schematic processing is prepotent. Siegle and colleagues (41) found that nearly all depressed patients have reduced prefrontal function and about one-half have increased amygdala activity. Thus, the balance of their respective activity is relevant to cognitive control. Banks and colleagues (58) found that the reduced amygdala coupling with the orbitofrontal cortex and the dorsal medial prefrontal cortex predicts the extent of attenuation of negative affect following reappraisal. Johnstone and colleagues (59) point out that a key feature underlying the pathophysiology of major depression is the dysfunctional engagement of the right prefrontal cortex and the lack of engagement of the left lateral ventral medial prefrontal circuitry, important for the down-regulation of amygdala responses to negative stimuli. They suggest that the top-down process of reappraisal is defective in depressed individuals; this may account for the importance of reappraisal in the cognitive therapy of this disorder. Thus, two concurrent processes are involved in emotional processing in depression: diminished cognitive control from prefrontal and cingulate regions and increased activity in the amygdala and other regions.

Deconstructing Depression

Interpretation of the research comparing components of the cognitive model with the neurophysiological investigations of depression poses a philosophical problem. How can one reconcile two totally different levels of abstraction: mentalism and materialism? The cognitive and neurophysiological approaches use different concepts, research strategies, and technical procedures. Given this philosophical problem, is there justification for mixing the two models in terms of causation or interaction (for example, reduction of serotonin causes an increase in dysfunctional attitudes; see reference 57) or are the neurophysiological and cognitive processes simply "different sides of the same coin," as I once argued (60)? According to my earlier notion, the cognitive processes are parallel to but do not interact with the biological processes.

Notwithstanding this philosophical problem, I believe that it is possible to present a pragmatic formulation of the interaction of the two levels (Figure 2). In deconstructing the phenomenon of depression, I propose a hypothetical pathway starting with genetic vulnerability (including predispositional but not protective genes). The 5-HTTLPR polymorphism leads to excessive reactivity of the amygdala (45). The heightened limbic reactivity to emotionally significant events triggers deployment of increased attentional resources to such events, manifested by negative attentional bias and recall (cognitive reactivity). The selective focus on the negative aspects of experience results in the familiar cognitive distortions such as exaggeration, personalization, and overgeneralization (6) and, consequently, in the formation of dysfunctional attitudes regarding personal adequacy, acceptability, and worth. Frequent reiterations of negative interpretations shape the content of the cognitive schemas (unlovable, inadequate, worthless). Concurrently, the negative interpretations of experience have an impact on the HPA axis and set in motion the previously described cycle involving the overreactive serotonergic system and consequently lead to depression. Care needs to be taken in the interpretation of gene-environment studies, including those of the 5-HTTLPR variant, given the numerous possible methodological pitfalls in these sorts of analyses (Kenneth Kendler, personal communication, May 11, 2008). Consequently, this particular formulation is tentative, subject to future research.

The theory of the consolidation of the negative attitudes and the core negative self-concept along with the associated affective, motivational, and behavioral factors into the depressive mode is speculative but is useful as an explanatory construct (20). The progression from depressive proneness to a full-blown depression would involve not only the hyperactivation of this conglomerate but also the diminution of reality testing. The biological counterpart of this theoretical model includes complex circuits involving multiple brain regions. Mayberg (61), for example, defines a major depressive episode as a "pattern of dysfunctional interactions among specific cingulate, paralimbic, subcortical, and frontal regions critical to maintaining emotional homeostasis under conditions of exogenous or endogenous stress" (p. 258). At present the most direct parallel involves the predominance of negatively biased processing and reduced reality testing on the one hand and amygdala activation and disengagement of executive (especially prefrontal) regions on the other.

Future Perspectives

The accumulation of studies of the psychological and biological aspects of depression has reached a critical mass warranting a new synthesis. The findings of relationships among the diverse genetic, neurophysiological, environmental, and cognitive aspects of the vulnerability to and development of depression call for future studies integrating these findings into a comprehensible formulation. A series of multiple wave prospective studies could identify the relevant variables and their interrelationships. The studies ideally would be complementary to each other so that each finding would contribute to the overall formulation of the theory of depression. The clarification of specific associations among the relevant variables should yield valuable information. In order to simplify the suggested plan, I have limited the genetic diathesis to the 5-HTTLPR gene. Obviously, other genes, including those that have a protective effect, as well as the individuals' social support should be included in any formulations. Moreover, as indicated previously, the research based on this gene is not totally reliable.

The proposed psychobiological model of depression poses a number of problems and questions that need to be addressed. The developmental model presupposes that the 5-HTTLPR gene in some as yet unidentified way leads to hyperreactivity of the amygdala to external stimuli. This activity is associated with a negative cognitive bias. In addition, increased reactivity of the HPA axis is also associated with this genetic variant (52). A longitudinal study starting in childhood could investigate the causal sequence. In one pathway, the hyperactive amygdala leads initially to attentional bias that gradually progresses into significant negative cognitive distortions of daily experiences that engage the HPA axis. Alternatively, the amygdala and HPA overactivity may contribute independently to the cognitive and physiological impact of life events.

A number of other problems warrant further investigation. The association of increased dysfunctional attitudes with serotonin depletion poses an interesting question: is the association due to a common linkage to some undefined third factor, such as amygdala reactivity? Does serotonin deficiency *cause* an increase in dysfunctional attitudes (55), is the converse true, or is there another explanation for this association? The finding that depressed individuals treated with cognitive therapy, compared to pharmacotherapy treated patients, do not show an increase in depressive symptoms (generally associated with dysfunctional attitudes) following tryptophan depletion calls for further investigation (62). These results indicate a more complex relationship between serotonin depletion and dysfunctional attitudes. The neurobiological mechanisms involved in the reduced reality testing of negative beliefs deserve further attention. The specific brain areas involved in dysconnectivity need to be spelled out. Is the preemption of amygdala activity over prefrontal and cingular executive functions related to reduction of serotonin inhibition of the amygdala (63)? Work relating poor error detection in depression to specific dysfunctions in various brain regions (64) needs to be followed.

The integrative developmental model postulates that various genetic variants sensitize individuals to life experiences that make them vulnerable to depression. Specifically, the studies would address the biological mechanisms that contribute to depression through the tendency to construe events in an excessively negative way. A series of waves, starting in early childhood, should examine the variables associated with the polymorphism: assessments of information processing biases (36, 37, 40), negative cognitions (38), and dysfunctional attitudes (65) following negative mood inductions. These findings would then be compared with studies of brain activity to determine their associations with the limbic system as well as prefrontal cingular and other regions. The early studies would determine whether automatic cognitive processing precedes the development of negative cognitions and dysfunctional attitudes. Another wave could examine diary records of daily dysfunctional cognitions in response to stressful situations and relate these to cortisol responses to specific stimuli situations. Overall, these assessments over a long time span would integrate findings from neuroimaging and neuroendocrine responses to stressors with cognitive responses to daily stressful activities as well as to major life events. The association of increased dysfunctional attitudes with serotonin depletion would also be determined in these studies, and in addition the attempt to find the specific relationships among these variables could be determined.

I have reason to hope that future research will perhaps provide a new paradigm which for the first time can integrate findings from psychological and biological studies to build a new understanding of depression.

Received May 15, 2008; accepted May 20, 2008 (doi: 10.1176/appi.ajp.2008.08050721). From the Department of Psychiatry, University of Pennsylvania. Address correspondence and reprint requests to Dr. Beck, Department of Psychiatry, University of Pennsylvania, 3535 Market St., Rm. 2032, Philadelphia, PA 19104; abeck@mail.med.upenn.edu (e-mail).

Dr. Beck reports no competing interests.

The author thanks Brad Alford, Andrew Butler, Brandon Gibb, Kenneth Kendler, Helen Mayberg, John O'Reardon, and Greg Siegle for criticism, comments, and suggestions and Brianna Mann and Allison Fox for technical support.

References

1. Beck AT: Depression: Clinical, Experimental, and Theoretical Aspects. New York Harper & Row, 1967.

2. Rush AJ, Beck AT, Kovacs M, Hollon SD: Comparative efficacy of cognitive therapy and pharmacotherapy in the treatment of depressed outpatients. Cognit Ther Res 1977; 1:7–37

3. Beck AT: Cognitive models of depression. J Cogn Psychother: An Int Quarterly 1987; 1:5–37

4. Clark DA, Beck AT: Scientific Foundations of Cognitive Theory and Therapy of Depression. New York, John Wiley & Sons, 1999

5. Beck AT, Steer RA, Brown GK, Weissman A: Factor analysis of the Dsyfunctional Attitude Scale in a clinical population. Psychological Assessment 1991; 3:478–483

6. Beck AT, Sethi B, Tuthill R: Childhood bereavement and adult depression. Arch Gen Psychiatry 1963; 9:295–302

7. Sethi BB: The relationship of separation to depression. Arch Gen Psychiatry 1964; 10:486–496

8. Harkness KL, Lumley MN: Child abuse and neglect and the development of depression in children and adolescents, in Handbook of Depression in Children and Adolescents. Edited by Abela JR, Hankin BL. New York, Guilford, 2008, pp 466–488

9. Beck AT: Cognitive Therapy and the Emotional Disorders. New York, Meridian, 1976

10. Scher C, Ingram R, Segal Z: Cognitive reactivity and vulnerability: empirical evaluation of construct activation and cognitive diatheses in unipolar depression. Clin Psychol Rev 2005; 25:487–510

11. Kendler KS, Kuhn JW, Vittum J, Prescott CA, Riley B: The interaction of stressful life events and a serotonin transporter polymorphism in the prediction of episodes of major depression: a replication. Arch Gen Psychiatry 2005; 62:529–535

12. Abela JRZ, Hankin BL: Cognitive vulnerability to depression in children and adolescents: a developmental psychopathology perspective, in Handbook of Depression in Children and Adolescents. Edited by Abela JRZ, Hankin BL. New York, Guilford, 2008, pp 35–78

13. Kendler KS, Thornton LM, Gardner CO: Stressful life events and previous episodes in the etiology of major depression in women: an evaluation of the "kindling" hypothesis. Am J Psychiatry 2000; 157:1243–1251

14. Monroe SM, Harkness KL: Life stress, the "kindling" hypothesis, and the recurrence of depression: considerations from a life stress perspective. Psychol Rev 2005; 112:417–445

15. Jacobs RH, Reinecke MA, Gollan JK, Kane P: Empirical evidence of cognitive vulnerability for depression among children and adolescents: a cognitive science and developmental perspective. Clin Psychol Rev 2008; 28:759–728

16. Abela JRZ, D'Alessandro DU: Beck's cognitive theory of depression: a test of the diathesis-stress and causal mediation components. Br J Clin Psychol 2002; 41:111–128

17. Segal ZV, Gemar M, Williams S: Differential cognitive response to a mood challenge following successful cognitive therapy or pharmacotherapy for unipolar depression. J Abnorm Psychol 1999; 108:3–10

18. Butler AC, Hokanson JE, Flynn HA: A comparison of self-esteem lability and low trait self-esteem as vulnerability factors for depression. J Pers Soc Psychol 1994; 66:166–177

19. Hankin BL, Fraley C, Abela JRZ: Daily depression and cognitions about stress: evidence for a trait-like depressogenic cognitive style and the prediction of depressive symptoms in a prospective daily diary study. J Pers Soc Psychol 2005; 88:673–685

20. Beck AT: Beyond belief: a theory of modes, personality, and psychopathology, in Frontiers of Cognitive Therapy. Edited by Salkovskis P. New York, Guilford, 1996, pp 1–25

21. Freud S: Collected Works of Sigmund Freud. New York and Washington, DC, BiblioBazaar, originally published in 1920

22. Chaiken S, Trope Y: Dual-Process Theories in Social Psychology. New York, Guilford, 1999

23. Beevers CG: Cognitive vulnerability to depression: a dual process model. Clin Psychol Rev 2005; 25:975–1002

24. Crick NR, Dodge KA: A review and reformulation of social information-processing mechanisms in children's social adjustment. Psychol Bull 1994; 115:74–101

25. Dozois DJA, Beck AT: Cognitive schemas, beliefs and assumptions, in Risk Factors for Depression. Edited by Dobson KS, Dozois DJA. Oxford, UK, Elsevier (in press)

26. Caspi A, Sugden K, Moffitt TE, Taylor A, Craig IW, Harrington HL: Influence of life stress on depression: moderation by a polymorphism in the 5-HTT gene. Science 2003; 301:386–389

27. Uher R, McGuffin P: The moderation by the serotonin transporter gene of environmental adversity in the aetiology of mental illness: review and methodological analysis. Molecular Psychiatry 2008; 13:131–146

28. Kaufman J, Yang B, Douglas-Palumberi H, Grasso D, Lipschitz D, Houshyar S: Brain-derived neurotrophic factor 5-HTTLPR gene interactions and environmental modifiers of depression in children. Biol Psychiatry 2006; 59:673–680

29. Kilpatrick DG, Koenen KC, Ruggiero KJ, Acierno R, Galea S, Resnick HS: The serotonin transporter genotype and social support and moderation of posttraumatic stress disorder and depression in hurricane-exposed adults. Am J Psychiatry 2007; 164:1693–1699

30. Gillespie NA, Whitfield JB, Williams B, Heath AC, Martin NG: The relationship between stressful life events, the serotonin trans-

porter (5-HTTLPR) genotype and major depression. Psychol Med 2005; 35:101–111

31. Zubenko GS, Hughes HB III: Effects of the G(-656), a variant on CREB1 promoter activity in a neuronal cell line: interactions with gonadal steroids and stress. Mol Psychiatry 2008 (Epub ahead of print)

32. Wichers M, Aguilera M, Kenis G, Krabbendam L, Myin-Germeys I, Jacobs N, Peeters F, Derom C, Vlietinck R, Mengelers R, Delespaul P, van Os J: The catechol-O-methyl transferase Val(158)Met polymorphism and experience of reward in the flow of daily life. Neuropsychopharmacology 2007 (Epub ahead of print)

33. Kim J, Stewart R, Kim S, Yang S, Shin I, Kim Y: Interactions between life stressors and susceptibility genes (5-HTTPR and BDNF) on depression in Korean elders. Biol Psychiatry 2007; 62:423–428

34. Hilt LM, Sander LC, Nolen-Hoeksema S, Simen AA: The BDNF Val66Met polymorphism predicts rumination and depression differently in young adolescent girls and their mothers. Neurosci Lett 2007; 429:12–16

35. Jokela M, Keltikangas-Järvinen L, Kivimäki M, Puttonen S, Elovainio M, Rontu R: Serotonin receptor 2A gene and the influence of childhood maternal nurturance on adulthood depressive symptoms. Arch Gen Psychiatry 2007; 64:356–360

36. Joormann J, Talbot L, Gotlib IH: Biased processing of emotional information in girls at risk for depression. J Abnorm Psychol 2007; 116:135–143

37. Beevers CG, Gibb BE, McGeary JE, Miller IW: Serotonin transporter genetic variation and biased attention for emotional word stimuli among psychiatric inpatients. J Abnorm Psychol 2007; 116:208–212

38. Beevers CG, Scott WD, McGeary C, McGeary JE: Negative cognitive response to a sad mood induction: associations with polymorphisms of the serotonin transporter (5-HTTLPR) gene. Cognition and Emotion (in press)

39. Canli T, Lesch K: Long story short: the serotonin transporter in emotion regulation and social cognition. Nat Neurosci 2007; 10:1103–1109

40. Hayden EP, Dougherty LR, Maloney B, Olino TM, Durbin CE, Sheihk HI: Early-emerging cognitive vulnerability to depression and the serotonin transporter promoter region polymorphism. J Affect Disord 2008; 107:227–230

41. Siegle GJ, Thompson W, Carter CS, Steinhauer SR, Thase ME: Increased amygdala and decreased dorsolateral prefrontal bold responses in unipolar depression: related and independent features. Biol Psychiatry 2007; 61:198–209

42. Surguladze S, Brammer MJ, Keedwell P, Giampietro V, Young AW, Travis MJ: A differential pattern of neural response toward sad versus happy facial expressions in major depressive disorder. Biol Psychiatry 2005; 57:201–209

43. Mayberg HS: Modulating dysfunctional limbic-cortical circuits in depression: towards development of brain-based algorithms for diagnosis and optimised treatment. Br Med Bull 2003; 65:193–207

44. Phillips ML, Drevets WC, Rauch SL, Lane R: Neurobiology of emotion perception II: implications for major psychiatric disorders. Biol Psychiatry 2003; 54:515–528

45. Munafò M, Brown S, Hariri A: Serotonin transporter (5-HTTLPR) genotype and amygdala activation: a meta-analysis. Biol Psychiatry 2008; 63:852–857

46. Dannlowski U, Ohrmann P, Bauer J, Kugel H, Arolt V, Heindel W: Amygdala reactivity to masked negative faces is associated with automatic judgmental bias in major depression: a 3T fMRI study. J Psychiatry Neurosci 2007; 32:423–429

47. Monk CS, Klein RG, Telzer EH, Schroth EA, Mannuzza S, Moulton JL III, Guardino M, Masten CL, McClure-Tone EB, Fromm S,

Blair RJ, Pine DS, Ernst M: Amygdala and nucleus accumbens activation to emotional facial expressions in children and adolescents at risk for major depression. Am J Psychiatry 2008; 165:90–98

48. LeDoux JE: The Emotional Brain: The Mysterious Underpinnings of Emotional Life. New York, Simon & Schuster, 1996

49. Siegle GJ, Steinhauer SR, Thase ME, Stenger VA, Carter CS: Can't shake that feeling: fMRI assessment of sustained amygdala activity in response to emotional information in depressed individuals. Biol Psychiatry 2002; 51:693–707

50. Siegle GJ, Carter CS, Thase ME: Use of fMRI to predict recovery from unipolar depression with cognitive behavior therapy. Am J Psychiatry 2006; 163:735–738

51. Abler B, Erk S, Herwig U, Walter H: Anticipation of aversive stimuli activates extended amygdala in unipolar depression. J Psychiatr Res 2007; 41:511–522

52. Gotlib IH, Joormann J, Minor K, Hallmayer J: HPA axis reactivity: A mechanism underlying the associations among 5-HTTLPR, stress, and depression. Biol Psychiatry 2008; 63:847–851

53. Parker KJ, Schatzberg AF, Lyons DM: Neuroendocrine aspects of hypercortisolism in major depression. Hormones & Behavior 2003; 43:60–66

54. Dickerson SS, Kemeny ME: Acute stressors and cortisol responses: a theoretical integration and synthesis of laboratory research. Psychol Bull 2004; 130:355–391

55. Meyer JH, McMain S, Kennedy SH, Korman L, Brown GM, DaSilva JN, Wilson AA, Blak T, Eynan-Harvey R, Goulding VS, Houle S, Links P: Dysfunctional attitudes and 5-HT$_2$ receptors during depression and self-harm. Am J Psychiatry 2003; 160:90–99

56. Booij L, Van der Does AJW: Cognitive and serotonergic vulnerability to depression: convergent findings. J Abnorm Psychol 2007; 116:86–94

57. Meyer JH, Houle S, Sagrati S, Carella A, Hussey DF, Ginovart N: Brain serotonin transporter binding potential measured with carbon 11–labeled DASB positron emission tomography: effects of major depressive episodes and severity of dysfunctional attitudes. Arch Gen Psychiatry 2004; 61:1271–1279

58. Banks SJ, Eddy KT, Angstadt M, Nathan PJ, Phan KL: Amygdalafrontal connectivity during emotion regulation. Soc Cogn Affect Neurosc 2007; 2:303–312

59. Johnstone T, van Reekum CM, Urry HL, Kalin NH, Davidson RJ: Failure to regulate: counterproductive recruitment of top-down prefrontal-subcortical circuitry in major depression. J Neurosc 2007; 27:8877–8884

60. Beck AT: Cognitive therapy, behavior therapy, psychoanalysis, and pharmacotherapy: a cognitive continuum, in Psychotherapy Research: Where Are We and Where Should We Go? Edited by Williams JBW, Spitzer RL. New York, Guilford, 1984, pp 114–135

61. Mayberg HS: Defining neurocircuits in depression: insights from functional neuroimaging studies of diverse treatments. Psychiatr Ann 2006; 4:258–267

62. O'Reardon JP, Chopra MP, Bergan A, Gallop R, DeRubeis RJ, Crits-Christoph P: Response to tryptophan depletion in major depression treated with either cognitive therapy or selective serotonin reuptake inhibitor antidepressants. Biol Psychiatry 2004; 55:957–959

63. Stutzmann GE, McEwen BS, LeDoux JE: Serotonin modulation of sensory inputs to the lateral amygdala: dependency on corticosterone. J Neurosci 1998; 18:9529–9538

64. Holmes AJ, Pizzagalli DA: Spatiotemporal dynamics of error processing dysfunctions in major depressive disorder. Arch Gen Psychiatry 2008; 65:179–188

65. Abela JRZ, Skitch SA: Dysfunctional attitudes, self-esteem, and hassles: cognitive vulnerability to depression in children of affectively ill parents. Behav Res Ther 2007; 45:1127–1140

Meta-analysis of Major Depressive Disorder Relapse and Recurrence With Second-Generation Antidepressants

Richard Hansen, Ph.D.
Bradley Gaynes, M.D., M.P.H.
Patricia Thieda, M.A.
Gerald Gartlehner, M.D., M.P.H.
Angela Deveaugh-Geiss, M.S.
Erin Krebs, M.D.
Kathleen Lohr, Ph.D.

Objective: This meta-analysis reviewed data on the efficacy and effectiveness of second-generation antidepressants for preventing major depression relapse and recurrence during continuation and maintenance phases of treatment, respectively. _Methods:_ MEDLINE, EMBASE, and PsycINFO, the Cochrane Library, and International Pharmaceutical Abstracts were searched for the period of January 1980 through April 2007 for reviews, randomized controlled trials, meta-analyses, and observational studies on the topic. Two persons independently reviewed abstracts and full-text articles using a structured data abstraction form to ensure consistency in appraisal and data extraction. _Results:_ Four comparative trials and 23 placebo-controlled trials that addressed relapse or recurrence prevention were included. Results of comparative trials have not demonstrated statistically significant differences between duloxetine and paroxetine, fluoxetine and sertraline, fluvoxamine and sertraline, and trazodone and venlafaxine. Pooled data for the class of second-generation antidepressants compared with placebo suggested a relatively large effect size that persists over time. For preventing both relapse and recurrence, the number of patients needed to treat is five (95% confidence interval of 4 to 6). Differences in the length of open-label treatment before randomization, drug type, and trial duration did not affect pooled estimates of relapse rates. Across all trials, 7% of patients randomly assigned to receive active treatment and 5% of patients randomly assigned to receive a placebo discontinued treatment because of adverse events. _Conclusions:_ This review demonstrates the overall benefits of continuation- and maintenance-phase treatment of major depression with second-generation antidepressants and emphasizes the need for additional studies of comparative differences among drugs. (_Psychiatric Services_ 59:1121–1130, 2008)

Dr. Hansen is affiliated with the Division of Pharmaceutical Outcomes and Policy, Dr. Gaynes is with the Department of Psychiatry, Ms. Thieda is with Cecil G. Sheps Center for Health Services Research, and Ms. Deveaugh-Geiss is with the Department of Epidemiology, all at the University of North Carolina–Chapel Hill. Dr. Gartlehner is with the Department for Evidence-Based Medicine and Clinical Epidemiology, Danube University, Krems, Austria. Dr. Krebs is with the Department of Medicine, Indiana University, Indianapolis. Dr. Lohr is with RTI International, Research Triangle Park, North Carolina. Send correspondence to Dr. Hansen at the School of Pharmacy, University of North Carolina–Chapel Hill, 2205 Kerr Hall, Campus Box 7360, Chapel Hill, NC 27599 (e-mail: rahansen@unc.edu).

Antidepressants are used commonly as a first-line treatment for major depressive disorder. In particular, second-generation antidepressants such as selective serotonin reuptake inhibitors (SSRIs), serotonin-norepinephrine reuptake inhibitors, and other drugs that selectively affect the activity of neurotransmitters play a prominent role in treatment. Although these drugs are believed to have similar efficacy to first-generation agents (for example, tricyclic antidepressants and monoamine oxidase inhibitors), they are recommended over the first-generation agents because of their relatively favorable side effect profile and reduced risk of harm in overdose or in combination with certain medications or food (1).

Current treatment guidelines for major depression (2,3) suggest an acute-phase treatment duration of six to 12 weeks. For patients who demonstrate an adequate response (usually defined as remission) to acute-phase treatment, continuation-phase treatment of four to nine months is recommended. The goal of continuation-phase treatment is to prolong the absence of depressive symptoms such that the patient's episode can be considered completely resolved. Effective continuation-phase treatment prevents relapse, defined as the return of depressive symptoms during the current depressive episode. After successful continuation-phase treatment, a maintenance phase of treatment to prevent recurrence of a new, distinct episode is considered. For patients with a history of recurrent depression, maintenance-phase treatment can frequently last for years.

For acute treatment of depression, approximately 60% of patients respond to second-generation antidepressants (4). Evidence from the one-year naturalistic follow-up phase of the Sequenced Treatment Alternatives to Relieve Depression (STAR*D) trial indicates that at least 40% of acute-phase responders relapse during continuation treatment (5). Randomized, double-blinded, controlled trials have assessed how treatments compare with placebo and with each other for preventing relapse and recurrence, but results for second-generation antidepressants have not been systematically reviewed. Two reviews have systematically assessed relapse prevention during continuation-phase treatment or recurrence prevention during maintenance-phase treatment (6,7), but these reviews included all antidepressants rather than just second-generation antidepressants. They are limited by the dates of their literature searches—searches censored at 1987 (6) and 2000 (7)—and thus exclude more recent studies. More recently, Zimmerman and colleagues (8) focused on second-generation antidepressants, although the intent of their review was to illustrate how conclusions differ between extension trials and placebo substitution trials.

Because second-generation drugs are now the most frequently prescribed antidepressants, our goal was to systematically evaluate data on the efficacy of second-generation antidepressants for preventing relapse and recurrence. We conducted a systematic review and meta-analysis of comparative and placebo-controlled evidence for 12 second-generation antidepressants (bupropion, citalopram, duloxetine, escitalopram, fluoxetine, fluvoxamine, mirtazapine, nefazodone, paroxetine, sertraline, trazodone, and venlafaxine). We refer to these agents collectively as antidepressants. We had two key questions for this review. First, for adults with a

depressive syndrome, do antidepressants differ in their efficacy or effectiveness for maintaining remission (specifically, preventing relapse during the continuation phase and preventing recurrence during the maintenance phase)? Second, for adults with depressive syndrome, what is the overall effect size for active treatment compared with placebo, and is this effect size persistent over time?

Methods

Key questions
Key questions designed to address efficacy, effectiveness, and tolerability of antidepressants for maintaining remission guided our work. The key questions were formulated through a process involving the public, the Scientific Resource Center for the Effective Health Care program of the Agency for Healthcare Research and Quality (AHRQ), and various stakeholder groups. AHRQ provided funding for the initial review, although this update and analysis were unfunded.

Literature search
To identify articles relevant to each key question, we searched MEDLINE, EMBASE, the Cochrane Library, PsycINFO, and International Pharmaceutical Abstracts. Searches covered studies published during the period of January 1980 through April 2007. In addition, we manually searched reference lists of relevant review articles and letters to the editor. We also manually searched the Center for Drug Evaluation and Research (CDER) database to identify unpublished research submitted to the U.S. Food and Drug Administration (FDA).

Study selection
Two persons independently reviewed article titles and abstracts. We included head-to-head trials comparing one antidepressant with another and placebo-controlled trials. Studies included adult inpatient and outpatient populations with depressive illness in which individuals demonstrated response to treatment or remission. Head-to-head trials were included if they reported relapse or recurrence rates, regardless of whether participants were randomly assigned

to treatment groups after successful acute-phase or continuation-phase treatment (that is, extension versus randomized substitution trials). For our meta-analysis, inclusion criteria were more stringent for placebo-controlled evidence; only studies that randomly assigned participants after demonstrating either an acute-phase response or lack of relapse during the continuation phase were included (randomized placebo-substitution trials).

Data abstraction
Trained reviewers abstracted data from each study; a senior reviewer read each abstracted article and evaluated completeness of data extraction. We recorded intention-to-treat results if available. When intention-to-treat results were not explicitly presented, we derived intention-to-treat results by using as the numerator the number of patients who experienced the outcome (relapse for continuation phase or recurrence for maintenance phase) and using as the denominator the number randomly assigned to that arm of the trial.

Quality and strength assessment
In terms of quality, we assessed the internal validity of trials on the basis of predefined criteria—ratings of good, fair, or poor—from the U.S. Preventive Services Task Force (9) and the National Health Service Centre for Reviews and Dissemination (10). Elements of internal validity assessment included randomization, allocation concealment, similarity of compared groups at baseline, use of intention-to-treat analysis, and overall and differential loss to follow-up. Discrepancies in quality assessment were resolved by discussion and, when necessary, consultation with a third party.

Data synthesis
We qualitatively summarized all studies. For placebo-controlled trials—a majority of the included studies—we also conducted quantitative analyses. We calculated the relative risk of loss of response for active treatment compared with placebo. The primary outcome measure was defined as loss of response or remission (in other words, continuation-phase relapse or

maintenance-phase recurrence). In most trials this was defined as an increase in the Hamilton Rating Scale for Depression (HAM-D) or Montgomery-Asberg Depression Rating Scale (MADRS) score above a predefined cutoff point. We conducted relative risk meta-analysis of relapse rates for trials stratified by duration of follow-up: less than one year and one year or more. Stratification of trials lasting one year or more was intended to represent a conservative delineation of maintenance-phase treatment (thus referring to recurrence), whereas trials lasting less than one year were assumed to represent relapse prevention during the continuation phase. Risk-difference meta-analyses were used to calculate numbers of patients needed to treat to prevent one relapse or recurrence overall and for each time period.

Our analyses included trials with multiple placebo comparisons. For example, for trials that compared multiple dosing arms with a single-placebo group, we combined the dosing arms for a single comparison as long as doses were within the range of FDA-approved doses. In trials that compared more than one drug with placebo, we included each drug-placebo comparison as an observation but reduced the sample size of the placebo group proportionately so as not to overrepresent the placebo group (11). For example, if 300 patients were randomly assigned to receive drug A (N=100), drug B (N=100), or placebo (N=100), our analysis compared drug A (N=100) with placebo (N=50) and drug B (N=100) with placebo (N=50). Although the proportion of placebo-treated participants having the outcome does not change, this approach inflates the variance of the log relative risk and ultimately results in a more conservative confidence interval. For each meta-analysis, we tested for heterogeneity of treatment effects, using I^2 statistics. We report the results of the more conservative random effects models (12). To estimate possible publication bias, we used funnel plots, the Beggs adjusted rank correlation test, and the Egger regression approach (13,14). However, because these tests have low statistical power when the number of trials is small (15), undetected bias may still be present.

The most common trial design was an open-label acute treatment phase of six to 15 weeks, followed by a randomized, double-blind, placebo-controlled continuation phase, maintenance phase, or both for acute-phase responders or remitters. Because trials differed in the length of open-label treatment before randomization and in the duration of treatment after randomization, we conducted a meta-regression to explore how heterogeneity in design influenced estimates of relative risk of relapse or recurrence. Similarly, we used meta-regression to explore whether pooling antidepressants as a class was a reasonable approach. For simplicity, this analysis explored heterogeneity by comparing SSRI trials (citalopram, escitalopram, fluoxetine, fluvoxamine, paroxetine, and sertraline) with other second-generation antidepressant trials (bupropion, duloxetine, mirtazapine, nefazodone, trazodone, and venlafaxine).

To balance our assessment of benefits, we examined reported rates of adverse events and rates of loss to follow-up that were attributed to adverse events. We qualitatively compared the rates from studies on relapse prevention and recurrence prevention with rates reported in acute-phase trials (4,16). We also conducted a relative risk meta-analysis for active treatment compared with placebo for both overall loss to follow-up and loss to follow-up attributed to adverse events. However, because of variability in study populations and in adverse event assessment and reporting among trials, caution should be taken in interpreting this evidence.

All statistical analyses were conducted with Stata 9.1 software.

Results

Our search identified 2,318 article titles and abstracts. [A flow diagram of the study selection for the meta-analysis is available as an online supplement to this article at ps.psychiatryonline. org.] Of these, we reviewed 902 full-text articles and retained 29 articles describing 27 unique trials that addressed relapse or recurrence prevention (Tables 1 and 2). The most com-

mon reason for exclusion was "wrong study design"; many excluded studies assessed acute-phase treatment. Included studies differed in their design (such as timing of randomization and eligibility criteria), although most studies randomly assigned acute-phase responders or remitters to ongoing treatment with active drug or placebo. Most trials used a predefined cutoff point on a standardized scale (such as the HAM-D or MADRS) to determine eligibility for randomization, although the cutoff point varied among trials. Likewise, operational definitions of relapse and recurrence varied among trials.

We gave most of the included trials a quality rating of fair. They represent a broad range of methodological quality.

The mean age of trial participants was generally between 40 and 50 years. We excluded trials of children and adolescents (under 18 years of age). Two trials were conducted in older populations (age range 65–87); the age of participants was 75 in one trial comparing citalopram with placebo (17) and 77 in one trial comparing sertraline with placebo (18).

Comparative trials

Four head-to-head trials (five publications) directly compared the efficacy of one second-generation antidepressant with another for maintaining remission (Table 1) (19–23). Comparisons included duloxetine with paroxetine (23), fluoxetine with sertraline (19), fluvoxamine with sertraline (20,21), and trazodone with venlafaxine (22). Relapse and recurrence rates did not differ significantly. Although none of these studies were designed to test an equivalence hypothesis, absolute differences in relapse and recurrence rates were consistently modest and likely not to be of clinical significance. Further, these comparative trials did not use a substitution design to randomly assign participants after successful acute-phase or continuation-phase treatment.

Placebo-controlled trials

Twenty-three randomized controlled trials provided placebo-controlled evidence to support the general efficacy of second-generation drugs for pre-

Table 1

Comparative studies reporting relapse or recurrence rates during continuation-phase or maintenance-phase treatment after a major depressive episode[a]

Study[b]	Eligibility criteria for relapse or recurrence of major depression[c]	Treatment phase	Duration (weeks)	N	Recurrent depression		Medication	Dose (mg per day)	Relapse or recurrence		p
					N	%			N	%	
Perahia et al., 2006 (23)	≥30% reduction in HAM-D total score	Acute	8	93	nr		Duloxetine	80	na		na
		Acute	8	102	nr		Duloxetine	120	na		na
		Acute	8	96	nr		Paroxetine	20	na		na
		Acute	8	99	nr		Placebo	—	na		na
		Continuation	24	71	nr		Duloxetine	80	6	9	nr
		Continuation	24	81	nr		Duloxetine	120	12	15	
		Continuation	24	70	nr		Paroxetine	20	2	3	
		Continuation	24	70	nr		Placebo	—	11	16	
Van Moffaert et al., 1995 (19)	≥50% reduction in MADRS or HAM-D score, or HAM-D score <10 and CGI-I score ≤2	Acute	8	82	25	30	Fluoxetine	20–40	na		na
		Acute	8	83	23	28	Sertraline	50–100	na		na
		Continuation	24	56	nr		Fluoxetine	20–40	7	13	nr (ns)
		Continuation	24	49	nr		Sertraline	50–100	5	10	
Franchini et al., 1997 (20); 2000 (21)	Absence of *DSM-IV* depressive symptoms; absence of functional impairment; HAM-D score <8	Acute	nr	nr	nr		nr		na		na
		Continuation	16	nr	nr		nr		na		na
		Maintenance, 2 year	104	32	32	100	Fluvoxamine	200	6	19	.88
		Maintenance, 2 year	104	32	32	100	Sertraline	100	7	22	
		Maintenance, 4 year	208	25	nr		Fluvoxamine	200	5	20	.92
		Maintenance, 4 year	208	22	nr		Sertraline	100	3	14	
Cunningham et al., 1994 (22)	CGI-I score ≤2	Acute	6	77	93[d]		Trazodone	150–400	na		na
		Acute	6	72	93[d]		Venlafaxine	75–200	na		na
		Acute	6	76	93[d]		Placebo	—	na		na
		Maintenance	52	30	nr		Trazodone	150–400	4	13	nr (ns)
		Maintenance	52	37	nr		Venlafaxine	75–200	3	8	
		Maintenance	52	29	nr		Placebo	—	4	14	

[a] nr, not reported; na, not applicable; ns, not significant

[b] Each study had a quality rating of fair.

[c] HAM-D, Hamilton Rating Scale for Depression (possible scores on the first 17 items range from 0 to 52, with higher scores indicating greater severity of symptoms); MADRS, Montgomery-Asberg Depression Rating Scale (possible scores range from 0 to 60, with higher scores indicating greater severity of symptoms); CGI-I, Clinical Global Impression of Improvement (possible scores range from 1 to 7, with lower scores indicating more improvement and higher scores indicating worsening; values of 4 represent no change)

[d] Values reported overall rather than by treatment

venting relapse or recurrence among patients with depressive disorders (Table 2) (17,18,24–44). For 12 trials (13 placebo comparisons) the randomized follow-up was shorter than one year, and the trials were deemed to represent relapse prevention during continuation-phase treatment (24–34,44). These trials provide consistent evidence in favor of active drug over placebo. The unadjusted frequency of relapse was 22% for active treatment, compared with 42% for placebo. An additional 11 randomized controlled trials had follow-ups of one year or longer and were deemed to represent recurrence prevention during maintenance-phase treatment (17,18,35–43). These trials also provide consistent evidence in favor of active treatment over placebo. The unadjusted frequency of recur-

rence was 26% for active treatment, compared with 48% for placebo.

Meta-analysis

Trials shorter than one year: relapse prevention. Our relative risk meta-analysis comprised 12 trials lasting less than one year (Figure 1): one on bupropion (24), three on citalopram (25,33,44), one on escitalopram (26), three on fluoxetine (27,28,34), and one each on mirtazapine (29), nefazodone (30), sertraline (31), and venlafaxine (32). The pooled relative risk of relapse was .54 (95% confidence interval [CI]=.46–.62), and the number of patients needed to treat to prevent one additional relapse over a mean time of eight months was five (CI=4–6). Heterogeneity among these trials was moderate (I^2=47%). Tests for publication

bias were not statistically significant.

Trials one year or longer: recurrence prevention. Eleven trials provided data points for follow-up of one year or more (Figure 2): one on citalopram (17), one on escitalopram (42), one on fluvoxamine (35), one on nefazodone (36), two on paroxetine (37,41), four on sertraline (18,38,39,43), and one on venlafaxine (40). Trials consistently favored active treatment over placebo for preventing recurrence, although differences were not always statistically significant. For example, during a 100-week comparison of sertraline 50–100 mg per day with placebo, 45% of sertraline-treated participants and 54% of placebo-treated participants had a recurrence, but differences were not statistically significant (18). The pooled relative risk of recurrence was

.56 (CI=.48–.66) and the number of patients needed to treat to prevent one additional recurrence over a mean time of 16 months was five (CI=4–6). Heterogeneity among these trials was moderate (I^2=30%). Tests for publication bias were not statistically significant.

Meta-regression
Our meta-regression explored heterogeneity among included trials with regard to the duration of open-label treatment before random assignment of responders, the length of the postrandomization phase, and drug type (SSRI or other type of second-generation antidepressant). None of these variables influenced our estimates of effect size at a statistically significant level.

Adverse events
The most common adverse event documented in continuation- and maintenance-phase studies was headache, followed by nausea (weighted mean incidence=15.5% and 7.4%, respectively). Compared with the incidence of adverse events in acute-phase studies (4,45), the relative incidence of these events during long-term treatment was slightly lower. On the basis of 22 trials that provided sufficient data, loss to follow-up in general and loss to follow-up because of adverse events represented an average of 50% and 7%, respectively, of patients randomly assigned to receive active treatment and 68% and 4%, respectively, of patients randomly assigned to receive placebo. Based on data pooled from 17 placebo-controlled trials, the relative risk of dropping out for any reason was statistically significantly lower for active treatment than for placebo (relative risk=.75, CI=.69–.83). Data pooled from 18 placebo-controlled trials demonstrated that loss to follow-up because of adverse events was not statistically significantly different between active treatment and placebo (relative risk=1.42, CI=.92–2.20).

Discussion
We systematically assessed the efficacy and tolerability of second-generation antidepressants for the prevention of relapse and recurrence during treatment in the continuation and maintenance phases of major depression, respectively. Only a small number of trials directly compared one antidepressant with another. Results of these trials did not demonstrate statistically significant differences between duloxetine and paroxetine (23), fluoxetine and sertraline (19), fluvoxamine and sertraline (20,21), or trazodone and venlafaxine (22) for preventing relapse or recurrence.

Although results are relatively consistent, we consider the strength of comparative evidence to be moderate because additional well-conducted studies could change our conclusions. Pooled data for second-generation antidepressants as a class compared with placebo suggest a relatively large effect size that persists over time, reflecting high-strength evidence for continued treatment beyond the acute phase. The number needed to treat to prevent one additional relapse during continuation-phase treatment or recurrence during maintenance-phase treatment is in the range of four to six patients.

The tolerability profile of continuation- and maintenance-phase treatment is fair to good. In clinical trials, 7% of patients randomly assigned to receive active treatment and 5% of patients assigned to receive placebo discontinued their continuation or maintenance phase of treatment because of adverse events. Although loss to follow-up was high (that is, 50% for active drug and 68% for placebo), the relative risk of discontinuing treatment because of adverse events did not differ significantly between active treatment and placebo. Overall loss to follow-up in acute-phase studies has been estimated at approximately 24% (16), which is considerably lower than our estimates from continuation- and maintenance-phase studies. Our estimates likely are high because of longer trial duration, the preventive aim of this treatment, and misclassification of clinical endpoints (relapse or recurrence) as loss to follow-up.

Current practice guidelines for major depression recommend continuation-phase treatment for four to nine months for patients who demonstrate an adequate response to acute-phase treatment (2,3). For patients with recurrent depression, maintenance treatment is recommended. Our systematic review and meta-analysis provide relatively strong support for these guidelines.

On the basis of consistency of effect sizes over time, our review illustrates stable benefits of active treatment over placebo for up to two years of treatment. Although we demonstrated continued benefits of drug treatment over time, we were unable to draw inferences as to the most appropriate duration of antidepressant treatment. We identified only one randomized controlled trial that compared relapse rates for differing lengths of antidepressant treatment (27), but the sample size of the longest treatment arm in this trial may have been insufficiently powered. Still, fluoxetine was shown to be more efficacious than placebo for up to 38 weeks (or approximately nine months) in this trial. More research is needed to determine the most appropriate length of therapy.

In a well-conducted systematic review of relapse prevention with first- and second-generation antidepressants in depressive disorders, Geddes and colleagues (7) reported a 70% reduction in the odds of relapse for patients continuing antidepressant treatment compared with patients discontinuing treatment. The effect sizes reported in their analysis were "similar for all classes of antidepressants," but such unadjusted indirect comparisons may not be valid. To explore this further, we used data reported in the Geddes and colleagues review and converted their odds ratio to a relative risk ratio, specifically .45 for active drug compared with placebo (CI=.41–.49) and .41 for second-generation antidepressants compared with placebo (CI=.35–.48). The confidence intervals for the relative risk of relapse that we calculated for only second-generation antidepressants (less than one year, CI=.46–.62; one year or longer, CI=.48–.66) overlapped this relative risk estimate from the Geddes and colleagues study, and our analysis included nearly twice as many trials of newer antidepressants.

Even though a small number of comparative studies found no statis-

Table 2

Placebo-controlled, randomized studies of prevention of relapse or recurrence of a major depressive episode[a]

Study[b]	Depression severity eligibility criteria for random assignment[c]	Treatment phase	Duration (weeks)	N	Recurrent depression N	Recurrent depression %	Medication	Dose (mg per day)	Relapse or recurrence N	Relapse or recurrence %	p
Weihs et al., 2002 (24)	CGI-I score ≤2	Acute	8	816	816	100	Bupropion SR[d]	300	na		na
		Continuation	44	210	210	100	Bupropion SR	300	78	37	.004
		Continuation	44	213	213	100	Placebo	—	111	52	
Montgomery et al., 1993 (44)	MADRS score ≤12	Acute	6	nr	nr		Citalopram	20–40	na		na
		Continuation	24	48	nr		Citalopram	20	4	8	.02[e]
		Continuation	24	57	nr		Citalopram	40	7	12	
		Continuation	24	42	nr		Placebo	—	13	31	
Robert & Montgomery, 1995 (25)	MADRS score ≤12	Acute	8	391	nr		Citalopram	20–60	na		na
		Continuation	24	152	nr		Citalopram	20–60	21	14	.04
		Continuation	24	74	nr		Placebo	—	18	24	
Hochstrasser et al., 2001 (33)	MADRS score ≤11	Acute	6–9	427	427	100	Citalopram	20–60	na		na
		Continuation	16	327	327	100	Citalopram	20–60	na		na
		Continuation	48	132	132	100	Citalopram	20–60	24	18	.001
		Continuation	48	137	137	100	Placebo	—	59	43	
Klysner et al., 2002 (17)	MADRS score ≤11	Acute	8	230	35	15	Citalopram	20–40	na		na
		Continuation	16	172	nr		Citalopram	20–40	na		na
		Continuation	48	60	nr		Citalopram	20–40	19	32	nr
		Continuation	48	61	nr		Placebo	—	41	67	
Kornstein et al., 2006 (42)	MADRS score ≤12	Acute	8	131	nr		Citalopram	20–60	na		na
		Acute	8	129	nr		Fluoxetine	20–80	na		na
		Acute	8	128	nr		Paroxetine	20–50	na		na
		Acute	8	127	nr		Sertraline	50–200	na		na
		Continuation	18	234	nr		Escitalopram	10–20	na		na
		Maintenance	52	73	nr		Escitalopram	10–20	20	27	nr
		Maintenance	52	66	nr		Placebo	—	43	65	
Rapaport et al., 2004 (26)	MADRS score ≤12	Acute	8	502	331	66	Escitalopram	10–20	na		na
		Continuation	36	181	nr		Escitalopram	10–20	47	26	.01
		Continuation	36	93	nr		Placebo	—	37	40	
Reimherr et al., 1998 (27)	Absence of *DSM-III* depressive symptoms; HAM-D score <7	Acute	12–14	839	nr		Fluoxetine	20	na		na
		Continuation	14	299	nr		Fluoxetine	20	77	26	.001
		Continuation	14	95	nr		Placebo	—	47	49	
		Continuation[f]	38	105	nr		Fluoxetine	20	9	9	.04
		Continuation[f]	38	52	nr		Placebo	—	12	23	
		Continuation[f]	50	28	nr		Fluoxetine	20	3	11	.54
		Continuation[f]	50	34	nr		Placebo	—	5	6	
Schmidt et al., 2000 (28)	Absence of *DSM-IV* depressive symptoms, CGI-S score ≤2, and HAM-D score ≤9	Acute	13	932	nr		Fluoxetine	20	na		na
		Continuation	25	189	143	76	Fluoxetine	20	49	26	.01[d]
		Continuation	25	190	137	72	Fluoxetine	90/week	70	37	
		Continuation	25	122	80	66	Placebo	—	61	50	
Gilaberte et al., 2001 (34)	Absence of *DSM-III* depressive symptoms, CGI-S score ≤2, and HAM-D score ≤8	Acute	8	253	253	100	Fluoxetine	20–40	na		na
		Continuation	24	179	179	100	Fluoxetine	20–40	na		na
		Maintenance	52	70	70	100	Fluoxetine	20	14	20	.01
		Maintenance	52	70	70	100	Placebo	—	28	40	
Terra & Montgomery, 1998 (35)	CGI-S score ≤2 and MADRS score <12	Acute	6	436	436	100	Fluvoxamine	100	na		na
		Continuation	18	283	283	100	Fluvoxamine	100	na		na
		Maintenance	52	110	110	100	Fluvoxamine	100	14	13	.001
		Maintenance	52	94	94	100	Placebo	—	33	35	
Thase et al., 2001 (29)	CGI-S score ≤2 and HAM-D score ≤7	Acute	8–12	410	211	52	Mirtazapine	15–45	na		na
		Continuation	40	76	nr		Mirtazapine	15–45	15	20	.001
		Continuation	40	80	nr		Placebo	—	35	44	
Feiger et al., 1999 (30)	HAM-D score ≤10	Acute	16	467	nr		Nefazodone	400–600	na		na
		Continuation	36	65	40	62	Nefazodone	400–600	1	2	.009
		Continuation	36	66	41	62	Placebo	—	12	18	
Gelenberg et al., 2003 (36)	≥50% reduction in HAM-D score	Acute	12	681	681	100	Nefazodone	300–600	na		na
		Continuation	16	269	269	100	Nefazodone	300–600	na		na
		Maintenance	52	76	76	100	Nefazodone	300–600	23	30	.043
		Maintenance	52	84	84	100	Placebo	—	40	48	
Montgomery & Dunbar, 1993 (37)	HAM-D score ≤8	Acute	8	172	172	100	Paroxetine	20–30	na		na
		Maintenance	52	68	68	100	Paroxetine	20–30	11	16	.01
		Maintenance	52	67	67	100	Placebo	—	29	43	

Continues on next page

Table 2

Continued from previous page

Study[b]	Depression severity eligibility criteria for random assignment[c]	Treatment phase	Duration (weeks)	N	Recurrent depression		Medication	Dose (mg per day)	Relapse or recurrence		p
					N	%			N	%	
Reynolds et al., 2006 (41)	HAM-D score 0–10 for 3 consecutive weeks, plus 16 weeks of stable continuation	Acute	nr	195	88	45	Paroxetine	10–40	na		na
		Continuation	16	151	nr		Paroxetine	10–40	na		na
		Maintenance[g]	110	35	15	43	Paroxetine	10–40	12	34	.06
		Maintenance[g]	110	18	7	39	Placebo	—	10	56	
Doogan & Caillard, 1992 (31)	Response satisfactory to both patient and investigator	Acute	8	480	306	64	Sertraline	50–200	na		na
		Continuation	44	185	nr		Sertraline	50–200	24	13	.001
		Continuation	44	110	nr		Placebo	—	48	46	
Keller et al., 1998 (38)	CGI-I score ≤2 and HAM-D score ≤7 or ≥50% reduction in HAM-D score, plus HAM-D score ≤15, CGI-I score ≤2, and CGI-S score ≤3	Acute	12	309	145	47	Sertraline	50–200	na		na
		Continuation	16	209	nr		Sertraline	50–200	na		na
		Maintenance	76	77	nr		Sertraline	50–200	5	6	.002
		Maintenance	76	84	nr		Placebo	—	19	23	
Lepine et al., 2004 (39)	Absence of depressed mood and markedly diminished interest according to *DSM-IV*, and ≤2 of other 7 *DSM-IV* criteria, and ≤2 for sum of first 2 MADRS items	Continuation	≥16	371	371	100	Not sertraline[h]	na	na		na
		Remission or stability	8	371	371	100	Placebo	—	na		na
		Maintenance	72	189	189	100	Sertraline	50–100	32	17	.002
		Maintenance	72	99	99	100	Placebo	—	33	33	
Lustman et al., 2006 (43)	4 consecutive twice-monthly BDI scores ≤9	Acute	16	351	351	100	Sertraline	50–200	na		na
		Maintenance	52	79	79	100	Sertraline	50–200	27	34	nr
		Maintenance	52	73	73	100	Placebo	—	38	52	
Wilson et al., 2003 (18)	≥50% reduction in HAM-D score	Acute	8	318	nr		Sertraline	50–200	na		na
		Continuation	16–20	254	nr		Sertraline	50–200	na		na
		Maintenance	100	56	16	29	Sertraline	50–150	25	45	.21
		Maintenance	100	57	15	26	Placebo	—	31	54	
Simon et al., 2004 (32)	CGI-S score ≤3 and HAM-D score ≤10	Acute	8	490	nr		Venlafaxine XR[i]	75–225	na		na
		Continuation	26	161	nr		Venlafaxine XR	75–225	45	28	.001
		Continuation	26	157	nr		Placebo	—	82	52	
Montgomery et al., 2004 (40)	HAM-D score ≤12 at day 56 with no HAM-D score ≤20 and no 2consecutive HAM-D scores >10	Acute or continuation	26	495	495	100	Venlafaxine	100–200	na		na
		Maintenance	52	109	109	100	Venlafaxine	100–200	24	22	.001
		Maintenance	52	116	116	100	Placebo	—	64	55	

[a] na, not applicable; nr, not reported

[b] With the exception of the studies of Lepine and colleagues (39) and Lustman and colleagues (43), which each had a quality rating of good, each study had a quality rating of fair.

[c] CGI-I, Clinical Global Impression of Improvement (possible scores range from 1 to 7, with lower scores indicating more improvement and higher scores indicating worsening; values of 4 represent no change); CGI-S, Clinical Global Impression of Severity (possible scores range from 1 to 7, with lower scores indicating normalcy or mild illness and higher scores indicating more severe illness); MADRS, Montgomery-Asberg Depression Rating Scale (possible scores range from 0 to 60, with higher scores indicating greater severity of symptoms); HAM-D, Hamilton Rating Scale for Depression (possible scores range from 0 to 52, with higher scores indicating greater severity of symptoms); BDI, Beck Depression Inventory (possible scores range from 0 to 63, with higher scores indicating greater severity of symptoms)

[d] SR, sustained release

[e] Active treatment versus placebo

[f] Not included in meta-analysis; compared with placebo switchers in the specified time interval

[g] Paroxetine plus clinical management and placebo plus clinical management groups only; psychotherapy groups were excluded.

[h] Patients were eligible for the study if their depression was in remission with any antidepressant other than sertraline.

[i] XR, extended release

tically significant differences between second-generation antidepressants, we were unable to draw firm conclusions as to whether one drug may be better than another for long-term treatment. These comparative trials were extension trials and did not reassign patients randomly to continuation or maintenance treatment but rather gave them the option to continue on with their blinded acute-phase treatment. This trial design has been shown to produce overall lower relapse rates, but it also yields larger differences between active treatment and placebo than placebo-substitution trials that randomly assign participants at the time of successful completion of acute-phase or continuation-phase treatment (8). For this reason, we limited

Figure 1

Meta-analysis of placebo-controlled trials with less than one year of double-blinded randomized follow-up for relapse prevention

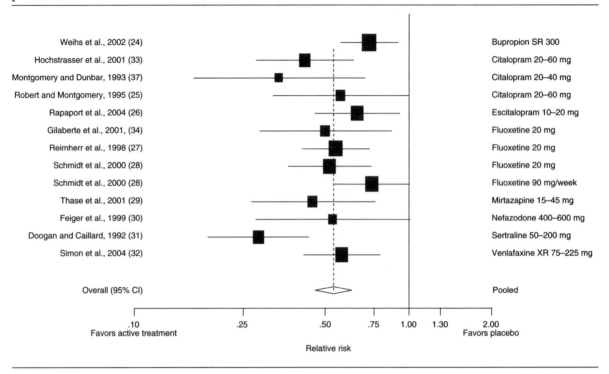

Figure 2

Meta-analysis of placebo-controlled trials with one year or more of double-blinded randomized follow-up for recurrence prevention

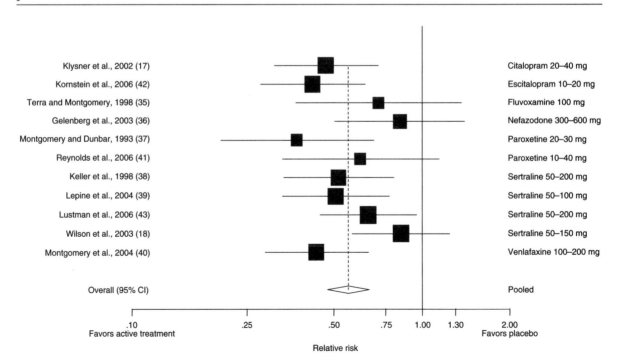

our meta-analyses to placebo-substitution trials. Although this refinement did not answer the question of whether the extension or placebo-substitution design provides a more accurate assessment of the benefits of drug treatment, we believe our results provide strong evidence for the benefits of continuing versus discontinuing antidepressant treatment after successful acute- or continuation-phase treatment.

Although it is tempting to draw inferences about one drug compared with another by indirectly comparing effect sizes among placebo-controlled trials (Figures 1 and 2), we caution against such inferences because included trials differed in design and because unadjusted comparisons may be inaccurate. Adjusted indirect comparisons usually agree with results of head-to-head comparisons, but only when the trials being indirectly compared are similar (46,47). Because of differences in trial design and in operational definitions (such as definition of relapse or recurrence) used by investigators, we chose not to conduct adjusted indirect comparisons. More research is needed to verify whether second-generation antidepressants differ in relapse rates.

Our analysis is limited chiefly by the sparse quantity and quality of available evidence addressing our research questions. Only a handful of comparative studies have been published, making it difficult to generalize about one drug compared with any other. Selective publication of relapse and recurrence prevention trials could influence our conclusions, as has been shown with acute-phase treatment trials of antidepressants (48). Although our statistical tests did not detect significant bias toward the publication of positive results, such bias may nevertheless be present, which would lead to an overestimation of the treatment effect. This possibility is especially important given that most of the included studies were sponsored by pharmaceutical companies. Evidence for some drugs was limited to a single study. Although we conducted a meta-regression to explore heterogeneity, data were insufficient to assess all important differences among trials. One

important distinction that we could not address is whether presenting with a history of a single depressive episode versus recurrent episodes made a difference in relapse or recurrence rates. Because this is a primary decision point for psychiatrists in deciding whether to continue with maintenance-phase treatment, more work is needed in this area.

Finally, we could not determine whether demographic factors such as patients' age influenced relapse rates, although results from trials with older participants were generally consistent with evidence from younger adult populations. Evidence from children was not considered.

Conclusions

This review confirms the benefits of continuation- and maintenance-phase treatment of major depression with second-generation antidepressants. Our review supports current clinical practice guidelines. In addition, our meta-regression provides some evidence that the efficacy of different types of second-generation antidepressants does not differ in clinically significant ways, although more research is needed to confirm this conclusion. Given that ongoing treatment can prevent a relapse or recurrence of depression for approximately one in five patients, clinicians should continue to encourage treatment beyond the acute phase and work with patients to find the most suitable drug.

Acknowledgments and disclosures

No funding was provided for the literature search and analysis. However, this review is based in part on work funded through contract 290-02-0016 from the Agency for Healthcare Research and Quality (AHRQ).

Dr. Gaynes has received financial support from GlaxoSmithKline, Ovation Pharmaceuticals, Pfizer, Shire Pharmaceuticals, and Wyeth Ayerst. Ms. Deveaugh-Geiss also has received funding from GlaxoSmithKline. The other authors report no competing interests.

References

1. Anderson IM, Ferrier NI, Baldwin CR, et al: Evidence-based guidelines for treating depressive disorders with antidepressants: a revision of the 2000 British Association for Psychopharmacology guidelines. Journal of Psychopharmacology 22:330–332, 2008

2. American Psychiatric Association: Practice guideline for the treatment of patients with major depressive disorder (revision). American Journal of Psychiatry 157:1–45, 2000

3. Depression Guideline Panel: Depression in Primary Care: Vol 2—Treatment of Major Depression. AHCPR pub no 93-0550. Rockville, Md, US Department of Health and Human Services, Public Health Service, Agency for Health Care Policy and Research, 1993

4. Hansen RA, Gartlehner G, Lohr KN, et al: Efficacy and safety of second-generation antidepressants in the treatment of major depressive disorder. Annals of Internal Medicine 143:415–426, 2005

5. Rush AJ, Trivedi MH, Wisniewski SR, et al: Acute and longer-term outcomes in depressed outpatients requiring one or several treatment steps: a STAR*D report. American Journal of Psychiatry 163:1905–1917, 2006

6. Loonen AJ, Peer PG, Zwanikken GJ: Continuation and maintenance therapy with antidepressive agents: meta-analysis of research. Pharmaceutisch Weekblad, Scientific Edition 13:167–175, 1991

7. Geddes JR, Carney SM, Davies C, et al: Relapse prevention with antidepressant drug treatment in depressive disorders: a systematic review. Lancet 361:653–661, 2003

8. Zimmerman M, Posternak MA, Ruggero CJ: Impact of study design on the results of continuation studies of antidepressants. Journal of Clinical Psychopharmacology 27:177–181, 2007

9. Harris RP, Helfand M, Woolf SH, et al: Current methods of the US Preventive Services Task Force: a review of the process. American Journal of Preventive Medicine 20:21–35, 2001

10. Undertaking Systematic Reviews of Research on Effectiveness: CRD's Guidance for Those Carrying Out or Commissioning Reviews. CRD report no 4, 2nd ed. York, United Kingdom, Centre for Reviews and Dissemination, 2001

11. Higgins JPT, Green S (eds): Cochrane Handbook for Systematic Reviews of Interventions, version 5.0.0. Oxford, United Kingdom, Cochrane Collaboration, Feb 2008

12. Egger M, Smith GD, Altman DG: Systematic Reviews in Health Care (2nd ed). London, BMJ Publishing, 2001

13. Begg CB, Mazumdar M: Operating characteristics of a rank correlation test for publication bias. Biometrics 50:1088–1101, 1994

14. Egger M, Davey Smith G, Schneider M, et al: Bias in meta-analysis detected by a simple, graphical test. British Medical Journal 315:629–634, 1997

15. Sterne JA, Gavaghan D, Egger M: Publication and related bias in meta-analysis: power of statistical tests and prevalence in the literature. Journal of Clinical Epidemiology 53:1119–1129, 2000

16. Gartlehner G, Hansen RA, Carey TS, et al: Discontinuation rates for selective serotonin reuptake inhibitors and other second-generation antidepressants in outpatients

with major depressive disorder: a systematic review and meta-analysis. International Clinical Psychopharmacology 20:59–69, 2005

17. Klysner R, Bent-Hansen J, Hansen HL, et al: Efficacy of citalopram in the prevention of recurrent depression in elderly patients: placebo-controlled study of maintenance therapy. British Journal of Psychiatry 181: 29–35, 2002

18. Wilson KC, Mottram PG, Ashworth L, et al: Older community residents with depression: long-term treatment with sertraline—randomised, double-blind, placebo-controlled study. British Journal of Psychiatry 182:492–497, 2003

19. Van Moffaert M, Bartholome F, Cosyns P, et al: A controlled comparison of sertraline and fluoxetine in acute and continuation treatment of major depression. Human Psychopharmacology 10:393–405, 1995

20. Franchini L, Gasperini M, Perez J, et al: A double-blind study of long-term treatment with sertraline or fluvoxamine for prevention of highly recurrent unipolar depression. Journal of Clinical Psychiatry 58:104–107, 1997

21. Franchini L, Gasperini M, Zanardi R, et al: Four-year follow-up study of sertraline and fluvoxamine in long-term treatment of unipolar subjects with high recurrence rate. Journal of Affective Disorders 58:233–236, 2000

22. Cunningham LA, Borison RL, Carman JS, et al: A comparison of venlafaxine, trazodone, and placebo in major depression. Journal of Clinical Psychopharmacology 14:99–106, 1994

23. Perahia DG, Wang F, Mallinckrodt CH, et al: Duloxetine in the treatment of major depressive disorder: a placebo- and paroxetine-controlled trial. European Psychiatry 21:367–378, 2006

24. Weihs KL, Houser TL, Batey SR, et al: Continuation phase treatment with bupropion SR effectively decreases the risk for relapse of depression. Biological Psychiatry 51:753–761, 2002

25. Robert P, Montgomery SA: Citalopram in doses of 20–60 mg is effective in depression relapse prevention: a placebo-controlled 6 month study. International Clinical Psychopharmacology 10(suppl 1):29–35, 1995

26. Rapaport MH, Bose A, Zheng H: Escitalopram continuation treatment prevents relapse of depressive episodes. Journal of Clinical Psychiatry 65:44–49, 2004

27. Reimherr FW, Amsterdam JD, Quitkin FM, et al: Optimal length of continuation therapy in depression: a prospective assessment during long-term fluoxetine treatment. American Journal of Psychiatry 155: 1247–1253, 1998

28. Schmidt ME, Fava M, Robinson JM, et al: The efficacy and safety of a new enteric-coated formulation of fluoxetine given once weekly during the continuation treatment of major depressive disorder. Journal of Clinical Psychiatry 61:851–857, 2000

29. Thase ME, Nierenberg AA, Keller MB, et al: Efficacy of mirtazapine for prevention of depressive relapse: a placebo-controlled double-blind trial of recently remitted high-risk patients. Journal of Clinical Psychiatry 62:782–788, 2001

30. Feiger AD, Bielski RJ, Bremner J, et al: Double-blind, placebo-substitution study of nefazodone in the prevention of relapse during continuation treatment of outpatients with major depression. International Clinical Psychopharmacology 14:19–28, 1999

31. Doogan DP, Caillard V: Sertraline in the prevention of depression. British Journal of Psychiatry 160:217–222, 1992

32. Simon JS, Aguiar LM, Kunz NR, et al: Extended-release venlafaxine in relapse prevention for patients with major depressive disorder. Journal of Psychiatric Research 38:249–257, 2004

33. Hochstrasser B, Isaksen PM, Koponen H, et al: Prophylactic effect of citalopram in unipolar, recurrent depression: placebo-controlled study of maintenance therapy. British Journal of Psychiatry 178:304–310, 2001

34. Gilaberte I, Montejo AL, de la Gandara J, et al: Fluoxetine in the prevention of depressive recurrences: a double-blind study. Journal of Clinical Psychopharmacology 21:417–424, 2001

35. Terra JL, Montgomery SA: Fluvoxamine prevents recurrence of depression: results of a long-term, double-blind, placebo-controlled study. International Clinical Psychopharmacology 13:55–62, 1998

36. Gelenberg AJ, Trivedi MH, Rush AJ, et al: Randomized, placebo-controlled trial of nefazodone maintenance treatment in preventing recurrence in chronic depression. Biological Psychiatry 54:806–817, 2003

37. Montgomery SA, Dunbar G: Paroxetine is better than placebo in relapse prevention and the prophylaxis of recurrent depression. International Clinical Psychopharmacology 8:189–195, 1993

38. Keller MB, Kocsis JH, Thase ME, et al: Maintenance phase efficacy of sertraline for chronic depression: a randomized controlled trial. JAMA 280:1665–1672, 1998

39. Lepine JP, Caillard V, Bisserbe JC, et al: A randomized, placebo-controlled trial of sertraline for prophylactic treatment of highly recurrent major depressive disorder. American Journal of Psychiatry 161:836–842, 2004

40. Montgomery SA, Entsuah R, Hackett D, et al: Venlafaxine versus placebo in the preventive treatment of recurrent major depression. Journal of Clinical Psychiatry 65: 328–336, 2004

41. Reynolds CF III, Dew MA, Pollock BG, et al: Maintenance treatment of major depression in old age. New England Journal of Medicine 354:1130–1138, 2006

42. Kornstein SG, Bose A, Li D, et al: Escitalopram maintenance treatment for prevention of recurrent depression: a randomized, placebo-controlled trial. Journal of Clinical Psychiatry 67:1767–1775, 2006

43. Lustman PJ, Clouse RE, Nix BD, et al: Sertraline for prevention of depression recurrence in diabetes mellitus: a randomized, double-blind, placebo-controlled trial. Archives of General Psychiatry 63:521–529, 2006

44. Montgomery SA, Rasmussen JG, Tanghoj P: A 24-week study of 20 mg citalopram, 40 mg citalopram, and placebo in the prevention of relapse of major depression. International Clinical Psychopharmacology 8: 181–188, 1993

45. Gartlehner G, Hansen RA, Thieda P, et al: Comparative Effectiveness of Pharmacologic Treatment of Depression. Rockville, Md, Agency for Healthcare Research and Quality, April 2006. Available at www.effectivehealthcare.ahrq.gov/reports/final.cfm

46. Song F, Altman DG, Glenny AM, et al: Validity of indirect comparison for estimating efficacy of competing interventions: empirical evidence from published meta-analyses. British Medical Journal 326:472, 2003

47. Glenny AM, Altman DG, Song F, et al: Indirect comparisons of competing interventions. Health Technology Assessment 9(special issue):1–134, 2005

48. Turner EH, Matthews AM, Linardatos E, et al: Selective publication of antidepressant trials and its influence on apparent efficacy. New England Journal of Medicine 358:252–260, 2008

MOC Part 4: Sample Peer and Patient Feedback Forms

Feedback Modules

The American Board of Psychiatry and Neurology (ABPN) requires Feedback Modules (Patient/Peer Second Party External Review) for MOC Part 4. MOC Peer Feedback and MOC Patient Feedback forms are available at the ABPN website, www.abpn.com/forms. Sample forms, as provided on the ABPN website (http://abpn.com/forms.html#moc) as of December 30, 2011, are provided in this section. These forms are for the physicians own use in identifying areas of improvement and are not to be forwarded either to the American Psychiatric Association or to the ABPN. The ABPN specifies on its website (as of July 12, 2012) that for the Peer and Patient Feedback Requirements for Part 4 MOC:

- Each diplomate must solicit personal performance feedback from at least five peers[1] and five of their own patients[2] concerning the diplomate's clinical activity over the previous 3 years.
- Each diplomate must then identify opportunities for improvement in the effectiveness and/or efficiency in his or her practice as related to the core competencies and take steps to implement suggested improvements.
- *Remeasurement:* within 24 months, each diplomate must collect the same data from at least another five peers and five patients to see if improvements in practice have occurred. Feedback may be obtained from the same patients and peers as in the original and follow-up feedback.

---

[1]Peers may include other professional healthcare staff such as, psychologists, social workers, physicians, counselors, and nurses.
[2]Patients can include those for which the diplomate supervises the care of another provider (e.g., resident).

Peer Feedback Form v1

Name of reviewer		**Date**	
Title		**Hospital**	
PEER Feedback for: Please print full name of physician being reviewed.		**Address**	
		City, State, Zip code	

Please rate the above-named physician on the six core competencies as identified by the Accreditation Council for Graduate Medical Education (ACGME) and the American Board of Medical Specialties (ABMS).

PERFORMANCE RATINGS

The following guidelines are to be used in selecting the appropriate rating:

1	2	3	4	5	6
Never	Rarely	Occasionally	Frequently	Always	Not Applicable

Patient Care   ○1 ○2 ○3 ○4 ○5 ○6

Implements the highest standards of practice in the effective and timely treatment of all patients regardless of gender, ethnicity, location, or socioeconomic status.

Medical Knowledge   ○1 ○2 ○3 ○4 ○5 ○6

Keeps current with research and medical knowledge in order to provide evidence-based care.

Interpersonal and Communication Skills   ○1 ○2 ○3 ○4 ○5 ○6

Communicates effectively and works vigorously and efficiently with all involved parties as patient advocate and/or consultant.

Practice-based Learning and Improvement   ○1 ○2 ○3 ○4 ○5 ○6

Assesses medical knowledge and new technology and implements best practices in clinical setting.

Professionalism   ○1 ○2 ○3 ○4 ○5 ○6

Displays personal characteristics consistent with high moral and ethical behavior.

Systems-based Practice   ○1 ○2 ○3 ○4 ○5 ○6

Efficiently utilizes health-care resources and community systems of care in the treatment of patients.

Please Return Completed Form To Physician For His/Her Confidential Records - Do Not Send to the ABPN

American Board of Psychiatry and Neurology, Inc., 2150 E. Lake Cook Road, Suite 900, Buffalo Grove, IL 60089
Ph: 847.229.6500 Fax: 847.229.6600 www.abpn.com

Patient Feedback Form v1

Patient review of Dr. [ ]   **Date** [ ]

Physician Specialty - Please select one: ○ Psychiatry   ○ Neurology   ○ Child Neurology

PERFORMANCE RATINGS

The following guidelines are to be used in selecting the appropriate rating:

Please select a performance rating for your doctor for each of the following statements:	1 Never	2 Rarely	3 Occasionally	4 Frequently	5 Always	6 Not Applicable
1) Physician listens carefully to your symptoms.	○ 1	● 2	○ 3	○ 4	○ 5	○ 6
2) Physician asks questions regarding your health history.	○ 1	○ 2	○ 3	○ 4	○ 5	○ 6
3) Physician explains tests that he/she ordered.	○ 1	○ 2	○ 3	○ 4	○ 5	○ 6
4) Physician discusses treatment options with you, including the expected course of treatment.	○ 1	○ 2	○ 3	○ 4	○ 5	○ 6
5) Physician explains drugs and other treatments (for example, psychotherapy), their expected effects, and possible side effects.	○ 1	○ 2	○ 3	○ 4	○ 5	○ 6
6) Physician discusses the treatment costs, insurance, and payment options with you.	○ 1	○ 2	○ 3	○ 4	○ 5	○ 6
7) Physician encourages you to ask questions about your treatment.	○ 1	○ 2	○ 3	○ 4	○ 5	○ 6
8) Physician answers questions to your satisfaction.	○ 1	○ 2	○ 3	○ 4	○ 5	○ 6
9) Physician gives you advice on what to do if symptoms persist or worsen.	○ 1	○ 2	○ 3	○ 4	○ 5	○ 6
10) Physician refers you to another specialist when necessary.	○ 1	○ 2	○ 3	○ 4	○ 5	○ 6
11) Physician tells you when to schedule a return visit.	○ 1	○ 2	○ 3	○ 4	○ 5	○ 6
12) Physician treats you in a professional manner.	○ 1	○ 2	○ 3	○ 4	○ 5	○ 6

Please Return Completed Form To Physician For His/Her Confidential Records - Do Not Send to the ABPN

American Board of Psychiatry and Neurology, Inc., 2150 E. Lake Cook Road, Suite 900, Buffalo Grove, IL 60089
Ph: 847.229.6500 Fax: 847.229.6600 www.abpn.com

Appendix:
ABPN Requirements for Maintenance of Certification

American Board of Psychiatry and Neurology, Inc.

A Member Board of the American Board of Medical Specialties (ABMS)

MAINTENANCE OF CERTIFICATION PROGRAM

Note: all policies, components, and requirements of the ABPN's Maintenance of Certification (MOC) Program are subject to change. It is the responsibility of each individual ABPN diplomate to remain apprised of the current applicable MOC Program. As such, diplomates are encouraged to consult the ABPN's website (www.abpn.com/moc) regularly to ascertain whether any changes have been made.

v.4 (February 2012)

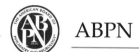

The ABPN Maintenance of Certification (MOC) Program

NOTE: All policies, components, and requirements of the ABPN's Maintenance of Certification (MOC) Program are subject to change. It is the responsibility of each individual ABPN diplomate to remain apprised of the current applicable MOC Program. As such, diplomates are encouraged to consult the ABPN's website (www.abpn.com/moc) regularly to ascertain whether any changes have been made.

Introduction

The ABPN MOC Program reflects the Board's commitment to lifelong learning throughout one's profession. The mission of the ABPN's Maintenance of Certification (MOC) Program is to advance the clinical practice of psychiatry and neurology by promoting the highest evidence-based guidelines and standards to ensure excellence in all areas of care and practice improvement. The MOC program requires diplomates to participate in sanctioned self-assessment performance measures, identify perceived weaknesses in their knowledge, pursue learning activities tailored to areas that need to be strengthened, and develop quality improvement programs based on their clinical practice. The goal is for diplomates to reflect on their personal knowledge and performance and commit to a process of improvement and reevaluation of performance measures over a specified time frame that will ultimately lead to improved care for their patients.

Diplomates are responsible for their own self-assessment activities, continuing education credits, and practice improvement plans, and they can choose the learning tools that will best address their perceived needs, expand their expertise, and enhance the effectiveness and efficiency of their practice.

Physicians who are certified in both psychiatry and neurology and who desire to maintain their certificates in both disciplines must only meet the CME, Self-assessment, and PIP requirements for one specialty. However, they will be required to pass cognitive examinations in both psychiatry and neurology.

Diplomates with certificates in the subspecialties of addiction psychiatry, clinical neurophysiology, forensic psychiatry, geriatric psychiatry, hospice and palliative medicine, neuromuscular medicine, pain medicine, psychosomatic medicine, sleep medicine, and vascular neurology must also maintain certification in their specialty in order to apply for recertification in the area of subspecialization. Diplomates in neurodevelopmental disabilities must maintain certification in neurology with special qualification in child neurology. *If certification in the specialty lapses, certification in the subspecialty is no longer valid.*

Diplomates in child and adolescent psychiatry do not need to maintain current certification in general psychiatry for their subspecialty certification to remain valid and to recertify in child and adolescent psychiatry.

There is no time limit on regaining certification status through maintenance of certification. It is the responsibility of diplomates to obtain application materials for maintenance of certification. *Information for Applicants* publications are available to download from www.abpn.com.

The ABPN encourages all diplomates to update their Clinically Active Status through ABPN Physician Folios at http://www.abpn.com/folios

As mandated by the American Board of Medical Specialties, the Board has developed a Maintenance of Certification (MOC) program that includes four components:
1. Professional Standing;
2. Self-Assessment and CME;
3. Cognitive Expertise;
4. Performance in Practice.

MOC Program participation includes meeting **all** MOC requirements, not just passing the MOC cognitive examination.

American Board of Psychiatry and Neurology, Inc., 2150 E. Lake Cook Road, Suite 900, Buffalo Grove, IL ◊ Ph: 847.229.6500 ◊ www.abpn.com

164   FOCUS Major Depressive Disorder Maintenance of Certification (MOC) Workbook

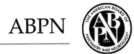

ABPN

The ABPN Maintenance of Certification Program (10YR-MOC) *(Nov. 2009)*
For Time-Limited Diplomates Certified or Recertified in 2011 or Earlier

As of October 1, 1994, all individuals achieving Board certification by the ABPN are issued 10-year, time-limited certificates. Certificates issued in the subspecialties of addiction psychiatry, clinical neurophysiology, epilepsy, forensic psychiatry, geriatric psychiatry, hospice and palliative medicine, neurodevelopmental disabilities, neuromuscular medicine, pain medicine, psychosomatic medicine, sleep medicine, and vascular neurology, including those issued prior to October 1, 1994, are 10-year, time-limited certificates. Time-limited certificates for child and adolescent psychiatry began in 1995.

Diplomates who are not recertified before their certificates expire are no longer Board certified in that area of certification. Once a former diplomate completes all MOC requirements and passes the MOC examination, however, he or she will regain certification status.

Record Keeping, Attestation, Multiple Certificates, and Auditing
Diplomates of the ABPN are required to maintain records of their self-assessment (SA) activities, Continuing Medical Education (CME) credits, and Performance in Practice (PIP) Units. Diplomates must provide their signature attesting to completion of these activities (as determined by the phase-in schedule) on their applications for the MOC examinations. When the MOC Program is fully operational, attestation to all components will be required on applications for the MOC examinations.

Diplomates are responsible for choosing their self-assessment activities, CME activities, and performance in practice components. **Completed activities can be applied to multiple certifications thus fulfilling MOC criteria for one or more specialty or subspecialty areas.**

Phase-In Schedule for ABPN Ten-Year MOC Component Requirements									
Original Certification or Recertification Year	MOC Application Year	MOC Exam Year	TOTAL CME Credits Required	CME From SA	First SA Activity Required	Second SA Activity Required	First PIP Unit Required	Second PIP Unit Required	Third PIP Unit Required
2002	2011	2012	180	0	X				
2003	2012	2013	210	0	X				
2004	2013	2014	240	20	X	X	X		
2005	2014	2015	270	40	X	X	X		
2006	2015	2016	300	60	X	X	X	X	
2007	2016	2017	300	80	X	X	X	X	X
2008	2017	2018	300	80	X	X	X	X	X
2009	2018	2019	300	80	X	X	X	X	X
2010	2019	2020	300	80	X	X	X	X	X
2011	2020	2021	300	80	X	X	X	X	X
2012	See **Continuous Pathway to Lifelong Learning** MOC Program (CP-MOC) at www.abpn.com/cp-moc								

Notes:
- MOC Program component requirements fully implemented for 2017 MOC Examination Year.
- Every ABPN diplomate must possess an active medical license in the U.S. or Canada, and all licenses must be unrestricted.
- At least an average of 8 of the CME credits per year (averaged over 2-5 years) should involve self-assessment.
- Only after completing licensure, CME, SA and PIP requirements are diplomates qualified to complete the ABPN MOC Cognitive Examination.

American Board of Psychiatry and Neurology, Inc., 2150 E. Lake Cook Road, Suite 900, Buffalo Grove, IL ◊ Ph: 847.229.6500 ◊ www.abpn.com

ABPN

The ABPN will audit approximately five percent of the applications submitted for the cognitive examination. Candidates whose applications are audited will receive a letter detailing the documentation required as evidence of completion of stipulated components (professional standing, self-assessment program, CME activities, and Performance in Practice Units) **as determined by the phase-in schedule.** Failure to return this documentation may result in the denial of the application for the MOC cognitive examination.

1. Professional Standing (continuously effective)

To show evidence of professional standing, the ABPN requires that diplomates must hold an active and unrestricted license to practice medicine in at least one state, commonwealth, territory, or possession of the United States or province of Canada. Such license must be maintained even if the physician is out of the country for extended periods of time. All medical licenses must be unrestricted.

2. Self-Assessment and CME

A. Self-Assessment Activities

Diplomates of the ABPN are required to participate in at least two major, broad-based self-assessment activities during the 10-year MOC cycle. The self-assessment activities can come from multiple self-assessment programs. Each self-assessment activity must cover new knowledge and/or current best practices in one or more of the competency areas, and provide feedback to the diplomate that can be used as the basis for focused CME, lifelong learning, and/or career development. That feedback must include the correct answer and recommended literature resources for each question, and (by 2014) comparative performance to peers. This requirement began in 2010 for those applying for 2011 MOC examinations. **Beginning in 2014, diplomates are required to use only ABPN-approved products for self-assessment activities.**

When this component is fully implemented in 2014:

- At least an average of 8 of the CME credits per year (averaged over 2-5 years) should involve self-assessment.
- The first self-assessment activity must be completed in years 1-3 of the 10-year MOC cycle.
- The second self-assessment activity must be completed in years 6-8 of the 10-year MOC cycle.
- Feedback must include comparative performance to peers.
- Self-assessment examinations must include no fewer than 25 questions per examination and 2 CME credits per activity.
- The self-assessment examination must take place before any subsequent CME educational activity.

The Board may approve additional programs over time. The ABPN reserves the right to approve or reject any course or guideline submitted for approval.

B. CME Activities

Diplomates of the ABPN are required to complete an average of 30 specialty or subspecialty Category 1 CME credits per year over the 10-year MOC cycle. CME activities must be accredited by ACCME or by the Royal College of Physicians and Surgeons of Canada, and CME must be relevant to the specialty in which the diplomate is certified. Diplomates certified in more than one area only need to accrue an average of 30 CME credits per year, as the same CME credits can be used to satisfy the MOC requirements for multiple specialties and subspecialties. This requirement was phased in beginning in 2006 for those applying for 2007 MOC examinations.

When this component is fully implemented in 2014:

- At least an average of 8 of the CME credits per year (averaged over 2-5 years) should involve self-assessment.
- 150 CME credits must be earned during the first 5-year block of the 10-year MOC cycle,
- 150 CME credits must be earned during the second 5-year block of the 10-year MOC cycle,
- Diplomates must accrue 300 Category 1 CME credits over the 10-year MOC cycle.

Examples of MOC activities approved by the Board may be found on the ABPN web site, www.abpn.com/moc.
The Board may approve additional programs over time. *The ABPN reserves the right to approve or reject any course or guideline submitted for approval.*

American Board of Psychiatry and Neurology, Inc., 2150 E. Lake Cook Road, Suite 900, Buffalo Grove, IL ◊ Ph: 847.229.6500 ◊ www.abpn.com

ABPN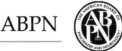

3. Cognitive Expertise (effective 1994)

Diplomates of the ABPN fulfill the cognitive expertise component by passing a cognitive examination prior to the expiration date on their certificates. To sit for a cognitive examination, all current MOC requirements must be satisfied at the time the MOC application is submitted. A passing score on the cognitive examination extends the renewal date of the certificate to December 31, 10 years from the year of the cognitive examination. Practice-relevant, clinically oriented, multiple-choice, computer-administered examinations are delivered in over 200 Pearson VUE testing centers throughout the country. To prepare for the MOC cognitive examinations, a diplomate should keep current with research and developments in the respective field, read specialty-specific journals and practice guidelines, and attend relevant CME programs.

MOC Program participation includes meeting **all** MOC requirements, not just passing the MOC cognitive examination.

4. Performance in Practice (PIP)

The Performance in Practice (PIP) component is a two-part quality improvement program designed for "clinically active" physicians (see definitions below) to participate in practice improvement activities over the 10-year MOC cycle by both chart review and second-party external review. Diplomates will be required to complete three (3) PIP Units, each consisting of both a Clinical Module (chart review) and a Feedback Module (Patient/Peer* second-party external review).

If a diplomate participates in an institutional quality improvement program that involves collection of chart data and comparison, and establishment of a plan to improve clinical activity for the individual physician, that institutional participation may also fulfill the Clinical module. If a diplomate participates in peer review in his/her clinical setting, that institutional activity may also fulfill the PIP Feedback Module criteria. This requirement is currently slated to begin in 2013 for those applying for 2014 MOC examinations. **Beginning in 2014, diplomates are required to use only ABPN-approved products for Performance in Practice Activities.**

When this component is fully implemented in 2017:
- The first PIP Unit must be completed in years 1-3 of the 10-year MOC cycle;
- The second PIP Unit must be completed in years 4-6 of the 10-year MOC cycle;
- The third PIP Unit must be completed in years 7-9 of the 10-year MOC cycle.

A) Clinical Modules (Chart Review)
- Each diplomate is required to collect data from at least five patient cases in a specific category (e.g., diagnosis, type of treatment, treatment setting) obtained from the diplomate's personal practice over the previous 3-year period.
- A minimum of 4 quality measures must be collected for each Clinical Module.
- Each diplomate must then compare data from the five patient cases with published best practices, or practice guidelines, or peer-based standards of care (e.g., hospital quality improvement programs), and develop a plan to improve effectiveness or efficiency of his/her clinical activities.
- Remeasurement: within 24 months, each diplomate must collect the same data from at least another five clinical cases in the same specific category, to see if improvements in practice have occurred. The same patients may be assessed in the original and follow-up data.

B) Feedback Modules (Patient** and Peer* Second Party External Reviews)
- Each diplomate must solicit personal performance feedback from at least five peers* and five of their own patients** concerning the diplomate's clinical activity over the previous three years.
- Each diplomate must then identify opportunities for improvement in the effectiveness and/or efficiency in their practice as related to the core competencies and take steps to implement suggested improvements.
- Remeasurement: within 24 months, each diplomate must collect the same data from at least another five peers* and five patients to see if improvements in practice have occurred. Feedback may be obtained from the same patients and peers as in the original and follow-up feedback.

* Peers may include other professional healthcare staff such as, psychologists, social workers, physicians, counselors, and nurses.
** Patients can include those for which the diplomate supervises the care of another provider (e.g., resident).
- *Model MOC PIP Peer Feedback and MOC PIP Patient Feedback forms are available on the web site, www.abpn.com/forms.*

American Board of Psychiatry and Neurology, Inc., 2150 E. Lake Cook Road, Suite 900, Buffalo Grove, IL ◊ Ph: 847.229.6500 ◊ www.abpn.com

FOCUS Major Depressive Disorder Maintenance of Certification (MOC) Workbook   167

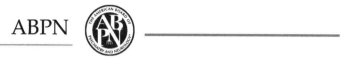

The ABPN recommends that diplomates allow ample time for completion of PIP units. It may take diplomates 24 months from the date that the original data is collected from patients and peers to complete one PIP unit. The Board may approve additional programs over time. The ABPN reserves the right to approve or reject any course or guideline submitted for approval.

Clinically Active Status

The American Board of Medical Specialties (ABMS) has issued definitions of "Clinically Active" and "Clinically Inactive" and requires that all diplomates self-report their status once every 24 months in each area of certification. This information will be available to the public.

1. "Clinically Active": Any amount of direct and/or consultative patient care has been provided in the preceding 24 months. This includes the supervision of residents.

    A. Engaged in direct and/or consultative care *sufficient* to complete Performance in Practice (PIP) Units.

    B. Engaged in direct and/or consultative care *not sufficient* to complete PIP Units.

2. "Clinically Inactive": No direct and/or consultative patient care has been provided in the past 24 months.

3. "Status Unknown": No information available on the clinical activity of this diplomate.

Diplomates who are in category 1.A. above are required to complete all components of the MOC Program including PIP Units.

Diplomates who are in categories 1.B. or 2 above are required to complete all components of the MOC Program, except for PIP Units.

A change in diplomate status from 1.B. or 2 to 1.A. requires the completion of at least one PIP Unit.

American Board of Psychiatry and Neurology, Inc., 2150 E. Lake Cook Road, Suite 900, Buffalo Grove, IL ◊ Ph: 847.229.6500 ◊ www.abpn.com

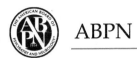 ABPN

Phase in Schedule for ABPN MOC Program (10YR-MOC) Component Requirements
For Time-Limited Diplomates Certified or Recertified in 2011 or Earlier

WHAT DO YOU NEED TO DO AND WHEN?

Diplomates of the ABPN fulfill the cognitive expertise component by passing a cognitive examination prior to the expiration date on their certificates. To sit for a cognitive examination, all current MOC requirements must be satisfied at the time the MOC application is submitted. A passing score on the cognitive examination extends the renewal date of the certificate to December 31, 10 years from the year of the cognitive examination. Practice-relevant, clinically oriented, multiple-choice, computer-administered examinations are delivered in over 200 Pearson VUE testing centers throughout the country. To prepare for the MOC cognitive examinations, a diplomate should keep current with research and developments in the respective field, read specialty-specific journals and practice guidelines, and attend relevant CME programs.

IF YOU WERE CERTIFIED IN 2002...
Apply for the 2012 MOC examination in 2011.
Requirements: 180 Category 1 CME credits (150 in past 5-yr block)
                  1 completed self-assessment activity

IF YOU WERE CERTIFIED IN 2003...
Apply for the 2013 MOC examination in 2012.
Requirements: 210 Category 1 CME credits (150 in past 5-yr block)
                  1 completed self-assessment activity

IF YOU WERE CERTIFIED/RECERTIFIED IN 2004...
Apply for the 2014 MOC examination in 2013.
Requirements: 240 Category 1 CME credits (150 in past 5-yr block), at least 20 of the CME credits should involve self-assessment*
                  2 completed self-assessment activities
                  1 completed PIP Unit

IF YOU WERE CERTIFIED/RECERTIFIED IN 2005...
Apply for the 2015 MOC examination in 2014.
Requirements: 270 Category 1 CME credits (150 in past 5-yr block), at least 40 of the CME credits should involve self-assessment*
                  2 completed self-assessment activities
                  1 completed PIP Unit

IF YOU WERE CERTIFIED/RECERTIFIED IN 2006...
Apply for the 2016 MOC examination in 2015.
Requirements: 300 Category 1 CME credits (150 in past 5-yr block), at least 60 of the CME credits should involve self-assessment*
                  2 completed self-assessment activities
                  2 completed PIP Units

IF YOU WERE CERTIFIED/RECERTIFIED IN 2007...
Apply for the 2017 MOC examination in 2016.
Requirements: 300 Category 1 CME credits (150 in past 5-yr block), at least 80 of the CME credits should involve self-assessment*
                  2 completed self-assessment activities
                  3 completed PIP Units

IF YOU WERE CERTIFIED/RECERTIFIED IN 2008...
Apply for the 2018 MOC examination in 2017.
Requirements: 300 Category 1 CME credits (150 in 1st 5-yr block, 150 in 2nd 5-yr block), at least 80 of the CME credits should involve self-assessment*
                  2 self-assessment activities (complete 1st SA 2009-2011; 2nd SA 2014-2016)
                  3 completed PIP Units

IF YOU WERE CERTIFIED/RECERTIFIED IN 2009...
Apply for the 2019 MOC examination in 2018.
Requirements: 300 Category 1 CME credits (150 in 1st 5-yr block, 150 in 2nd 5-yr block), at least 80 of the CME credits should involve self-assessment*
                  2 self-assessment activities (complete 1st SA 2010-2012; 2nd SA 2015-2017)
                  3 completed PIP Units

IF YOU WERE CERTIFIED/RECERTIFIED IN 2010...
Apply for the 2020 MOC examination in 2019.
Requirements: 300 Category 1 CME credits (150 in 1st 5-yr block, 150 in 2nd 5-yr block), at least 80 of the CME credits should involve self-assessment*
                  2 self-assessment activities (complete 1st SA 2011-2013; 2nd SA 2016-2018)
                  3 PIP Units (complete 1st PIP 2011-2013; 2nd PIP 2014-2016; 3rd PIP 2017-2019)

IF YOU WERE CERTIFIED/RECERTIFIED IN 2011...
Apply for the 2021 MOC examination in 2020.
Requirements: 300 Category 1 CME credits (150 in 1st 5-yr block, 150 in 2nd 5-yr block), at least 80 of the CME credits should involve self-assessment*
                  2 self-assessment activities (complete 1st SA 2012-2014; 2nd SA 2017-2019)
                  3 PIP Units (complete 1st PIP 2012-2014; 2nd PIP 2015-2017; 3rd PIP 2018-2020)

FOR THOSE CERTIFIED/RECERTIFIED IN 2012 OR LATER...
Requirements: See Continuous Pathway to Lifelong Learning (CP-MOC) found on page 10.

* self-assessment CME credit may be averaged over 2 to 5 years.

American Board of Psychiatry and Neurology, Inc., 2150 E. Lake Cook Road, Suite 900, Buffalo Grove, IL ◊ Ph: 847.229.6500 ◊ www.abpn.com

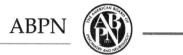

FREQUENTLY ASKED QUESTIONS ABOUT MOC (10YR-MOC)   *(Nov. 2009)*

1. What is Maintenance of Certification (MOC)?
Maintenance of Certification (MOC) is an initiative of the American Board of Medical Specialties (ABMS) aimed at insuring that physician specialists, certified by one of the 24 member boards of the ABMS, offer quality patient care through an ongoing process of self-improvement. MOC entails four basic components: professional standing, self-assessment and continuing medical education (CME), cognitive expertise, and performance in practice.

2. Why should I participate?
It is likely that the public and political emphasis on the continuous documentation of clinical competence and quality improvement by physicians will only increase over the years ahead, making a program like MOC essential.

3. What is ABPN trying to accomplish with MOC?
The American Board of Psychiatry and Neurology (ABPN) has strived to develop a credible MOC program for our diplomates that strikes a balance between what will likely be required by organizations that license, credential, and pay physicians and what is reasonable and straight-forward enough to be accomplished by busy physicians. Many of our diplomates are already participating in various components of MOC through institutional or practice group quality improvement programs and the MOC Program will try to recognize those efforts. ABPN has tried to develop a clear MOC program that will enable a diplomate to demonstrate their competence throughout a 10-year certificate cycle.

4. What is the MOC Program timetable?
The MOC program is being phased in incrementally, and diplomates should become familiar with the current requirements and phase-in schedule for the 4-part ABPN MOC Program.

5. Is participation in the MOC Program mandatory?
While participation in the MOC Program is voluntary, it is a requirement in order to maintain certification for diplomates with time-limited certificates. Holders of time-limited certificates must complete all components of the ABPN MOC Program in order to maintain their Board certification.

6. Should I participate in the MOC Program if I have a "lifetime" certificate?
Participation in the MOC Program is not required for diplomates with "lifetime" certificates; however, credentialing requirements for hospitals, practice groups, and third-party payers may require evidence of continuous certification efforts. In addition, some states are considering the implementation of Maintenance of Licensure Programs, similar to the MOC Program. If a life-time certificate holder voluntarily participates in the MOC Program and does not pass the cognitive examination, that individual will not lose their "lifetime" certificate.

7. How do I keep track of completed MOC components during the MOC cycle?
Maintain a file that documents the completion of all Self-Assessment, CME, and PIP activities in the event one is audited by the ABPN.

American Board of Psychiatry and Neurology, Inc., 2150 E. Lake Cook Road, Suite 900, Buffalo Grove, IL ◊ Ph: 847.229.6500 ◊ www.abpn.com

ABPN

The ABPN has developed a new online ABPN Physician web portal for our diplomates at http://www.abpn.com/folios. A diplomate is able to securely log on to the ABPN Physician Folios to apply and pay online for examinations and keep a record of completed MOC components. The system will also monitor progress of completion according to an individual's MOC cycle.

8. When do I begin with the MOC process?

You are automatically enrolled in the MOC Program after achieving board certification. A diplomate should log on to the ABPN Physician Folios to activate their online account and keep updated on MOC Program requirements.

9. What should I do now to make sure I keep current with the MOC requirements?

- Maintain an unrestricted license to practice medicine.
- Complete a Self-Assessment activity that provides CME credit such as those listed on our web site, www.abpn.com.
- Earn at least an average of 8 hours of CME credit per year from Self-Assessment activities.
- Use the results of completed Self-Assessment activities to design a plan for subsequent CME.
- Complete at least an average of 30 hours of CME credit per year (this includes the 8 hours of CME credit per year from Self-Assessment activities).
- Become familiar with practice guidelines relevant to one's area of clinical practice in anticipation of the requirement (in 2013) to compare data from one's own clinical cases to those practice guidelines in the PIP Clinical Modules.
- Become familiar with the peer and patient feedback forms on the ABPN website (www.abpn.com) in anticipation of the requirement (in 2013) to solicit feedback from one's patients and peers about one's clinical practice in the PIP Feedback Modules.
- Encourage the Quality Assurance Program of one's hospital, clinic, practice plan, etc. to design its programs to provide the type of information that will fulfill the requirements of the PIP Clinical and Feedback Modules.
- Meet the required deadlines on the ABPN web site (www.abpn.com) to apply for the ABPN MOC Examination.

10. What happens if my certificate expired already?

Diplomates who are not recertified before their certificates expire are no longer Board certified in that area. Once a former diplomate completes all of the MOC Program requirements and passes the MOC examination, however, he or she will regain certification status. It is not necessary to sit for the initial certification examination again or complete additional training.

11. If I hold more than one certification, do I need to accrue CME credits and perform other MOC activities for each certification?

If a diplomate is certified in two or more areas, any CME, self-assessment, and PIP activities completed in one area of specialization/subspecialization may accrue and count for multiple certifications. However, if the diplomate is certified in more than one specialty/subspecialty (e.g. psychiatry and neurology) and wants to maintain certificates in both, the diplomate must pass cognitive examinations in both areas, (e.g. psychiatry and neurology).

American Board of Psychiatry and Neurology, Inc., 2150 E. Lake Cook Road, Suite 900, Buffalo Grove, IL ◊ Ph: 847.229.6500 ◊ www.abpn.com

FOCUS Major Depressive Disorder Maintenance of Certification (MOC) Workbook   171

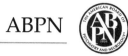

ABPN

Continuous Pathway to Lifelong Learning (CP-MOC) *(February 2012)*
For Diplomates Certified or Recertified in 2012 or Later

The Continuous Pathway to Lifelong Learning Program (CP-MOC) is a four-part MOC program, where all component requirements must be met to maintain certification. Beginning in 2012, diplomates who pass their initial certification or MOC examination will enter into the Continuous Pathway to Lifelong Learning. Diplomates who passed their initial certification or MOC examination prior to 2012 may elect to participate.

The Program will assist diplomates to comply with Maintenance of Certification (MOC) requirements and timeframes and facilitate the required annual recording and reporting of diplomate MOC participation. Instead of a single fee at the time of the MOC examination, participants in the Continuous Pathway to Lifelong Learning will pay a small annual fee. This annual fee covers participation in the ABPN Physician Folios and includes one MOC cognitive examination in a ten-year period. Less than 10 years of participation, or applying for a modular examination, may require an additional fee.

The focal point of the Continuous Pathway to Lifelong Learning Program is the ABPN Physician Folios, which offers a single source for personalized information regarding certification and MOC status. You must activate a ABPN Physician Folios account on the ABPN website to begin the MOC process.

While passing a cognitive examination is still required at least every ten years, a diplomate's certification status is dependent upon fulfillment of all four MOC Program components (Professional Standing, Self-Assessment and CME, Cognitive Expertise, and Performance in Practice), along with annually logging completed MOC activities into ABPN's Physician Folios and payment of an annual MOC registration fee.

Continuous Pathway to Lifelong Learning Program Requirements
* Maintaining an unrestricted license(s) and no restrictions on any license.
* Passing an MOC cognitive examination at least **every 10 years** for every time-limited certificate.
* Completing MOC activities **every 3 years** (one stage):
    * 24 CME hours of self-assessment activities
    * 90 Category 1 CME hours total (including 24 CMEs from SA activities)
    * 1 Performance in Practice (PIP) Unit (one clinical module & one feedback module)

1. Professional Standing (continuously effective)
To show evidence of professional standing, the ABPN requires that diplomates must hold an active and unrestricted license to practice medicine in at least one state, commonwealth, territory, or possession of the United States or province of Canada. Such license must be maintained even if the physician is out of the country for extended periods of time. All medical licenses must be unrestricted.

2. Self-Assessment and CME

A. Self-Assessment Program
Diplomates of the ABPN are required to participate in broad-based self-assessment activities. Self-Assessment Activities can come from multiple self-assessment programs. Each self-assessment activity must cover new knowledge and/or current best practices in one or more of the competency areas, and provide feedback to the diplomate that can be used as the basis for focused CME, lifelong learning, and/or career development. That feedback must include the correct answer and recommended literature resources for each question, and comparative performance to peers. **Beginning in 2014, diplomates are required to use only ABPN-approved products for self-assessment activities.**

- At least an average of 8 of the CME credits per year (averaged over 3 years) should involve self-assessment.
- Feedback must include comparative performance to peers.
- Self-assessment examinations must include no fewer than 25 questions per examination and 2 CME credits per activity.
- The self-assessment examination must take place before any subsequent CME educational activity.

American Board of Psychiatry and Neurology, Inc., 2150 E. Lake Cook Road, Suite 900, Buffalo Grove, IL ◊ Ph: 847.229.6500 ◊ www.abpn.com

172   FOCUS Major Depressive Disorder Maintenance of Certification (MOC) Workbook

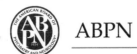

The Board may approve additional programs over time. The ABPN reserves the right to approve or reject any course or guideline submitted for approval.

B. CME Activities
Diplomates of the ABPN are required to complete an average of 30 specialty or subspecialty Category 1 CME credits per year. CME activities must be accredited by ACCME or by the Royal College of Physicians and Surgeons of Canada, and CME must be relevant to the specialty in which the diplomate is certified. Diplomates certified in more than one area only need to accrue an average of 30 CME credits per year, as the same CME credits can be used to satisfy the MOC requirements for multiple specialties and subspecialties.
- Diplomates must accrue an average of 30 specialty or subspecialty Category 1 CME credits per year (averaged over 3 years).
- At least an average of 8 of the CME credits per year (averaged over 3 years) should involve self-assessment.

3. Cognitive Expertise (effective 1994)

Diplomates of the ABPN fulfill the cognitive expertise component by passing a cognitive examination. To sit for a cognitive examination, all current MOC requirements must be satisfied at the time the MOC application is submitted. A passing score on the cognitive examination extends the examination renewal date to December 31, 10 years from the year of the examination. Practice-relevant, clinically oriented, multiple-choice, computer-administered examinations are delivered in over 200 Pearson VUE testing centers throughout the country. To prepare for the MOC cognitive examinations, a diplomate should keep current with research and developments in the respective field, read specialty-specific journals and practice guidelines, and attend relevant CME programs.

MOC Program participation includes meeting **all** MOC requirements, not just passing the MOC cognitive examination.

4. Performance in Practice (PIP)
The Performance in Practice (PIP) component is a two-part quality improvement program designed for "clinically active" physicians (see definitions below) to participate in practice improvement activities through both chart review and second-party external review. Diplomates will be required to complete one PIP Unit every 3 years, consisting of both a Clinical Module (chart review) and a Feedback Module (Patient/Peer* second-party external review).

If a diplomate participates in an institutional quality improvement program that involves collection of chart data and comparison, and establishment of a plan to improve clinical activity for the individual physician, that institutional participation may also fulfill the Clinical module. If a diplomate participates in peer review in his/her clinical setting, that institutional activity may also fulfill the PIP Feedback Module criteria. **Beginning in 2014, diplomates are required to use only ABPN-approved products for Performance in Practice Activities.**

A) Clinical Modules (Chart Review)
- Each diplomate is required to collect data from at least five patient cases in a specific category (e.g., diagnosis, type of treatment, treatment setting) obtained from the diplomate's personal practice over the previous 3-year period.
- A minimum of 4 quality measures must be collected for each Clinical Module.
- Each diplomate must then compare data from the five patient cases with published best practices, or practice guidelines, or peer-based standards of care (e.g., hospital quality improvement programs), and develop a plan to improve effectiveness or efficiency of his/her clinical activities.
- Remeasurement: within 24 months, each diplomate must collect the same data from at least another five clinical cases in the same specific category, to see if improvements in practice have occurred. The same patients may be assessed in the original and follow-up data.

B) Feedback Modules (Patient** and Peer* Second Party External Reviews)
- Each diplomate must solicit personal performance feedback from at least five peers* and five of their own patients** concerning the diplomate's clinical activity over the previous three years.
- Each diplomate must then identify opportunities for improvement in the effectiveness and/or efficiency in their practice as related to the core competencies and take steps to implement suggested improvements.

American Board of Psychiatry and Neurology, Inc., 2150 E. Lake Cook Road, Suite 900, Buffalo Grove, IL ◊ Ph: 847.229.6500 ◊ www.abpn.com

FOCUS Major Depressive Disorder Maintenance of Certification (MOC) Workbook   173

ABPN

•Remeasurement: within 24 months, each diplomate must collect the same data from at least another five peers* and five patients to see if improvements in practice have occurred. Feedback may be obtained from the same patients and peers as in the original and follow-up feedback.

* Peers may include other professional healthcare staff such as, psychologists, social workers, physicians, counselors, and nurses.
** Patients can include those for which the diplomate supervises the care of another provider (e.g., resident).
•*Model MOC PIP Peer Feedback and MOC PIP Patient Feedback forms are available on the Forms page at www.abpn.com/forms.*

The ABPN recommends that diplomates allow ample time for completion of PIP Units. It may take diplomates 24 months from the date that the original data is collected from patients and peers to complete one PIP Unit.

The Board may approve additional programs over time. The ABPN reserves the right to approve or reject any course or guideline submitted for approval.

One stage of MOC activities will be waived for diplomates who complete ACGME-accredited/ABPN-approved subspecialty training and sit for and pass an ABPN subspecialty examination in 2012 or later.

Clinically Active Status
The American Board of Medical Specialties (ABMS) has issued definitions of "Clinically Active" and "Clinically Inactive" and requires that all diplomates self-report their status once every 24 months in each area of certification. This information will be available to the public.
1."**Clinically Active**": Any amount of direct and/or consultative patient care has been provided in the preceding 24 months. This includes the supervision of residents.
    A. Engaged in direct and/or consultative care *sufficient* to complete Performance in Practice (PIP) Units.
    B. Engaged in direct and/or consultative care *not sufficient* to complete PIP Units.
2."**Clinically Inactive**": No direct and or/consultative patient care has been provided in the past 24 months.
3."**Status Unknown**": No information available on the clinical activity of this diplomate.
    •Diplomates who are in category 1.A. above are required to complete all components of the MOC Program including PIP Units.
    •Diplomates who are in categories 1.B. or 2 above are required to complete all components of the MOC Program, except for PIP Units.
    •A change in diplomate status from 1.B. or 2 to 1.A. requires the completion of at least one PIP Unit.

American Board of Psychiatry and Neurology, Inc., 2150 E. Lake Cook Road, Suite 900, Buffalo Grove, IL ◊ Ph: 847.229.6500 ◊ www.abpn.com

174   FOCUS Major Depressive Disorder Maintenance of Certification (MOC) Workbook

ABPN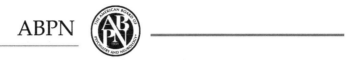

FREQUENTLY ASKED QUESTIONS ABOUT MOC (CP-MOC)   *(February 2012)*

1. Why is ABPN moving to a Continuous MOC Program?
The Continuous Maintenance of Certification Program (CP-MOC) will facilitate the required annual recording and reporting of diplomate MOC participation.

2. What are the advantages of participating in the Continuous MOC Program?
You only pay one small annual fee instead of a large amount every ten years. The ABPN Physician Folios gives you a personalized list of all your MOC activities that you can provide to your employer/hospital/licensing board, if required. You will be informed on a regular basis of what you must do to meet the MOC requirements so you don't fall behind with requirements.

3. Does everyone have to join?
Beginning in 2012, all diplomates who pass their initial certification or MOC examination must enter into the Continuous Pathway to Lifelong Learning.
Diplomates who pass their initial certification or MOC examination prior to 2012 will not be required to participate in this program unless they elect to do so.

4. What about lifetime certificate holders?
Lifetime certificate holders will not be required to participate in this program unless they elect to do so. However, all time-limited certificate holders will be required to participate in this program beginning with the 2012 initial certification and MOC examinations.

5. How will I be reported to the public if I am a lifetime certificate holder & I choose not enter the CP-MOC Program?
Physicians who hold certificates issued prior to October 1, 1994 (lifetime certificate holders) are not required to participate in maintenance of certification. Those physicians who choose to not enter the CP-MOC program will be listed as Certified, but not meeting MOC requirements and not required to do so.

6. How does a lifetime certificate holder enter the CP-MOC Program?
The ABPN understands that some physicians holding lifetime certificates may wish to complete maintenance of certification requirements and enter the CP-MOC program. By passing an MOC examination, lifetime certificate holders will automatically be enrolled into the CP-MOC program and the physician will be listed as voluntarily meeting MOC requirements. *Failure to pass the MOC examination will have no impact on the lifetime certificate.*

7. What if I have multiple certificates?
The annual fee covers one cognitive MOC examination in a ten-year period. There is only one annual fee collected per diplomate. An annual fee is not collected for every certificate. You will be responsible for the full payment for any cognitive MOC examination taken in addition to the first one.

8. What if I take a modular MOC examination (a combination of up to 3 specialty/subspecialties in one examination administration)?
The modular MOC examination fee is higher than the standard MOC examination fee; therefore, you will be required to pay the difference in fees at the time of registration for the examination.

9. I am participating in an ACGME-accredited/ABPN subspecialty program. Can I get MOC credit for the fellowship?
Yes. Physicians becoming certified in their primary specialty may count completion of fellowship training <u>and</u> certification in a subspecialty as one Continuous Pathway to Life-Long Learning (CP-MOC) unit. Completion of this requirement will take the place of one stage of MOC activities (three year cycle) including self-assessment, CME, and PIP requirements.

American Board of Psychiatry and Neurology, Inc., 2150 E. Lake Cook Road, Suite 900, Buffalo Grove, IL ◊ Ph: 847.229.6500 ◊ www.abpn.com

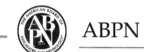 **ABPN**

10. Why is there an annual MOC program fee?

The annual MOC program fee covers participation in the ABPN Physician Folios and includes one MOC cognitive examination in a ten-year period. The fee also includes regular email reminders and updates from ABPN so that a diplomate does not fall behind with requirements.

11. What happens if I do not pay the annual fee?

A diplomate will be reported as 'Not Meeting MOC Requirements' if they do not pay the annual fee.

12. What happens if I do not sign on to the ABPN Physician Folios?

A diplomate is required to pay their annual fees and enter their MOC activity through ABPN Physician Folios, therefore a diplomate will be reported as 'Not Meeting MOC Requirements' if they do not sign on to the ABPN Physician Folios.

13. What happens if I do not complete all of the MOC requirements?

A diplomate will be reported as 'Not Meeting MOC Requirements' if they have not met all of the MOC requirements.

14. What happens if I fail the cognitive MOC examination?

A diplomate will be reported as 'Not Meeting MOC Requirements' if they fail or miss the cognitive MOC examination. Diplomates will be allowed to retake the examination within one year of the failed/missed examination. If the diplomate fails or misses the cognitive MOC examination on the second attempt, he/she will be reported as 'Not Certified'.

15. How can I change my status from 'Not Meeting MOC Requirements' to 'Meeting MOC Requirements'?

A diplomate will be reported as 'Not Meeting MOC Requirements' if they have not met all MOC requirements for one stage (three years). A diplomate may change their status to 'Meeting MOC Requirements' by completing insufficient stage activities, current stage activities, and payment of all required fees.

16. What if I miss more than 6 years (2 stages) of MOC activities?

A diplomate will be reported as 'Not Certified' if they miss more than 6 years (2 stages) of MOC activities. Diplomates may change their status back to 'Certified and Meeting MOC Requirements' upon successful completion of all MOC activities included in one stage:
- An unrestricted license(s) and no restrictions on any license
- 24 CME hours of self-assessment (SA) activities
- 90 Category-1 CME hours total (including CMEs from SA activities)
- 1 Performance in Practice (PIP) Unit (one clinical module and one feedback module)
- Pass MOC cognitive examination (pay full fee)

17. I have an active 10-year certificate and wish to join the CP-MOC Program. How do I do that?

Diplomates with active 10 year certificates may log onto their Physician Folio account and enter the Continuous Pathway to Life Long Learning program. By following a simple series of step-by-step instructions physicians may enroll in the CP-MOC program. MOC requirements will be prorated according to the expiration date of the certificate.

18. I have an expired 10-year certificate and wish to join the CP-MOC Program. How do I do that?

Physicians with expired 10 year certificates may enter the CP-MOC program by meeting the requirements for admission to the current year's examination and passing the MOC examination.

American Board of Psychiatry and Neurology, Inc., 2150 E. Lake Cook Road, Suite 900, Buffalo Grove, IL ◊ Ph: 847.229.6500 ◊ www.abpn.com

ABPN

ABPN Continuous Pathway to Lifelong Learning (CP-MOC)
For Diplomates Certified or Recertified in 2012 or Later

MOC Cycle	Year 1	Year 2	Year 3	Year 4	Year 5	Year 6	Year 7	Year 8	Year 9	Year 10	Year 11	Year 12
Examination (Part III)										MOC Exam		
License (Part I)	License Maintained & Verified Continuously											
Self Assessment (Part II)	24 CME credits from Self-Assessment Activities — Deadline			24 CME credits from Self-Assessment Activities — Deadline			24 CME credits from Self-Assessment Activities — Deadline			24 CME credits from Self-Assessment Activities — Deadline		
CME (Part II)	30 Cat-1	30 Cat-1	30 Cat-1 — Deadline — 90 CME credits per Stage	30 Cat-1	30 Cat-1	30 Cat-1 — Deadline — 90 CME credits per Stage	30 Cat-1	30 Cat-1	30 Cat-1 — Deadline — 90 CME credits per Stage	30 Cat-1	30 Cat-1	30 Cat-1 — Deadline — 90 CME credits per Stage
Performance in Practice (Part IV)	Minimum One (1) PIP — Deadline			Minimum One (1) PIP — Deadline			Minimum One (1) PIP — Deadline			Minimum One (1) PIP — Deadline		
Annual MOC Registration Fee	Annual Fee	Annual Fee	Annual Fee — 3 Annual Fee Payments — Milestone	Annual Fee	Annual Fee	Annual Fee — 3 Annual Fee Payments — Milestone	Annual Fee	Annual Fee	Annual Fee — 3 Annual Fee Payments — Milestone	Annual Fee	Annual Fee	Annual Fee — 3 Annual Fee Payments — Milestone

American Board of Psychiatry and Neurology, Inc., 2150 E. Lake Cook Road, Suite 900, Buffalo Grove, IL ◊ Ph: 847.229.6500 ◊ www.abpn.com